Sports and Exercise Medicine

Sports and Exercise Medicine

Edited by **Pablo De Souza**

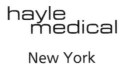

New York

Published by Hayle Medical,
30 West, 37th Street, Suite 612,
New York, NY 10018, USA
www.haylemedical.com

Sports and Exercise Medicine
Edited by Pablo De Souza

© 2015 Hayle Medical

International Standard Book Number: 978-1-63241-356-7 (Hardback)

Printed in the United States of America.

Contents

Preface

A descriptive account on novel areas of current knowledge in the vast field of sports and exercise medicine has been provided in this insightful book. Experts from across the world have contributed in this book. It discusses the physiology behind sports injuries and describes novel and intriguing approaches to manage such injuries. It also explores the relation between health, performance and exercise by elucidating novel information in areas such as the use of iron supplementation for performance, exercise and immunity, impacts of exercise on reactive oxygen species, and the proposed advantages of authentic and simulated altitude training. It is a well-researched and comprehensive book which will serve as a valuable source of information for physiologists, physical conditioners, sports medicine specialists, coaches, students and physiotherapists.

The researches compiled throughout the book are authentic and of high quality, combining several disciplines and from very diverse regions from around the world. Drawing on the contributions of many researchers from diverse countries, the book's objective is to provide the readers with the latest achievements in the area of research. This book will surely be a source of knowledge to all interested and researching the field.

In the end, I would like to express my deep sense of gratitude to all the authors for meeting the set deadlines in completing and submitting their research chapters. I would also like to thank the publisher for the support offered to us throughout the course of the book. Finally, I extend my sincere thanks to my family for being a constant source of inspiration and encouragement.

Editor

Sports Medicine

The Physiology of Sports Injuries and Repair Processes

Kelc Robi, Naranda Jakob, Kuhta Matevz and
Vogrin Matjaz

Additional information is available at the end of the chapter

1. Introduction

Sports injuries are among the most common injuries and therefore present a significant public health problem. Physiologic processes after injuries are often neglected while much more attention is being paid to the management of symptoms. However, comprehension of these processes is becoming more and more important as therapies are getting increasingly focused on specific molecular and cellular processes. In recent decades, extensive research of tissue regeneration after injury and degeneration, including molecular pathways in healing, helped towards better understanding of this process and led to discoveries of new potential therapeutic targets. In this chapter physiology of sports injuries and the latest advances in understanding pathophysiological processes after injury will be discussed.

2. Physiology of tendon and ligament injury and repair

For skeletal muscles to act properly they must be attached to the bone. Tendons serve as mediators of force transmission that results in joint motion, but they also enable that the muscle belly remains at an optimal distance from the joint on which it acts. Tendons act as springs, which allows them to store and recover energy very effectively. Ligaments on the other hand attach bone to bone and therefore provide mechanical stability of the joint, guide joint motion through their normal range of motion when a tensile load is applied and prevent excessive joint displacement. Although tendons and ligaments differ in function, they share similar physiological features with a similar hierarchical structure and mechanical behavior.

2.1. Histoanatomical features of tendons and ligaments

Tendons are made up predominantly of collagen fibers embedded in proteoglycan matrix that attracts water and elastin molecules with a relatively small number of fibroblasts.

Fibroblasts are the predominant cell type in tendons. They are spindle shaped and arranged in fascicles with surrounding loose areolar tissue called peritenon. Cells are orientated in the direction of muscle loading. In mature tendon tissue they are arranged in parallel rows along the force transmitting axis of the tendon. Long cytoplasmic processes extend between the intratendinous fibroblasts, enabling cell-to-cell contact by gap-junctions.

Fibroblasts are connected to the extra cellular matrix (ECM) via integrins that permit the cells to sense and respond to mechanical stimuli which appears vital for their function because this way the mechanical continuum is established along which forces can be transmitted from the outside to the inside of the cell and vice versa. Integrins are also likely candidates for sensing tensile stress at the cell surface. It is also speculated that integrin-associated proteins are involved in signaling adaptive cellular responses upon mechanical loading of the tissue [1-5].

Type I collagen is the major constituent of tendons, accounting for about 95% of the dry tendon weight. Collagen type III accounts for about 5% of the dry tendon weight, but smaller quantities of other collagens are also present, including types V, VI, XII and type II collagen. The latter is primarily found in regions that are under compression [1-3].

Fibroblasts secrete a precursor of collagen, called procollagen, which is cleaved extracellularly to form type I collagen. The synthesis of collagen fibrils occurs in two stages: intracellular and extracellular. The pro α-chains are initially synthesized with an additional signal peptide at the aminoterminal end with the function to direct movement of the polypeptides into the rough endoplasmic reticulum where it is cleaved off. Triple helix with three polypeptide chains wound together to form a stiff helical structure is formed intracellularly. Then the procollagen is secreted into the extracellular matrix where it is converted to collagen. Finally, collagen molecules aggregate and the cross-links responsible for its stable structure are formed [1-4].

The parallel arrangement of the collagen fibers in tendons enables them to sustain high tensile loads. Collagen molecules group together to form microfibrils, which are defined as 5 collagen molecules stacked in a quarter-stagger array. Microfibrils combine to form subfibrils, and those combine further to form fibrils (50-200 nm in diameter). Fibrils combine together to form fibers (3-7 μm in diameter) which further combine to form fascicles, and these group together to form a tendon. Fascicles are separated by endotenon and surrounded by epitenon. At the level of fascicles, the characteristic »crimp« pattern can be seen histologically (discussed later in this chapter) (Figure 1) [1-4].

Proteoglycans (PGs) account for 1-5% of the dry weight of the tendon. PGs are highly hydrophilic they attract water molecules. The predominant proteoglycans in the tendon are decorin and lumican. Biglycan and decorin (and collagen type V) regulate collagen fiber diameter in fibrillogenesis. Because decorin molecules form cross-links between collagen fibers they may increase the stiffness of the fibrils. Proteoglycans are also responsible for lubricating collagen fibers and thus allowing them to glide over each other [2-4]. Aggrecan, a normal structure of articular cartilage, in found in tendons that are under compression [5].

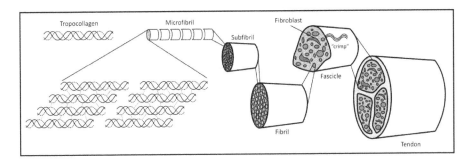

Figure 1. Structure of a tendon. See text for details. Adopted from Kastelic et al. [6]

Although tendons and ligaments are very similar in structure, there are some differences between them. (1) Ligaments consist of lower percentage of collagen molecules, but a higher percentage of the proteoglycans and water. (2) Collagen fibers are more variable and have higher elastin content and (3) fibroblasts appear rounder. (4) Furthermore, ligaments receive blood supply from insertion sites (Table 1) [1, 2].

Content / Feature	Ligaments	Tendons
Fibroblasts	20%	20%
Ground substance	20-30%	lower
Collagen	70-80%	Slightly higher
Collagen type I	90%	95-99%
Collagen type III	10%	1-5%
Elastin	Up to 2x collagen	scarce
Water	60-80%	60-80%
Organisation	More random	Organized
Orientation	Weaving pattern	Long axis orientation

Table 1. Differences between tendon and ligament structure

2.1.1. Vascular supply

There are two types of tendons: (1) tendons covered with paratenon, and (2) sheathed tendons. They mainly differ in vascular supply. In sheathed tendons a mesotenon (vincula) carries a vessel that supplies only one part of the tendon. Therefore, parts of the tendon are relatively avascular and their nutrition depends on diffusion. On the other hand, paratenon-covered tendons receive their blood supply from vessels entering the tendon surface and forming a rich capillary system. Because of the difference in the vasculature, paratenon-covered tendons heal better. As stated above, ligaments receive their blood supply from insertion sites [2, 3].

There is still an ongoing debate about the efficiency of the blood supply to tendons during exercise. Experiments showed that although the increase in tendon blood flow is somehow restricted during exercise, there is no indication of any major ischemia in the tendon region. The question remains how blood flow to the tendon region is regulated. Several candidates as regulators of blood flow in skeletal muscle have been proposed, and it is possible that similar substances and metabolites are vasoactive also in the tendon region suca as bradykinin [2].

2.1.2. Insertion sites

As tendons attach skeletal muscles to bony structures, two types of tendinous junction are to be distinguished – osteotendinous where tendon attaches to the bone and musculotendinous where it attaches to the muscle. Four distinct zones have been observed at the osteotendinous junction, with a gradual change between them (Figure 2). (1) The first zone is structurally similar to the tendon propter, but with smaller amounts of PG decorin. This zone is followed by (2) fibrocartilage, where mostly collagen type II and III are found, but also small amounts of types I, IX and X. Furthermore, there is less PGs aggrecan and decorin. In the third zone, (3) mineralized fibrocartilage is made up of mainly collagen type II, but large quantities of collagen X and aggrecan are also present. The fourth zone is (4) bone, build up mainly of collagen type I and minerals [1-3].

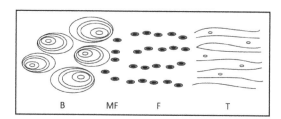

Figure 2. Diagram of a osteotendinous junction; B – bone; MF – minarelized fibrocartilage; F – fibrocartilage; T – tendon.

At musculotendinous junction, muscle cells are involuted and folded to provide maximal surface for attachment where fibrils attach. Sarcomeres of the fast contracting muscles are shortened at the junction, which may reduce the force intensity within the junction [3].

Ligaments insert into bone in two ways: through indirect or direct insertions. In indirect insertions the superficial layer is continued at with the periosteum and the deeper layer anchores to bone via Sharpey's fibers. In direct insertions, fibers attach to bone at 90° angle. Four distinct zones have been observed, with a gradual change between ligament midsubstance, fibrocartilage, mineralized fibrocartilage, and bone [2].

2.1.3. Biomechanics of tendons and ligaments

Typical parameters describing the tendon/ligament mechanical properties are *strain*, which describes the elongation/deformation of the tendon (ΔL) relative to the normal length (L0); *stress*, the tendon force (Ft) relative to the tendon cross-sectional area (CSA), *stiffness*, the change in tendon length (ΔL) in relation to the force applied (ΔFt) and *modulus*, which describes the relation between tendon stress and tendon strain and represents the properties independently of the CSA (Figure 3 and 4). High modulus indicates stiffer tissue [7-9].

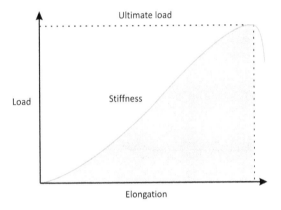

Figure 3. Structural properties of the bone-ligament-bone complex - A load/elongation curve; stiffness is represented by the slope of the curve; ultimate load is the highest load applied to the bone-ligament-bone complex before failure; the dashed area under the curve is the maximum energy stored by the complex [7, 9].

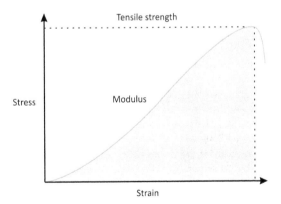

Figure 4. Mechanical properties of the bone-ligament-bone complex – A stress/strain curve; modulus is represented by the slope of the curve; tensile strength is the maximum stress of the bone-ligament-bone complex before failure; the dashed area under the curve represents the strain energy density [7, 9].

The biomechanics of ligaments is similar to tendon biomechanics. The biomechanical properties of ligaments are described as either structural properties of the bone-ligament–bone complex or the material properties of the ligament midsubstance itself. Structural properties of the bone-ligament-bone complex depend on the size and shape of the ligament, therefore they are extrinsic measures. They are obtained by loading a ligament to failure and therefore represented as a load-elongation curve between two defined limits of elongation. Mechanical properties are intrinsic measures of the quality of the tissue substance and are represented by a stress-strain curve [7, 8].

A tendon is the strongest component in the muscle-tendon-bone unit. It is estimated that tensile strength is about one-half of stainless steel (e.g. 1 cm^2 cross-section of a tendon can bear weight of 500-1000 kg) [3, 9].

2.1.4. Non-linear elasticity and viscoelasticity

There are three distinct regions of the stress/strain curve: (1) the toe region, (2) the linear region, and (3) the yield and failure region (Figure 5). In normal activity, most ligaments and tendons exist in the toe and somewhat in the linear region. This region is responsible for nonlinear stress/strain curve, because the slope of the toe region is not linear. The toe region represents "un-crimping" of the collagen fibrils. Since it is easier to stretch out the crimp of the collagen fibrils, this part of the stress strain curve shows a relatively low stiffness compared to linear portion. The toe region ends at about 2% strain when all crimpled fibers straighten. When all collagen fibrils become uncrimped, the collagen fibers stretch. The tendon deforms in a linear fashion due to the inter-molecular sliding of collagen triple helices. If strain is less than 4%, the tendon will return to its original length when unloaded, therefore this portion is elastic and reversible and the slope of the curve represents an elastic modulus. When a tendon/ligament is stretched beyond physiological limits, some fibrils begin to fail. Micro failure accumulates, stiffness is reduced and the ligament/tendon begins to fail. This occurs when intramolecular cross-links between collagen fibers fail. The tendon therefore undergoes irreversible plastic deformation. When the tendon/ligament is stretched to more than 8-10% of its original length, macroscopic failure follows [2, 3, 7].

Viscoelasticity refers to time dependent mechanical behavior. In other words, the relationship between stress and strain is not constant but depends on the time of displacement or load. There are three major characteristics of a viscoelastic material of ligaments and tendons: creep, stress relaxation, and hysteresis or energy dissipation. *Creep* indicates increasing deformation under constant load. This is in contrast with the usual elastic material, which does not elongate, no matter how long the load is applied (Figure 6). *Stress relaxation* is a feature of a ligament or tendon meaning that stress acting upon them will be eventually reduced under a constant deformation (Figure 7). When a viscoelastic material is loaded and unloaded, the unloading curve is different from the loading curve. This is called *hysteresis*. The difference between the two curves represents the amount of energy that is dissipated or lost during loading (Figure 8). If loading and unloading are repeated several times, different curves are obtained. However, after about 10 cycles, the loading and unloading curves do not change anymore, but they are still different. In other words, the amount of hysteresis un-

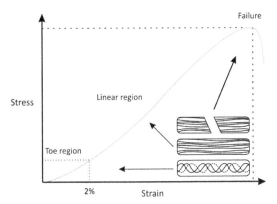

Figure 5. There are three distinct regions of the stress/strain curve: (1) the toe region, (2) the linear region, and (3) the yield and failure region. The *toe* region represents "un-crimping" of the collagen fibrils; toe region ends at about 2% of strain when all crimpled fibers straighten. It os followed by linear region, in which the collagen fibers respond linearly to load. If strain is less than 4%, the tendon will return to its original length when unloaded. Between 4 to 8 per cent of strain the collagen fibers begin to slide past one another as the cross-links start to fail which results in microscopic failure. If strain is more than 8%, macroscopic failure results.

der cyclic loading is reduced and the stress-strain curve becomes reproducible (Figure 9). This behavior is called *pseudo-elasticity* to represent the nonlinearity of ligament/tendon stress strain behavior [7].

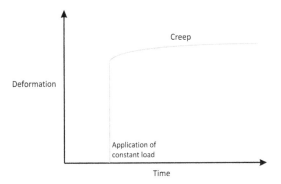

Figure 6. Creep is increasing deformation under constant load.

2.1.5. The influence of loading and gender on tendon and ligament size

Ligaments and tendons are adapted according to changes in mechanical stiffness. However, changes occur slowly, partly due to the fact that tendons and ligaments are relatively avascular tissues. There is strong evidence that tendons undergo hypertrophy, at least after long-term mechanical loading.

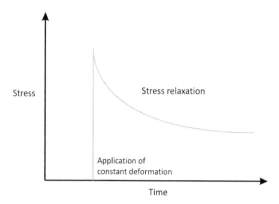

Figure 7. Stress relaxation - the stress will be reduced under a constant deformation.

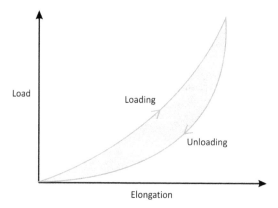

Figure 8. Hysteresis or energy dissipation – when tendon or ligament is loaded and unloaded, the unloading curve will not follow the loading curve. The energy is lost as heat (dashed area).

Male runners were found to have about larger Achilles tendon cross-sectional areas than non-runners. Furthermore, greater cross-sectional area (CSA) of patella tendons in the leading leg of male athletes competing for at least 5 years in sports with a side-to-side difference was demonstrated; an almost 30% difference in the cross-sectional area of the proximal part of the tendon between the leading and non-leading leg was observed [8, 10]. When subjected to short-term loading, only certain parts of tendons hypertrophied. It appears that tendons undergo hypertrophy in response to both long- and short-term loading, but that short-term changes in CSA are relatively small and seemingly occur only in specific regions of the tendon [8].

Interestingly, findings described above seem to be gender specific since marked differences in tendon CSA were not consistently found between female athletes and sedentary controls.

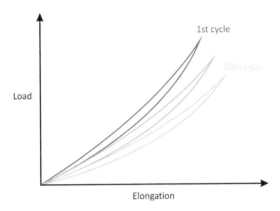

Figure 9. During cyclic loading and unloading, the stress/strain curve shifts to the right. After 10 repetitions, the curve becomes reproducible. The amount of hysteresis under cyclic loading is reduced.

Some other studies do in fact indicate that the exercise related adaptation of the tendon tissue is lower when levels of estrogen are high but the mechanism of this is not clear [8, 11]. Similary, premenopausal women were found to have lower risk for developing lower leg tendinopathies than men. The risk for developing lower leg tendinopathy in women increases in the post-menopausal period and is probably influenced by hormone-replacement therapy and activity levels. The mechanism behind this observations is not clear [12].

2.1.6. The effect of aging and immobilization ligament and tendon structure and function

With age there is an increase in the mechanical properties of ligaments and tendons up to the young adulthood when a decrease in the mechanical properties follows. Woo and colleagues tested femur-acl-tibia complex from young cadaver knees with the average age of 35 and older cadaver knees with the age of 76. They found that the linear structural stiffness of the ACL decreased both when tested at 30 degrees of knee flexion and when tested along the axis of the ligament complex [13].

Immobilization has a negative impact on tendons and ligaments [14]. Corresponding to the reduction in mechanical properties, there is a reduction in the ligament structure. Immobilization has a more rapid effect on mechanical properties than increased load from exercise. It was established that during immobilization,the cross sectional area of the ACL is reduced, which is believed to be a consequence of a loss in collagen fibrils as well as glycosaminoglycan that form the ground substance of the ligament. In addition, there might be alterations in collagen fibril orientation reducing the ligament properties. Upon remobilization, it appeared that the mechanical properties normalized first, followed by the structural properties. It is also believed that structural loss at the ligament insertion site may take longer to be removed than changes in ligament substance [7].

2.2. Tendon and ligament injury mechanisms

Tendon injury occurs because of direct trauma (i.e. penetrating, blunt, etc.) or indirect tensile overload. Acute tensile failure occurs if strain is more than 10%. However, lesser strain can cause tendon failure due to pre-existing chronic repeated insult and degeneration. Musculo-tendinous junction is the weakest link, especially during eccentric contractions. Maximum tension is created in forceful contractions. Furthermore, greater speed of eccentric contraction will increase the force developed. If the loading rate is slow, avulsion fracture is likely to occur. If loading is fast, tendon failure is more likely, especially if degenerated [3].

Tendon overuse injuries are a source of major concern in competitive and recreational athletes. It is estimated that 30% to 50% of all sport injuries are due to overuse [15, 16]. Studies from primary care show that 16% of general population suffers from shoulder pain, which rises to 21% in the elderly. The prevalence of Achilles tendinopathy in runners has been estimated at 11%. Tendinopathy of the forearm extensor tendons affects 1-2% of the population, most commonly occurring in the fourth and fifth decade of life. The overall prevalence of patellar tendinopathy among elite and non-elite athletes is high and varies between 3% and 45% [17]. Quadriceps tendon and tibialis posterior tendon are also often affected [15]. In the great majority of patients with spontaneous tendon rupture, the ruptured tendon shows degenerative lesions present before the rupture [16].

The term »tendinitis« has been widely used to describe a combination of tendon pain, swelling, and impaired performance. It is believed to be an inflammatory condition, although histopathological studies show degeneration rather than inflammation and therefore the term »tendinopathy« has been suggested as a more appropriate term [16, 18]. The term tendinopathy encompasses a spectrum of disorders, including lesions of the tenosynovium, the paratenon, the entesis, or tendon proper. Lesions can coexist and the tendon can tear partially or completely. Tendinopathies can be divided according to the duration of symptoms into acute (up to 2 weeks in duration), subacute (2-4 weeks), and chronic (over 6 weeks) [18].

There are multiple theories for the mechanism of tendon degeneration: (1) mechanical, (2) vascular, (3) neural, and (4) alternative theory.

In the *mechanical theory* of tendon injury, the overload of the tendon tissue is blamed for the pathologic process. Towards the higher end of the physiologic range, a microscopic failure may occur within a tendon and repetitive microtrauma can lead to matrix and cell changes, altered mechanical properties of the tendon, and symptoms development. Non-uniform stress within a tendon may produce localized fiber degeneration and damage without a history of a specific injury [15]. Studies have shown that cyclic mechanical stretching of cells can cause changes in cell morphology and alteration of both DNA and protein syntheses. In situ cell nucleus deformation does occur during tensile loading of tendons which may play a significant role in the mechanical signal transduction pathway in the affected tendon [19]. The production of prostaglandin E2 (PGE2) in tendon fibroblasts increases in a stretching magnitude-dependent manner for which cyclooxygenase (COX) is responsible [20]. Studies also showed that asymptomatic pathologic changes were common in the Achilles and patellar tendons in elite soccer players and that a greater number of hours per week resulted in a higher prevalence of patellar tendinopathy. However, »underuse« may also be the cause of tendon degeneration because the etiopathogenic stimulus for the degenerative cascade is the catabolic response of tendon cells to mechanobiological understimulation [19].

The *vascular theory* of tendinopathy suggests that tendons generally have poor blood supply, especially the Achilles tendon and those of tibialis posterior and supraspinatus muscle. The Achilles tendon should have a hypovascular region 2-6 cm proximal to its calcaneal insertion. In such tendons overuse may lead to injury.

However, studies on the Achilles blood flow show that blood supply along the whole tendon is in fact evenly distributed throughout the tendon, but is significantly lower at the distal insertion. Blood flow in the symptomatic tendons was significantly elevated as compared with the controls, demonstrated a similar vascular response to physical loading with a progressive decline in blood flow with increasing tension [21]. Male gender, advancing age, and mechanical loading of the tendon are associated with diminished tendon blood flow [22]. Therefore, vascular theory may be more important in the lesions of fibrocartilagenous entheses that are relatively avascular, and this may contribute to a poor healing response. Angiogenesis is mediated by angiogenic factors such as vascular endothelial growth factor (VEGF). VEGF is highly expressed in degenerative Achilles tendons, whereas its expression is nearly completely downregulated in healthy tendons. Several factors are able to upregulate VEGF expression in tenocytes: hypoxia, inflammatory cytokines, and mechanical load. Since VEGF has the potential to stimulate the expression of matrix metalloproteinases and inhibit the expression of tissue inhibitors of matrix metalloproteinases (TIMP), this cytokine might play a significant role in the pathogenetic processes during degenerative tendon disease [23].

The neural theory suggests that neurally mediated mast cell degranulation could release mediators such as substance P, which is contained in primary afferent nerves. Its quantity could be related to chronic pain. The increased amount of substance P in the subacromial bursa and nerve fibers immunoreactive to substance P were localized around the vessels of rotator cuff, especially in patients with the non-perforated rotator cuff injury [24]. Inflammatory cytokines, proteinases, and cyclooxygenase enzymes, have been shown to be present in the subacromial bursa of patients with rotator cuff tear [25]. However, neural theory does not explain why morphologically pathologic tendons are not always painful [15].

The alternative theory suggests that exercise induced localized hyperthermia may be detrimental to tendon cell survival. Tendons that store energy during locomotion, such as the equine superficial flexor digitorum tendon and the human Achilles tendon, suffer a high incidence of central core degeneration which is thought to precede tendon rupture. Studies have shown that the central core of equine tendon reaches temperatures as high as 45°C during high-speed locomotion, but temperatures above 42.5°C are known to result in fibroblast death *In vitro* [26]. Temperatures experienced in the central core of the tendon *In vivo* are unlikely to result in tendon cell death, but repeated hyperthermic insults may compromise cell metabolism of matrix components, resulting in tendon central core degeneration [27].

Although exact mechanism or their combination has not been determined yet, some factors influencing the development of tendinopathy have been. There is some evidence for genetic correlation, especially with target genes close to ABO gene on chromosome 9 like COL5A1 and TNC gene [28]. Women seem to have less tendinopathy than men, especially prior to menopause. Although tendons do not degenerate with age as such, a reduction in proteoglycans and an increase in cross-links with increasing age make tendon stiffer and less capable in tolerating load. Decreased flexibility, training on harder surface, and even drugs such as corticosteroids and quinolone antibiotics have been reported to be associated with the development of tendinopathy [15].

Ligament injuries are classified into three grades. (1) Grade I injury – mild sprain. Clinically, there is minimal pain present over the injured ligament and no joint instability can be detected by clinical examination despite the microfailure of collagen fibers. (2) Grade II injury – moderate sprain or partial tear of the ligament. There is severe pain present and minimal instability detected by clinical testing. Ligament strength and stiffness decrease by 50%. (3) Grade III injury – a complete ligament tear. Most collagen fibers have ruptured and the joint is completely unstable. Another type of injury is ligament avulsion from its bony insertion. Midsubstance ruptures are more common in45 adults; avulsion injuries are more common in children. Avulsion occurs between unmineralized and mineralized fibrocartilage layers [2, 3].

2.3. Pathophysiology of tendon and ligament repair

The process of tendon healing follows a pattern similar to that of other healing tissues. There are three phases of healing: (1) hemostasis/inflammation, (2) reparative phase, and (3) remodeling and maturation phase. Ligament healing goes through the same stages as tendon healing. However, there are differences among different ligaments. A classic model for ligament healing is the rupture of medial collateral ligament of the knee (MCL). MCL has a good tendency to heal spontanelously. In contrast, the anterior cruciate ligament of the knee (ACL) does not show any tendency to heal spontaneously, which is believed to be the consequence of synovial fluid interrupting the healing process between the ruptured ends of the ligament. Therefore, an ACL reconstruction is a treatment of choice [2, 3].

After the injury, the wound site is infiltrated by inflammatory cells. Platelets aggregate at the wound and create a fibrin clot to stabilize the torn tendon edges. The clot contains cells and platelets that immediately begin to release a variety of molecules, most notably growth factors (such as platelet-derived growth factor, transforming growth factor β, and insulin-like growth factor -I and –II) causing acute local inflammation. During this inflammatory phase that usually lasts three to five days, there is an invasion of extrinsic cells such as neutrophils and macrophages which clean up necrotic debris by phagocytosis and together with intrinsic cells (such as endotenon and epitenon cells) produce a second pool of cytokines to initiate the reparative phase [2-4].

In reparative phase (three to six weeks) large amounts of disorganized collagen are deposited at the repair site with granulation tissue formation, together with neovascularization, extrinsic fibroblast migration, and intrinsic fibroblast proliferation. After four days fibroblasts infiltrate the wound site and proliferate. They produce extracellular matrix, including large amounts of collagen III and glycosaminoglycan [2-4].

In the remodeling phase, there is a decrease in the cellular and vascular content of the repairing tissue, and an increase in collagen type I content and density. Eventually, the collagen becomes more organized, properly orientated, and cross-linking with the healthy matrix outside the injury takes place. Matrix metalloproteinase degrade the collagen matrix, replacing type II collagen with type I collagen. The remodeling stage can be divided into a consolidation and maturation phase. At the end of the consolidation phase, at about 10–12 weeks, and with the beginning of the maturation phase, the fibrous tissue is converted to a stronger scar tissue. Around the fourth week collagen fibers are being longitudinally reorganized so that they are aligned in the direction of muscle loading. During the next three months the individual collagen fibers form bundles identical to the original ones. After the healing process is complete, cellularity, vascularity, and collagen makeup will return to something approximating that of the normal tendon, but the diameters and cross-linking of the collagen will often remain inferior after healing. This phase lasts for months or years, usually between 6 weeks and 9 months or more. However, the tissue continues to remodel for up to 1 year. The structural properties of the repaired tendon typically reach only two thirds of normal, even years after injury [2-4].

There are slight differences in the way different tendons heal. Extrasynovial tendons can be easily influenced by growth factors and cytokines produced by extrinsic cells (e.g. paratenon), but intrasynovial tendons are more reliant on intrinsic cells (e.g. epitenon and endotenon) [3].

2.4. Treatment of tendon and ligament injuries

According to stages of healing response, a proper rehabilitation program time frame can be introduced. During the inflammatory phase of 3-5 days rehabilitation program should avoid excess motion because it can disrupt the healing process. During the repair phase a gradual introduction of motion can be introduced to prevent excessive muscle atrophy and prevent the diminishing of range of motion (ROM). Later progressive stress can be applied, however, tendons can require up to one year to get close to normal strength levels [3, 29].

Proper postsurgical rehabilitation strategies are being debated. Rehabilitation protocols differ due to anatomical site, because different tendons have different healing characteristics. There is even a difference in the rehabilitation protocol between sheathed tendons and tendons that are not enclosed in sheaths. In sheathed tendons, early mobilization is crucial to prevent scar formation between tendon sheath, therefore diminishing ROM. The response of healing tendons to mechanical load varies depending on anatomical location. Flexor tendons require motion to prevent adhesion formation, yet excessive force results in gap formation and subsequent weakening of the repair [2, 3].

2.4.1. Immobilization and early remobilization

Ruptured and immobilized ligaments heal with a fibrous gap between the ruptured ends, whereas sutured ligaments heal without fibrous gap. The mechanical properties of scars are inferior to normal ligaments, which may lead to joint dysfunction by abnormalities in joint kinematics [30]. In spite of this, many ligaments are not repaired routinely[3].

Protective immobilization may enhance tendon-to-bone healing compared with other post repair loading regimens like exercise or complete tendon unloading. In the repaired rotator cuff, immobilization has shown to be beneficial in tendon-to-bone healing. A complete removal of loading is detrimental to rotator cuff healing. However, immobilization is not a proper treatment for all repaired tendons; some require early passive motion [4].

Tendons requiring long excursions for function (e.g. the flexor tendons) are typically encased in synovial sheaths. To maintain gliding after injury, adhesions between the tendon surface and its sheath must be prevented. Passive mechanical rehabilitation methods have shown to be beneficial to prevent fibrotic adhesions [4, 31].

The optimal time for the initiation of such treatment is about 5 days after tendon repair [31]. Controlled loading can enhance healing in most cases, but a fine balance must be reached between loads that are too low (leading to a catabolic state) or too high (leading to micro damage).

2.4.2. Surgical reconstruction

There is still a debate when ligament or tendon injuries should be treated conservatively and when surgical repair is indicated. In practice the »50% rule« is commonly used [32]. The »50% rule« suggests that tendon/ligament injuries with structural involvement of less than 50% should be treated conservatively, but damage greater than 50% should be treated by surgical repair or reconstruction. This rule applies to a variety of orthopedic conditions, like partial fractural involvement of less than 50%, anterior cruciate ligament, partial-thickness injuries of the rotator cuff, and partial tears of the long head of the biceps tendon. However, there is very little evidence for accuracy, reproducibility, or predictive power and this rule has to be used with caution. It is maybe better to individualize the treatment according to a patient's clinical and physical status, expectations, and demands after the treatment [32].

2.5. The role of corticosteroid injection therapy

At the cellular level, anti-inflammatory and immunosuppressive actions of corticosteroids are the consequence of inhibition of cytokine-genes and pro-inflammatory mediators' synthesis, such as nitric oxide and prostaglandins. The immunosuppressive and anti-inflammatory actions of corticosteroids are mediated through the interference of two transcription factors: activating protein-1 (AP-1) and nuclear factor-κB (NF-κB) [16]. The exact mechanism by which corticosteroids inhibit the transcriptional activity of AP-1 is not fully understood. However, the activation of the cell by immune signals leads to degradation of IκB inhibitory protein from NF-κB, allowing nuclear translocation of NF-κB and consequently the transcription of multiple target genes. Corticosteroids induce the production of IκB and therefore provide efficient inactivation of NF-κB [16].

Besides the anti-inflammatory action, corticosteroids decrease the production of collagen and extracellular matrix proteins by the fibroblasts and enhance bone resorption. Furthermore, the production of extracellular matrix degrading enzymes MMP-3 (stromelysin-1), MMP-13 (collagenase-3), and MMP-1 (collagensae-1) in ligaments and other tissues is also suppressed. Whether this is beneficial when treating chronic tendon lesions is unknown, but some reports indicate the overexpression of MMPs in the Achilles tendinopathy [16].

Corticosteroids alter mechanical properties of tendons. Incubation of tendon fibrils in corticosteroids resulted in a significant reduction in tensile strength after only 3 days [33, 34]. It is possible, that corticosteroid injection affect the component of the extracellular matrix in a way that influences tensile strength. They may reduce decorin gene expression and inhibit the proliferation and activity of tenocytes, which leads to suppression in collagen production [34]. However, the magnitude of reduction in collagen type 1 and decorin gene expression appeared to be smaller when corticosteroid treatment was combined with mechanical strain [35].

Recommendations for the use of local corticosteroid injections are still not clear. Application should be peritendinous rather than intratendinous due to the demonstrated deleterious effect of corticosteroid on tendon tissue. Short or moderate acting, more soluble preparations are recommended because in theory they cause fewer side effects (hydrocortisone, methylprednisolone). Local anesthetics are usually mixed with the corticosteroid injection for wider dispersion and more comfortable procedure; but some manufacturers warn against mixing because of theoretical risk of precipitation. Corticosteroid injections in »high strain« tendons, especially the Achilles tendon or patellar tendon, are discouraged due to the possible and well documented risk of tendon rupture [18]. This therapy should be reserved only for chronic tendon injuries after the intensive use of other approaches for at least 2 months; injections should be peritendinous only. One study showed an increased rupture risk only when corticosteroids were injected intratendionously, but not when injected in peritendinous tissue. A maximum of three injections at one site should be given with a minimum interval between injections of 6 weeks. If two injections do not provide at least 4 week's relief, they should be discontinued [18].

2.6. Future therapies to improve tendon and ligament healing

Injection of growth factors, especially those derived from activated thrombocytes, and tissue-engineering strategies, such as (1) the development of scaffold microenvironment, (2) responding cells, and (3) signaling biofactors are generating potential areas for additional prospective investigation in tendon or ligament regeneration. Tissue engendering is a promising field to enhance tendon and ligament repair. Nevertheless, significant challenges remain to accomplish a complete and functional tendon or ligament repair that will lead to a clinically effective and commercially successful application. More will be discussed in the following sections.

3. Skeletal muscle damage and repair

Musculoskeletal injuries resulting in the necrosis of muscle fibers are frequently encountered in clinical and sports medicine [36] and are the most common cause of severe long-term pain and physical disability, affecting hundreds of millions of people around the world and accounting for the majority of all sport-related injuries [37].

The annual direct and indirect costs for musculoskeletal conditions in the United States were estimated at USD $849 billion or ~ 8% of the gross domestic product. Similarly, a study published in 2009 by Fit for Work Europe, examining musculoskeletal disorders in 23 European countries, reported that > 44 million members of the European Union workforce had a long-standing health problem or disability that affected their ability to work and that musculoskeletal disorders accounted for a higher proportion of sickness absence from work than any other health condition. In 2009, the total cost of musculoskeletal disorders in European workforce was estimated at €240 billion a year [38, 39].

Injured skeletal muscle can undergo repair spontaneously via regeneration; however, this process often is incomplete because the overgrowth of extracellular matrix and the deposition of collagen lead to significant fibrous scarring [40, 41].

Muscle injuries therefore frequently result in significant morbidity, including early functional and structural deficits, contraction injury, muscle atrophy, contracture, and pain.

By neutralizing pro-fibrotic processes in injured skeletal muscle, it is possible to prevent fibrosis and enhance muscle regeneration, thereby improving the functional recovery of the injured muscle [40].

3.1. Muscle structure and mechanism of action

A number of non-contractile connective tissue elements are necessary for the organization of the contractile muscle fibers into effective mechanical stress. Thus the fibers are bound together into fascicles by the fibroelastic perimysium; the ends of the muscle are attached to the bones by tendons and aponeuroses, and the whole muscle is held in its proper place by the connective tissue sheets called fasciae [42].

The arrangement of muscle fascicles, and the manner in which they approach the tendons, has many variations. In some muscles, the fascicles are parallel with the longitudinal axis and terminate at either end in flat tendons. In case of the converging fascicles to one side of a tendon the muscle is called *penniform*, like the semimembranosus muscle. If muscles converge to both sides of a tendon, they are called *bipenniform*, or if they converge to several tendons, they are called *multipenniform*, as in case of deltoid muscle. The nomenclature of striated muscle is based on different parameters describing their properties (Table 2).

The arrangement of fascicles and the power of muscles are positively correlated. Those with comparatively few fascicles, extending the length of the muscle, have a greater range of motion but not as much power. Penniform muscles, with a large number of fascicles distributed along their tendons, have a greater power but a smaller range of motion (ROM).

Molecular basis of muscle contraction is in the interaction between *actin* and *myosin*, fuelled by ATP and initiated by the increase in $[Ca^{2+}]_i$. Skeletal muscle possesses an array of transverse T-tubules extending into the cell from the plasma membrane, through which the action potential is spread into the inner portion of the muscle fiber (Figure 10), followed by releasing a short puff of Ca^{2+} from the sarcoplasmic reticulum (SR) into the sarcoplasm. Ca^{2+} binds to troponin, a protein that normally blocks the interaction between actin and myosin. When Ca^{2+} binds, troponin moves out of the way and allows the contractile machinery to operate.

Muscle, named by	Muscle
location	• brachialis • supraspinatus
direction	• rectus abdominis • obliquus abdominis
action	• flexor hallucis • extensor digitorum
shape	• deltoideus • trapezius
attachment points	• sternocleidomastoideus • omohyoideus

Table 2. Muscle nomenclature according to different parameters.

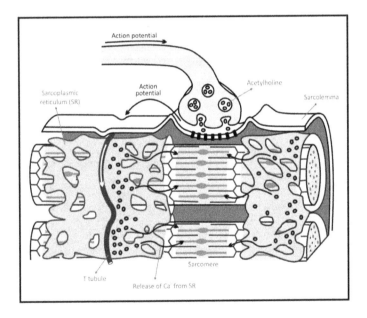

Figure 10. Molecular basis of muscle contraction.

3.2. Muscular injury mechanisms

Muscle injuries can be a consequence of a variety of causes: during the exercise, on the sports field, in the workplace, during surgical procedures, or in any kind of accidents. Regarding the mechanism, they are classified as direct and indirect. Direct injuries include lacerations and contusions, whereas the indirect class involves complete or incomplete muscle strain [43].

The current classification of muscle injuries distinguishes mild injuries from moderate and severe, based on the clinical symptoms. In a mild muscle injury, a strain or contusion is characterized by a tear of only a few muscle fibers with minor swelling and discomfort accompanied with no or only minimal loss of strength and restriction of movement. Moderate injury is represented by greater muscle damage with a clear loss of function, whereas a tear across the entire cross-section of the muscle resulting in a virtually complete loss of muscle function, is termed a severe injury [44, 45].

Muscle strain injuries after eccentric contractions are the most common type of muscle injury in athletes and are especially common in sports that require sprinting or jumping [46]. Submaximal lengthening contractions are used in everyday life, but it is well known that high-force lengthening contractions are associated with muscle damage and pain [47, 48]. Muscle strains are divided into three grades according to severity (Table 3) [43].

Muscle strains classification according to clinical severity	
Grade	Clinical Manifestation
I	Tear of new muscle fibers with minimal swelling and discomfort Minimal loss of strength with almost no limitation of movements
II	A greater damage of muscle Partial loss of strength and limitation of movements
III	A severe tear across the whole section of the muscle Total loss of the muscle function

Table 3. Classification of muscle strains according to clinical manifestation [43].

3.3. Pathophysiology of muscle damage and repair

The cellular and molecular mechanisms of muscle regeneration after injury and degeneration have been described extensively in recent decades [39, 49, 50]. Physiologically, healing progresses over a series of overlapping phases [43]. These stages include: (a) hemostasis, which usually starts with the formation of a blood clot and is followed by the local degranulation of platelets, which release several granule constituents; (b) the acute inflammatory phase is characterized by peripheral muscle fiber contraction, formation of edema and cell damagen and death; and (c) the remodeling phase that lasts from 48 hrs up to 6 wks; anatomic structures are restored and tissue regeneration occurs. Several cell types are involved in this phase and fibroblasts start to synthesize scar tissue.

Only local necrosis affects the injured ends of the myofibres because the torn sarcolemma is rapidly resealed, allowing the rest of the ruptured myofibres to survive [51]. Debris is removed by macrophages that secrete growth factors and activate the satellite cells. These are regenerative mononucleated stem cells of muscle tissue that normally lie between the basal lamina and plasma membrane of the muscle fiber [52]. First, they form myoblasts which then begin to produce muscle specific proteins and finally mature into muscle fibers with peripherally located nuclei [49].

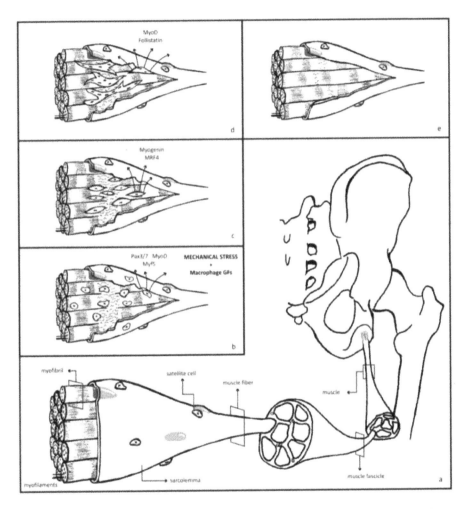

Figure 11. Role of satellite cells in muscle regeneration after acute injury. (a) quiescent satellite cells in a normal muscle just above sarcolemma; (b) mechanical stress and growth factors released from macrophages activate satellite cells that begin to express myogenic proteins which further stimulate proliferation; (c) in early differentiation phase, myoblasts express myogenin and MRF4, factors that promote further differentiation and the fusion of mononucleated cells; (d) in the late differentiation phase polynucleated myotubes begin to express factors that promote the final fusion and definite differentiation of myotubes into mature myofibres; (e) although muscle tissue is capable of self-regeneration, partial fibrosis contributes to function loss.

A typical feature during muscle differentiation is the variation in expression of various genes along with myogenic factors [53]. Sequence-specific myogenic regulatory factors (MRFs) are expressed exclusively in skeletal muscle and regulate the process of muscle development [54] (Figure 11). It is their role to govern the expression of multiple genes in myogenesis, from the engagement of mesodermal cells in the muscle lineage, to the differentiation of somatic cells and the terminal differentiation of myocytes into myofibres [55].

The MRFs consist of a group of transcription factors. They have been divided into two functional groups: The primary MRFs, MyoD, and Myf-5 required for the determination of skeletal myoblasts; and the secondary MRFs, myogenin and MRF4 that act later in the program, most likely as differentiation factors [54]. Activated satellite cells first express either Myf-5 or MyoD followed soon by co-expression of Myf-5 and MyoD. After the proliferation, myogenin and MRF4 are expressed in cells and begin their differentiation program [53].

The cellular process required for degeneration and regeneration may be affected by alterations in the inflammatory response. Although strained skeletal muscle is capable of self-regeneration, the healing process is slow and often incomplete, resulting in strength loss and a high rate of reinjury at the site of the initial injury [40]. Unfortunately, the muscle repair process involves a complex balance between muscle fiber regeneration and scar-tissue formation [39].

3.4. TGF-β and myostatin – a key factors in muscular scarring

TGF-β is a cytokine with numerous biologic activities related to wound-healing, including fibroblast and macrophage recruitment, stimulation of collagen production, downregulation of proteinase activity, and increases in metalloproteinase inhibitor activity. There are three mammalian isoforms of TGF-β: TGF-β1, TGF-β2, and TGF-β3. All three isoforms are potentially produced by most cells active in wound-healing, with platelets being a major contributor [56]. The major functions of TGF-β are listed in Table 4.

Activity of TGF-β
Stimulation of mesenchymal cell proliferation
Regulation of endothelial cells and fibroblasts
Promotion of extracellular matrix production
Stimulation of endothelial chemotaxis and angiogenesis
Inhibition of macrophage and lymphocyte proliferation
Inhibition of satellite cell differentiation

Table 4. Activity of TGF-β summarized by Borrione et al. [43]

TGF-β is a potent stimulator of fibrosis in the kidneys, liver, heart, and lungs [57-59] and is closely associated with skeletal muscle fibrosis as well where it plays a significant role in both the initiation of fibrosis and the induction of myofibroblastic differentiation of myogenic cells in injured skeletal muscle [41]. Many reports indicate that the overproduction of transforming growth factor TGF-β1 in response to injury and disease is a major cause of tissue fibrosis both in animals and humans [36, 57].

Muscle-derived stem cells (MDSDs) are populations of stem cells that appear to be distinct from satellite cells and can differentiate into myofibroblasts after muscle injury [41]. But myoblasts can also differentiate into fibrotic cells where TGF-β is a key factor that stimulates fibrotic differentiation [36].

Inhibition of TGF-β has been shown to decrease collagen deposition and scarring. For example, the application of neutralizing antibodies to TGF-β in rat incisional wounds successfully reduced cutaneous scarring [53].

However, it is not yet clear whether TGF-β acts alone or requires an interaction with other molecules during the development of muscle fibrosis. Recent studies have shown that myostatin may also be involved in fibrosis formation within skeletal muscle [60, 61].

Over the last years, the TGF-β member myostatin (MSTN) has gained particular relevance because of its ability to exert a profound effect on muscle metabolism, by regulating the myofibre size in response to physiological or pathological conditions [62]. Myostatin or GDF8 (Growth differentiation factor 8) is a TGF-β protein family member that inhibits muscle differentiation and growth [63] and is expressed specifically in developing and adult skeletal muscle [62]. It inhibits the activity of satellite cells during muscle regeneration due to its control of the movement of macrophages, and also inhibits the multiplication of myoblasts and their differentiation [64]. In myogenic cells, myostatin induces down-regulation of Myo-D, an early marker of muscle differentiation, and decreases the expression of Pax-3 and Myf-5, which encode transcriptional regulators of myogenic cell proliferation [65]. Its expression is restricted initially to the myotome compartment of developing somites and continues to be limited to the myogenic lineage at later stages of the development and in adult animals [53]. Major functions of myostatin are summarized in Table 5.

Activity of myostatin
Inhibition of satellite cell activity
Control of macrophage movement
Down-regulation of MyoD
Inhibition of transcriptional regulators of proliferation
Inhibition of myoblast multiplication in differentiation
Regulation of myofibre size

Table 5. Activity of myostatin.

Myostatin loss-of-function due to naturally occurring mutations into its gene triggers muscle mass increase in cattle [66], dogs [67], and humans as well [68]. Jarvnien et al. reported that the injection of a neutralizing monoclonal antibody to myostatin led to increased skeletal muscle mass in mice without side effects [51]. This method was found to be safe in a subsequent clinical trial, although dose escalation was limited by cutaneous hypersensitivity restricting potential efficacy [69]. Blocking of the MSTN signaling transduction pathway by specific inhibitors and genetic manipulations has been shown to result in a dramatic increase of skeletal muscle mass [70]. In principle, blocking of MSTN signaling can be achieved by three different pharmacological strategies: blocking MSTN gene expression (knocking out, inactivating the MSTN gene by viral-based gene overexpression, and antisense technologies); blocking the synthesis of the MSTN protein; and blocking of the MSTN receptor (small molecules, specific blocking antibodies) [71].

3.5. Therapeutic standards and controversies in treatment of muscle injuries

Despite the clinical significance of muscle injuries, the current treatment principles for injured skeletal muscle lack a firm scientific basis and are based on performing RICE (Rest, Ice, Compression, and Elevation). These four methods are supposed to limit the hematoma formation, though there are no randomized studies confirming their true value in the management of soft tissue injuries [72].

The most convincing is the effect of "rest" on muscle regeneration [73]. Limb immobilization prevents further retraction of the injured muscle and thereby greater discontinuity of the tissue, enlargement of hematoma, and the consequential scar tissue formation. Putting „ice"also so limits the formation of the hematoma, additionally impairs inflammation, and accelerates early tissue regeneration [74]. Concerns about the limited perfusion in the damaged muscle because of the limb „compression" are putting it under question while its „elevation" above the level of the heart follows the basic physiological principles as the hydrostatic pressure in the elevated tissue falls, followed by lesser interstitial fluid accumulation and the formation of edema. In this phase it is recommended to maintain the cardiovascular fitness without the risk for reinjury like cycling or swimming [51].

Although lacking scientific background, therapeutic ultrasound is a widely accepted adjuvant method for treating muscle injuries [75]. Micro massage with high-frequency waves has a pain relieving effect and it is supposed to act proregeneratory, especially in the early phase after an injury [51]. Despite promoting proliferation, therapeutic ultrasound does not seem to have a positive effect on the final outcome of muscle healing [76, 77].

Another adjuvant therapeutic option for improving muscle repair is hyperbaric oxygen therapy (HBO), which has shown to have positive effects during the early phase of repair by accelerating the recovery of the injured muscle [78]. However, not a single randomized prospective study has been performed on the treatment of severe skeletal muscle injuries by HBO, which might increase the sensation of pain in less severe forms of injuries like delayed onset muscle soreness (DOMS) [79]. In case of both mild and severe muscle injuries there is a lack of clinical studies confirming the real place of this therapeutic option in athletes.

The use of non-steroidal anti-inflammatory drugs (NSAID's) in the treatment of muscle injuries is common, but controversial. The most commonly prescribed are COX-2 inhibitors administered either via intramuscular, oral or transdermal route [39]. While the first studies reported on the positive effects of NSAID's on muscle regeneration without compromising muscle contractility or stem cell proliferation, the more recent showed the importance of the inflammatory process after injury and by inhibiting it the NSAID's promote scar tissue formation [80, 81]. Incomplete muscle fiber regeneration and fibrotic infiltration can lead to long-term functional deficits and physical incapacitation [39]. The use of glucocorticoids in case of muscle injuries is even more questionable as the elimination of the hematoma and necrotic tissue seems to be slower and biomechanical strength of the injured muscle reduced [66, 82].

The identification of MRFs allows researchers a new and more detailed insight into the processes of muscle regeneration which is crucial for developing novel therapeutic targets. In recent years many studies using antifibrotic agents have been performed in patients with different heart and kidney diseases or systemic sclerosis. *In vitro* and *In vivo* studies showed important antifibrotic effects of platelet-rich plasma derived growth factors, recombinant proteins such as decorin, follistatin, γ-interferon, suramin, relaxin, and other biologically active agents like mannose-6-phosphate, N-acetylcysteine, and angiotensin-receptor blockers. Although none of these has yet been tested on humans, their promising effects may significantly alter the therapeutic options of muscle injuries in the future. Furhter discussion on these bioactive agents will follow in Chapter XX (numer needed: Latest advances).

4. Articular cartilage damage and repair

Cartilage comprises of inherited limited healing potential and thus remains a challenging tissue to repair and reconstruct. Traumatic and degenerative cartilage defects occur frequently in the knee joint and represent difficult clinical dilemma. Articular cartilage has a limited capacity to self-repair principally due to its avascular nature and the limited ability of mature chondrocytes to produce a sufficient amount of extracellular matrix. Untreated cartilage injuries therefore lead to the development of arthritis. Current first line treatment options for smaller and mid-sized lesions in lower-demand patients are debridement or lavage and bone marrow-stimulating techniques (microfracture) which promote a fibrocartilage healing response. On the other hand, restorative treatment options such as osteochondral autologous graft transplantation (OATS) are limited by the amount of donor tissue availability and the size and depth of the defect. Regenerative treatment techniques such as autologous chondrocyte implantation (ACI) are promising treatment options for large full thickness articular cartilage defects where cells from healthy non-weight bearing areas are multiplied *In vitro* and implanted into such defects. Opposed to the traditional reparative procedures (e.g. bone marrow stimulation – microfracture), which promote a fibrocartilage formation with lower tissue biomechanical properties and poorer clinical results, ACI is capable to restore hyaline-like cartilage tissue in damaged articular surfaces. This technique has undergone several advances and is constantly improving. Indeed, there are numerous studies exploring new biomaterials; applications of various growth factors; the synergistic effects of mechanical stimulation in terms of tissue engineering *In vitro*, *In vivo*, and in animal models in order to stimulate the formation of hyaline-like cartilage.

4.1. Cartilage structure

Articular (hyaline) cartilage is a specific and well-characterized tissue with remarkable mechanical properties consisting of exclusively one cell type - chondrocytes which are embedded in the extracellular matrix (ECM). The principal function of articular cartilage is to withstand mechanical loads, facilitate smooth and perfect glide among articular surfaces, and enable painless and low friction movements of synovial joints. The articular cartilage is an aneural, avascular and alymphatic structure. The nutrition of chondrocytes occurs via diffusion between synovial fluid and cartilage matrix.

The only resident cells in articular cartilage (chondrocytes) contribute to only 1-5 % of tissue volume. The remaining 99 % represent the extracellular matrix (ECM) structural components that mainly consist of water, collagen, and proteoglycans (PGs). ECM works as a biphasic structure composed of a fluid phase (water and electrolytes) and solid phase consisting mainly of collagen and proteoglycans. The solid phase comprises of low permeability due to the high resistance of a fluid flow which causes a high rate of fluid pressurization and contributes to the load transmission of cartilage. Together, both solid and fluid phase establish the stiffness and viscoelastic properties of a cartilage [83, 84].

4.1.1. Structural layers

The structure of cartilage matrix varies with the depth; four different zones (superficial, transitional, radial, and calcified) are distinguished based upon the cell morphology, matrix composition, and collagen fibril orientation (Figure 12). Chondrocytes change their conformation from parallel to vertical in deep zones. Similarly, collagen fibers alignment becomes parallel in deeper zones of cartilage tissue. There is also an increase in the overall volume, water content, and overall biological activity in deeper zones [85].

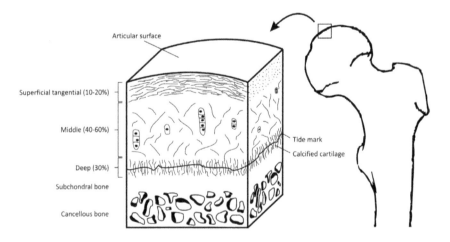

Figure 12. Structural layers of articualar cartilage.

Chondrocytes are specialized cells and basic structural cells in the articular cartilage, which are sparsely spread within the matrix and altogether form only 1-5 % of cartilage volume. They are deprived of blood supply and obtain the nutrients by diffusion from synovial fluid.

The formation of cartilage tissue and maturation of chondrocytes follows a multi-step process called chondrogenesis. In general it comprises of mesenchymal stem cell proliferation and their differentiation into mature chondrocytes capable to synthesize structural components of ECM (type II collagen, PG and non-collagenous proteins) and to maintain its continuous formation and restoration.

Each step of chondrogenesis can be classified according to the expression of different sets of transcription factors, cell adhesion molecules and extracellular matrix components. Chondrocytes have no cell-to-cell contacts, are highly metabolically active (however, due to low overall cell volume the total activity appears low) and are exposed to low oxygen environment and anaerobic metabolism. Mature chondrocytes are in the continuous communication with ECM and hence respond to changes in ECM and regulate its metabolism [85, 86].

Cartilage tissue is under constant impact of anabolic and catabolic cellular activity in response to extracellular environment and exposure to different cytokines and growth factors. Anabolic proteins such as tumor growth factor beta (TNF-beta), insulin growth factor (IGF-1), bone morphogenic protein (BMP), and fibroblast growth factor (FGF) stimulate matrix formation and promote the anabolic activity of chondrocytes. On the other hand, catabolic proteins such as tumor necrosis factor alpha (TNF-α) and interleukin 1 beta (IL-1β) inhibit protein synthesis and promote matrix degeneration. The constant equilibrium in the functioning of all signaling pathways is of crucial importance for the proper function and maintenance of cartilage tissue. The modern concept of cartilage tissue engineering is based on the imitation of the cartilage natural environment and the process of chondrogenesis to try to stimulate the formation of such a cartilage, which contains all the structural and biomechanical properties of native cartilage [87].

Extracellular matrix (ECM) is consists of water, collagen, and proteoglycans. All together water represents 60-85 % of the weight of the cartilage. The water content varies with the depth of the tissue; near the articular surface the water content is the highest and PG concentration is relatively low; vice versa is found in a deeper zone near subchondral bone, where the water content is the lowest but the PG concentration is the greatest. A high amount of water content in cartilage tissue is important for nutrition, lubrication, and for creating a low-friction gliding surface. In diseased cartilage such as osteoarthritis, the water content amounts to more than 90% as a result of matrix disruption and increased permeability. This leads to the decreased modulus of elasticity and reduction in load bearing capability.

Collagen is the main component of ECM. This fibrous protein represents 60 to 70% of the dry weight of the tissue. Type II collagen is the predominant collagen (90–95%) of ECM and provides a tensile strength to the articular cartilage. The high rate of cross-linkage between collagen molecules provides cartilages its resistance against traction forces. Other types of collagen molecules are also found in cartilage tissue in smaller amounts, these are types V, VI, IX, X and XI. Type IX and XI are most abundant in minor types collagen. Type XI participates in cross-linkage with type II collagen, integrins, and proteoglycans, whereas type XI is important in regulating the fibril diameter of type II collagen. Collagen architecture varies through the depth of the tissue. On the sliding surface of entire cartilage (tangential zone) collagen fibers are oriented parallel to the cartilage surface.

Proteoglycans (PGs) are protein polysaccharides and form 10–20% dry weight of the articular cartilage. Their primary function is to provide compressive strength to cartilage tissue. In articular cartilage they can be classified in two major classes, large aggregating proteoglycan monomers (aggrecans) and small proteoglycan molecules (decorin, biglycan, and fibromodulin). PG are composed of glycosaminoglycans (GAG) subunits (chondroitin and keratin sulfate) which are bound to a central core protein via sugar bonds to form proteoglycan aggrecan, which is highly characteristic for hyaline cartilage. Aggrecan, 250 kDa protein represents more than 80 % of all PG molecules in cartilage tissue. It binds to hyaluronic acid to form high molecular weight aggregates with more than 3.5 x 106 kDa. In the cartilage tissue these aggregates are located within the collagen type II fibril network resulting in densely packed negative charge which interacts with water via hydrogen bond and causing electrostatic repulsion. This key feature enables cartilage tissue to resist deformation under compression and to withstand and redistribute mechanical [83] [84].

4.2. Cartilage lesions

Injuries to articular cartilage are observed with an increasing frequency in athletes. In particular participation in pivoting sports such as football, basketball, and soccer they are associated with a rising number of sport-related cartilage injuries. The exact incidence of the cartilage damage is not known since they mostly appear asymptomaticly. However, during a review of 25,124 and 31.516 knee arthroscopies the injury of articular cartilage was found in 60 - 63 % [88, 89]. The incidence of 5 – 11 % was reported for full-thickness cartilage lesions (ICRS grade III and IV) [90]. Additionally, cartilage injuries of the knee joint are often accompanied with other acute injures such as ligament and meniscal injuries, traumatic patellar dislocation, osteochondral injuries, etc. [91].

The main symptom in patients with cartilage defects is the joint pain. Patients may also experience swelling and mechanical symptoms. Traumatic cartilage injury in the athletic population may progress to chronic pathological loading patterns such as joint instability and axis deviation. Although intact articular cartilage has the ability to adjust to the increasing weight bearing activity in athletes by increasing cartilage volume and thickness recent studies indicated that the degree of adaptation is limited [92]. Any activity beyond a threshold value may therefore result in maladaptation and cartilage damage. It has been shown that high impact joint loading above the adaptation limit causes decreased PGs content and leads to increase of degradative enzymes release and chondrocytes apoptosis [93]. Eventually, the integrity of functional weight bearing unit of cartilage is disrupted and leads to the loss of articular cartilage volume and stiffness, elevation of pressure and further articular cartilage damage in the long run.

Clinically, focal lesions are ranked according to the appearance of superficial zone of articular cartilage and are generally small (<1cm2) and sub-chondral and therefore asymptomatic.

It is difficult to predict whether the chondral lesion will progress to the more extensive deg-radation. However, in animal studies it was observed that smaller defects have the potential of spontaneous healing while the inverse relationship to repair potential was revealed in larger defects [94]. Once a patient becomes symptomatic due to cartilage damage, the lesion is likely to progress. A mechanical injury to articular cartilage can be acute, chronic, or acute and chronic. Cartilage loss often occurs after single or repeated impact loading due to trau-ma or misalignment. An increase in shear forces as a consequence of chronic abnormal load-ing of a joint surface results in irreversible changes in the biochemical composition of articular cartilage. Loading studies reported of significant swelling of articular cartilage (in-creased water content) and changes in the proteoglycans content only two weeks after ab-normal loading [95].

Cartilage tissue has a limited intrinsic capacity of healing response after cartilage damage, thus cannot fully regenerate and often leads to secondary degenerative disease. Early recog-nized and treated cartilage lesions might therefore prevent the secondary damage and pro-gression to the osteoarthritis. The main raisons for limited capacity to self-repair and regeneration seem to be the avascular nature of cartilage tissue and inability for clot forma-tion, which is the basic step in the healing cascade. That is why progenitor cells in blood and bone marrow and resident chondrocytes are unable to migrate to sites of the cartilage lesion [96]. Generally, intrinsic cartilage repair does not follow the main steps that usually occur after an injury in the other tissue: necrosis, inflammation, and repair or remodeling. Further-more, mature chondrocytes own limited proliferative capacity and have the limited ability to produce a sufficient amount of extracellular matrix to cover the defect. However, several cells are mobilized to the cartilage surfaces after an injury and can produce the repair ma-trix, although this matrix is morphologically and mechanically inferior to the original native cartilage tissue. Such a spontaneous healing was observed in small sub-chondral defects of fetal lambs and partial healing was also detected in small (less than 3 mm diameter) full-thickness lesions in rabbits [97]. However, larger cartilage defects of more than 6 mm rarely, if ever, show intrinsic healing potential but lead to progressive degenerative disease [94].

4.2.1. Partial and full thickness defects

Cartilage lesions can be divided into partial thickness defects which do not penetrate the subchondral bone and do not repair spontaneously, and full thickness defects which do pen-etrate subchondral bone have a partial repair potential, depending on the size and locations of the defect (Figure 13) [98]. The nature of the partial thickness defects has been studied and it was observed that the cells adjacent to the wound margin undergo cell death. Howev-er, there is an increase in cell proliferation, chondrocyte cluster formation, and matrix syn-thesis, but this repair is short-lived and eventually fails to repair the defect. It was also documented that the cells from synovia can migrate to the lesion in the presence of growth factors and can fill the defect with repair tissue. Due to anti-adhesive properties of PG and the absence of fibrin matrix these cells usually fail to adhere to the surface of defect [99].

The potential of cartilage repair in full thickness lesions is due to breaching of subchondral bony plate which leads to local influx of blood and undifferentiated mesencyhmal cells and hematoma formation containing fibrin clot, platelet, red and white blood cells. The blood clot can only fill the smaller defects < 2-3mm in diameter from the subchondral bone marrow. However, mobilized cells in the newly formatted blood clot are not capable to replace the defect with native hyaline cartilage, but produce fibrocartilage tissue, composed of higher collagen type I to collagen type II ratio and less proteoglycan, which has as mentioned already inferior properties compared to native hyaline cartilage. Several surgical techniques used the same attempt to treat full thickness defects such as micfrofracture which penetrate the subchondral bone in order to stimulate the clot formation and immobilize cells to the side of cartilage lesion [98].

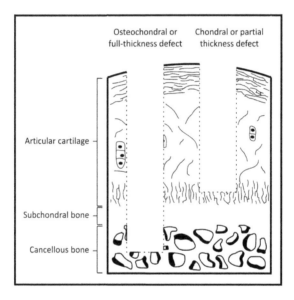

Figure 13. Partial and full thickness defects of articular cartilage.

4.2.2. Cartilage lesion classification

There are several classification systems to access cartilage lesion used in clinical practice. A number of elements are important in deciding what intervention might be the most helpful in trying to restore cartilage tissue such as: the size and area of cartilage damage, the depth of the damage, the degree of functional disability, patients' age, etc. However, not enough is known about a proper treatment of particular cartilage. Therefore, more objective data, methods and operative outcomes are required for good decision making regarding the treatment modalities since new procedures are rather expensive. Currently, the structural classifications such as Outerbridge and ICRS Classification (Table 6) are commonly used involving the examination of the extent and the depth of the cartilage lesion that helps surgeons to follow progression and improvement of the cartilage lesions.

	OUTERBRIDGE - description	ICRS - description
GRADE 0	normal cartilage	normal cartilage
GRADE 1	cartilage with softening and swelling	nearly normal: soft indentation and/or superficial fissures and cracks
GRADE 2	a partial-thickness defect (fibrillation or superficial fissures) less than 0.5-in diameter	a partial-thickness defect: extending down to <50% of cartilage depth
GRADE 3	deep fissuring of the cartilage to the level of subhondral bone without bone exposed greater than 0.5-in diameter	a partial-thickness defect: extending down to "/>50% of cartilage depth
GRADE 4	exposed subchondral bone.	severely abnormal (through the subchondral bone)

Table 6. Classification of articular cartilage lesions: Outerbridge and ICRS classification

The modified ICRS classification describes the defect macroscopically and correlates better with clinical outcome; grade 1 has good, grade 2-3 intermediate and grade 4 poor clinical result. However, along with the grade and depth, it is important to record the dimensions and position of the lesion (Modified ICRS Chondral Injury Classification System), to assess any bone loss or sclerotic change, the thickness of the surrounding cartilage and surrounding walls. Additionally, overall outcome depends also on patient's age, BMI index, the level of physical activity, etc.

4.3. Treatment of articular cartilage lesions

The main goals of surgical management of cartilage defects are to reduce symptoms, restore cartilage congruence, prevent additional cartilage deterioration, and to maintain the function of the joint without the insertion of artificial implants. Surgical treatment options may be divided upon their expected outcome as palliative, reparative or restorative [15]. Many procedures lead to the formation of fibrocartilaginous tissue with significantly inferior biochemical properties compared with those of hyaline cartilage. The newly formed scar tissue is unable to prevent a progression of a degenerative cartilage disease. The application of a specific surgical method is based on the patient's demand and the level of symptoms. For example, in lower demand patients with fewer symptoms the effective first-line treatments are palliative such as debridement and lavage. Similarly, reparative techniques are used in patients with moderate symptoms such as bone marrow stimulating procedures (drilling, abrasion arthroplasty, or microfracture) in effort to promote fibrocartilage formation. However, larger cartilage defects in higher demand patients (e.g. athletes with extreme weight bearing activity) with significant symptoms may not profit from standard treatment options, but should be advanced towards reparative treatment options such as autologous chondrocyte implantation (ACI) or osteochondral grafting [100].

4.3.1. Debridement and lavage

The goals of palliative treatment options (debridement and lavage) are the reduction of the inflammatory response due to mechanical irritation, functional improvement, and pain relief. Debridement involves the smoothing of cartilage and meniscal surfaces, removing necrotic tissue, and refreshing edges of cartilage lesions. Likewise, the beneficial effect of lavage implies the reduction of inflammation; removal of free cartilage fragments due to an injury and potential calcium phosphate crystals. Although the effectiveness of such a method is short-termed since it does not apply the restoration of cartilage defects, it significantly reduces pain symptomatic and improves the functionality of the articular joint compared to the conservative therapy. It is primarily recommended for patients with lower daily physical load and specifically localized mechanical symptoms (e.g. meniscal tear). Rehabilitation time after surgery is short and allows immediate loading activities without restrictions [101, 102].

4.3.2. Marrow stimulating techniques

Articular cartilage is deprived of its own blood supply; therefore traditional wound healing and clot formation is not possible. By opening up the subchondral bone plate, which separates the cartilage layer from the blood supply in bone marrow, hemorrhage can be induced to stimulate mesenchymal stem cells (MSCs), leukocytes, and growth on the side of the lesion as well as trigger remodeling and fibrocartilaginous cartilage repair. Bone marrow stimulating techniques are divided into drilling, microfracture, and abrasion, and are all based on the infiltration of blood products, fibrin clot formation, and fibrocartilage tissue repair [103].

Nowadays, microfracture is often used as a primary treatment option, and if not successful, more invasive cartilage repair methods are performed. The procedure is performed arthroscopically after a careful examination of articular cartilage surface and the quality of the cartilage. First, the focal chondral defects are debrided and the walls of the defect are smoothened. Any calcified cartilage is removed from the defect zone in order to prepare a better surface for the adherence of the clot and improved chondral nutrition through subchondral diffusion. Likewise, the walls of the lesion should be perpendicular to the defect to provide an area where the clot progenitor cell can form and adhere. After the initial preparation, the surgical awl is used to make multiple holes in the exposed subchondral bone. The holes should be placed 3-4mm from each other and should not connect. Subsequently, blood clot rich with bone marrow elements is formed which eventually undergoes the phase of remodeling and turns into fibrocartilage tissue [101-103]. Such cartilage resembles the native cartilage, but it differs significantly in the structural, biochemical, and mechanical properties and mostly contains type I collagen, which is cartilage non-specific and results in poor mechanical properties and poorly integrates into the adjacent cartilage.

A major concern is therefore the longevity of a fibrocartilage to withstand the stress and mechanical load on an active knee joint [104]. However, in follow-up studies 7-10 years after the surgery pain release and improved joint functionality was reported [105]. Moreover, microfracturing seems to have similar clinical results as ACI (look further chapter). Another problem was recently reported with microfracture procedure whether it can decrease the success of further alternative procedures such as ACI. In the study patients allocated to bone stimulating technique showed similar results following ACI as those where only debridement alone was performed [106]. Furthermore, in another study patients who previously underwent bone stimulating procedure showed a poorer outcome after ACI compared to those where only ACI alone had been performed [107].

Postoperative rehabilitation plays a key role in overall success of the treatment. Patients should undergo continuous passive motion physiotherapy for a period of 4 to 6 weeks and have the protected weight bearing. Following that period, patients are allowed an active range of motion exercises and progression to full weight bearing. However, no cutting, jumping or twisting sports are allowed until at least 4 – 6 months after surgery.

4.3.3. Osteochondral autograft transplantation (AOT)

Regeneration of damaged cartilage can be achieved with bone-cartilage transplants called osteochondral autograft transplantation (AOT). Nowadays, AOT is a well-established technique, but since the majority of the cartilage defects found in the knee joint are chondral rather than subchondral, there is a controversy regarding the overall usage of a osteochondral grafts and reaming in the healthy subchondral bone. The surgical procedure of AOT involves the removal of a full thickness hyaline cartilage attached to its underlying bone and the implantation of the osteochondral graft on the side of the lesion in a press-fit technique. Osteochondral autografts are usually harvested from non-weight bearing areas in order to avoid new damage or loss of function on the donor side. The site of the lesion should be prepared prior to implantation; any remaining cartilage is removed, the walls of the defect are made smooth and the tunnel of the same size as of the cartilage plug is drilled. However, the depth on the damage site should be 2 mm less than the plug size in order to achieve a favorable and stable position of the osteochondral graft and maintain an appropriate fit to the edges of the graft with surrounding intact cartilage. This helps to reduce shear stress on the border of the graft and ensures long-term success of the transplantation. Cartilage defects should not range more than 3cm2 due to a limited amount of donor tissue. For larger lesions several osteochondral plugs are used, therefore the procedure is called »mosaicoplasty«.

The main advantage of osteohondral grafting is that it possesses the normal native hyaline cartilage and does not include fibrocartilage which develops in the microfrature technique. However, the disadvantages include donor side morbidity (pain and cartilage defect), technical difficulty to match the shape of the plug to the contour of the articular joint, residual gap between adjacent plugs, and the risk of osteochondral collapse. Postoperative rehabilitation contains the use of continuous passive motion machine and weight bearing restrictions for a period up to 6 weeks. Clinical results are satisfactory; they reported good to excellent results even 10 years after surgery in 79 - 92% patients. The effectiveness of the method depends on the site of injury and is the most successful in isolated injuries of the femur condyles [101, 102].

4.3.4. Autologous cartilage implantation (ACI)

Autologous cartilage implantation represents a promising solution for the treatment of articular cartilage and enables permanent replacement of damaged cartilage tissue with its own native hyaline cartilage. The idea of an ACI is to harvest cartilage cells from the knee and grow them *In vitro* under specific laboratory conditions (Figure 14). Once millions of cells have been grown they are implanted into the area of cartilage defect. The procedure was first proposed by Brittberg in 1994 [108] and has become more widespread so that it currently represents the most developed articular cartilage repair technique.

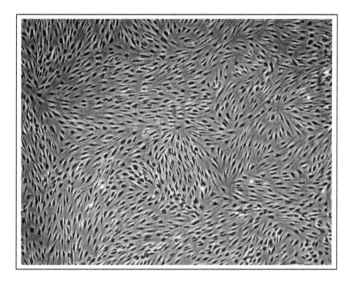

Figure 14. Proliferation of chondrocytes under monolayer culturing condition.

The original technique of ACI is a two-step procedure (Figure 15). The first step of ACI includes an arthroscopy to identify and access cartilage damage. Once the lesion is determined as suitable to perform the ACI procedure, the cartilage cells are harvested from the non-weight bearing zone in the knee. The chondrocytes are then isolated and grown in the tissue culture to allow them to multiply for several weeks. Once a sufficient number of cartilage cells has been obtained in the culture, the second surgery is scheduled. During the second surgery the cell suspension is re-injected into the cartilage defect underneath the periosteal patch. It is very important that the periosteal patch is carefully sutured in place and sealed with a fibrin glue in order to prevent any leakage of newly implanted cell suspension. ACI is usually used in intermediate and high-demand patients who have failed arthroscopic debridement or microfracture. The technique can also be used for larger 2 – 10 cm² symptomatic lesions. Prior to the surgery, patients must understand and be well prepared to participate in intensive postoperative rehabilitation and should fit the following profile: (1) the cartilage damage is focal and not widespread arthritis, (2)presence of pain or swelling that limits everyday activities, (4) a stable knee with no associated ligament damage and (5) normal body mass index (BMI). The postoperative rehabilitation consists of non-weight bearing in addition to range of motion (ROM) exercises with the use of a CPM machine for 6 weeks. Due to two surgical procedures and larger open arthrotomy, pain relief and restoration of function may take as long as 12 to 18 months [109, 110].

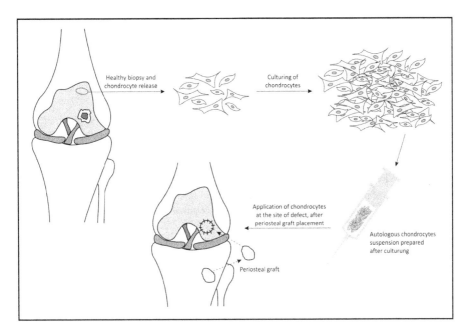

Figure 15. Schematic diagram showing the different stages involved in the process of autologous chondrocyte implantation.

The effectiveness of ACI varies and different levels of success were reported. Recently, ACI has been compared to microfracture technique. Both two and five years follow-up results, after patients were randomized for ACI or microfracture treatment of localized articular lesions of the knee joint, concluded that both methods had acceptable short-term results [111, 112]. There was no significant difference in macroscopic or histological results after two years. Similarly, after five years both methods provided satisfactory results in about 77 % of patients with no significant difference in clinical and radiographic results [112]. Currently, it seems as ACI is as good or a slightly better technique compared to a less invasive, simpler, and cheaper surgical technique in short-term. On the other hand, the significant superiority of ACI over mosaicoplasty for the repair of articular defects in the knee was reported in prospective randomized controlled trails [113, 114].

These results might not be surprising considering the traditional ACI (first generation ACI) encountered several problems. The most common complication with 10-25% incidence is periosteal hypertrophy due to scar tissue formation around the edge of the periosteal patch [115]. In addition, the need of periosteum widens the donor site morbidity and extends the operation time. The periosteum has to be tightly and waterproof sutured to prevent the potential leakage of the cell suspension from the defect. Another frequent disorder is patch delamination due to incomplete bonding of the patch with surrounding tissue. There are several other disadvantages regarding this method: the growth of cartilage tissue is age-dependent (lower potential in the elderly), difficulty to harvest and isolate sufficient numbers of cells from a small amount of tissue removed, fast differentiation of chondrocytes during *In vitro* cultivation in monolayers (loss of phenotype, differentiation in fibroblast-like cells), etc. Reoperation rate as high as 42 % was reported by several authors [116].

4.4. Future prospective for cartilage repair

Some of the problems have been avoided by using the collagen membrane instead of traditional periosteum patch. Anyway, the new technique (ACI-C) has still not solved the problem of watertight sutures and possible leakage. Nevertheless, in randomized control trial the comparison among the two procedures showed a lower re-operative rate in ACI-C, most probably due to the lesser extent of periosteum hypertrophy [117]. The new concept of cartilage tissue preservation was developed using tissue engineering technologies, combining new biomaterials as a scaffold, and applying growth factors, stem cells, and mechanical stimulation [118]. The recent development of so-called second regeneration ACI uses a cartilage-like tissue in a 3-dimensional culture system that is based on the use of biodegradable material which serves as a temporary scaffold for the *In vitro* growth and subsequent implantation into the cartilage defect. It has been shown *In vitro* that the application of 3-D environment promotes hyaline-like cartilage production and allows for mechanical stimulation [119, 120]. Several reports already described a superior role of the MACI (matrix/membrane autologous chondrocyte implantation) and CACI (collagen-covered autologous chondrocyte implantation) compared to the standard ACI procedure [121]. Additionally, the modern concept of tissue engineering uses various types of growth factors which are the endogenous regulators of chondrogenesis and their logical choice of use and relative ease of application have been reported to promote cartilage development [122]. Further studies are attempting to create the ideal scaffold and explore the synergistic effect of concomitant application of growth factors and mechanical loading [120] [123]. Finally, for clinical practice, single stage procedures appear attractive to reduce cost and patient morbidity. These procedures are promising, but there are only a few clinical studies and the results are in the process of publication and will be presented in the following chapter as they represent the most advanced and future therapeutic strategies for cartilage repair.

5. Conclusion

Locomotory system injuries are significant public health problems that contribute to a large burden of disability and suffering worldwide and are the most common injuries encountered in sports. The management of these injuries in athletes is particularly difficult as they have high demands and expectations. Achieving a fast recovery time and low possibility for reinjury is an ideal goal of each therapeutic team. Neglecting physiological processes in an injured tissue can often lead to inappropriate therapeutical interventions followed by unfunctional regeneration. The importance of keeping in mind the tissue processes at molecular level is therefore crucial and the only way to appropriate therapies.

Author details

Kelc Robi, Naranda Jakob, Kuhta Matevz and Vogrin Matjaz

Department of Orthopedic Surgery, University Medical Center Maribor, Slovenia

References

[1] Miller MD. Review of Orthopaedics, Fifth Edition. Philadelphia: Elsevier; 2008.

[2] Lieberman JR. Comprehensive Orthopaedic Review. Rosemont: American Academy of Orthopaedic Surgeons; 2009.

[3] Skinner HB. Current Diagnosis & Treatment in Orthopaedics, Third Edition. New York: Lange Medical Books; 2003.

[4] Killian ML, Cavinatto L, Galatz LM, Thomopoulos S. The role of mechanobiology in tendon healing. Journal of shoulder and elbow surgery / American Shoulder and Elbow Surgeons [et al]. 2012 Feb;21(2):228-37.

[5] Kumai T, Yamada G, Takakura Y, Tohno Y, Benjamin M. Trace elements in human tendons and ligaments. Biological trace element research. 2006 Winter;114(1-3): 151-61.

[6] Kastelic J, Galeski A, Baer E. The multicomposite structure of tendon. Connective tissue research. 1978;6(1):11-23.

[7] Woo SL, Debski RE, Zeminski J, Abramowitch SD, Saw SS, Fenwick JA. Injury and repair of ligaments and tendons. Annual review of biomedical engineering. 2000;2:83-118.

[8] Heinemeier KM, Kjaer M. In vivo investigation of tendon responses to mechanical loading. Journal of musculoskeletal & neuronal interactions. 2011 Jun;11(2):115-23.

[9] Suhodolcan L, Brojan M, Kosel F, Drobnic M, Alibegovic A, Brecelj J. Cryopreservation with glycerol improves the in vitro biomechanical characteristics of human patellar tendon allografts. Knee surgery, sports traumatology, arthroscopy : official journal of the ESSKA. 2012 Mar 15.

[10] Couppe C, Kongsgaard M, Aagaard P, Hansen P, Bojsen-Moller J, Kjaer M, et al. Habitual loading results in tendon hypertrophy and increased stiffness of the human patellar tendon. J Appl Physiol. 2008 Sep;105(3):805-10.

[11] Hansen M, Koskinen SO, Petersen SG, Doessing S, Frystyk J, Flyvbjerg A, et al. Ethinyl oestradiol administration in women suppresses synthesis of collagen in tendon in response to exercise. The Journal of physiology. 2008 Jun 15;586(Pt 12):3005-16.

[12] Thornton GM, Hart DA. The interface of mechanical loading and biological variables as they pertain to the development of tendinosis. J Musculoskelet Neuronal Interact. 2011 Jun;11(2):94-105.

[13] Woo SL, Hollis JM, Adams DJ, Lyon RM, Takai S. Tensile properties of the human femur-anterior cruciate ligament-tibia complex. The effects of specimen age and orientation. The American journal of sports medicine. 1991 May-Jun;19(3):217-25.

[14] Amiel D, Frank CB, Harwood FL, Akeson WH, Kleiner JB. Collagen alteration in medial collateral ligament healing in a rabbit model. Connective tissue research. 1987;16(4):357-66.

[15] Rees JD, Maffulli N, Cook J. Management of tendinopathy. The American journal of sports medicine. 2009 Sep;37(9):1855-67.

[16] Paavola M, Kannus P, Jarvinen TA, Jarvinen TL, Jozsa L, Jarvinen M. Treatment of tendon disorders. Is there a role for corticosteroid injection? Foot and ankle clinics. 2002 Sep;7(3):501-13.

[17] Zwerver J, Verhagen E, Hartgens F, van den Akker-Scheek I, Diercks RL. The TOP-GAME-study: effectiveness of extracorporeal shockwave therapy in jumping athletes with patellar tendinopathy. Design of a randomised controlled trial. BMC musculoskeletal disorders. 2010;11:28.

[18] Speed CA. Fortnightly review: Corticosteroid injections in tendon lesions. Bmj. 2001 Aug 18;323(7309):382-6.

[19] Arnoczky SP, Lavagnino M, Egerbacher M, Caballero O, Gardner K, Shender MA. Loss of homeostatic strain alters mechanostat "set point" of tendon cells in vitro. Clinical orthopaedics and related research. 2008 Jul;466(7):1583-91.

[20] Wang JH, Jia F, Yang G, Yang S, Campbell BH, Stone D, et al. Cyclic mechanical stretching of human tendon fibroblasts increases the production of prostaglandin E2 and levels of cyclooxygenase expression: a novel in vitro model study. Connective tissue research. 2003;44(3-4):128-33.

[21] Astrom M, Westlin N. Blood flow in chronic Achilles tendinopathy. Clinical orthopaedics and related research. 1994 Nov(308):166-72.

[22] Astrom M. Laser Doppler flowmetry in the assessment of tendon blood flow. Scandinavian journal of medicine & science in sports. 2000 Dec;10(6):365-7.

[23] Pufe T, Petersen WJ, Mentlein R, Tillmann BN. The role of vasculature and angiogenesis for the pathogenesis of degenerative tendons disease. Scandinavian journal of medicine & science in sports. 2005 Aug;15(4):211-22.

[24] Gotoh M, Hamada K, Yamakawa H, Inoue A, Fukuda H. Increased substance P in subacromial bursa and shoulder pain in rotator cuff diseases. Journal of orthopaedic research : official publication of the Orthopaedic Research Society. 1998 Sep;16(5): 618-21.

[25] Voloshin I, Gelinas J, Maloney MD, O'Keefe RJ, Bigliani LU, Blaine TA. Proinflammatory cytokines and metalloproteases are expressed in the subacromial bursa in patients with rotator cuff disease. Arthroscopy : the journal of arthroscopic & related surgery : official publication of the Arthroscopy Association of North America and the International Arthroscopy Association. 2005 Sep;21(9):1076.

[26] Birch HL, Wilson AM, Goodship AE. The effect of exercise-induced localised hyperthermia on tendon cell survival. The Journal of experimental biology. 1997 Jun;200(Pt 11):1703-8.

[27] Wilson AM, Goodship AE. Exercise-induced hyperthermia as a possible mechanism for tendon degeneration. Journal of biomechanics. 1994 Jul;27(7):899-905.

[28] September AV, Schwellnus MP, Collins M. Tendon and ligament injuries: the genetic component. British journal of sports medicine. 2007 Apr;41(4):241-6; discussion 6.

[29] Adutler-Lieber S, Ben-Mordechai T, Naftali-Shani N, Asher E, Loberman D, Raanani E, et al. Human Macrophage Regulation Via Interaction With Cardiac Adipose Tissue-Derived Mesenchymal Stromal Cells. Journal of cardiovascular pharmacology and therapeutics. 2012 Aug 15.

[30] Thornton GM, Leask GP, Shrive NG, Frank CB. Early medial collateral ligament scars have inferior creep behaviour. Journal of orthopaedic research : official publication of the Orthopaedic Research Society. 2000 Mar;18(2):238-46.

[31] Duzgun I, Baltaci G, Atay OA. Comparison of slow and accelerated rehabilitation protocol after arthroscopic rotator cuff repair: pain and functional activity. Acta orthopaedica et traumatologica turcica. 2011;45(1):23-33.

[32] Pedowitz RA, Higashigawa K, Nguyen V. The "50% rule" in arthroscopic and orthopaedic surgery. Arthroscopy : the journal of arthroscopic & related surgery : official publication of the Arthroscopy Association of North America and the International Arthroscopy Association. 2011 Nov;27(11):1584-7.

[33] Haraldsson BT, Langberg H, Aagaard P, Zuurmond AM, van El B, Degroot J, et al. Corticosteroids reduce the tensile strength of isolated collagen fascicles. The American journal of sports medicine. 2006 Dec;34(12):1992-7.

[34] Haraldsson BT, Aagaard P, Crafoord-Larsen D, Kjaer M, Magnusson SP. Corticosteroid administration alters the mechanical properties of isolated collagen fascicles in

rat-tail tendon. Scandinavian journal of medicine & science in sports. 2009 Oct;19(5): 621-6.

[35] Chen CH, Marymont JV, Huang MH, Geyer M, Luo ZP, Liu X. Mechanical strain promotes fibroblast gene expression in presence of corticosteroid. Connective tissue research. 2007;48(2):65-9.

[36] Li Y, Foster W, Deasy BM, Chan Y, Prisk V, Tang Y, et al. Transforming growth factor-beta1 induces the differentiation of myogenic cells into fibrotic cells in injured skeletal muscle: a key event in muscle fibrogenesis. The American Journal of Pathology. 2004;164(3):1007-19.

[37] Woolf AD, Pfleger B. Burden of major musculoskeletal conditions. B World Health Organ. 2003;81(9):646-56.

[38] Bevan S, Quadrello, T., McGee, R., et al. Fit for work? Musculoskeletal disorders in the European workforce. London2009.

[39] Gehrig SM, Lynch GS. Emerging drugs for treating skeletal muscle injury and promoting muscle repair. Expert Opin Emerg Dr. 2011 Mar;16(1):163-82.

[40] Huard J, Li Y, Fu FH. Current concepts review - Muscle injuries and repair: Current trends in research. J Bone Joint Surg Am. 2002 May;84A(5):822-32.

[41] Li Y, Huard J. Differentiation of muscle-derived cells into myofibroblasts in injured skeletal muscle. Am J Pathol. 2002 Sep;161(3):895-907.

[42] Gray H. Gray's anatomy. 29th ed. ed. Goss C, editor. Philadelphia: Lea & Febiger; 1973.

[43] Borrione P, Di Gianfrancesco A, Pereira MT, Pigozzi F. Platelet-Rich Plasma in Muscle Healing. Am J Phys Med Rehab. 2010 Oct;89(10):854-61.

[44] Ekstrand J, Gillquist J. Soccer Injuries and Their Mechanisms - a Prospective-Study. Med Sci Sport Exer. 1983;15(3):267-70.

[45] Jackson DW, Feagin JA. Quadriceps Contusions in Young Athletes - Relation of Severity of Injury to Treatment and Prognosis. J Bone Joint Surg Am. 1973;A 55(2): 421-2.

[46] Garrett WE. Muscle strain injuries. Am J Sport Med. 1996;24:S2-S8.

[47] Hammond JW, Hinton RY, Curl LA, Muriel JM, Lovering RM. Use of Autologous Platelet-rich Plasma to Treat Muscle Strain Injuries. Am J Sport Med. 2009 Jun;37(6): 1135-42.

[48] Proske U, Allen TJ. Damage to skeletal muscle from eccentric exercise. Exerc Sport Sci Rev. 2005 Apr;33(2):98-104.

[49] Carlson BM, Faulkner JA. The regeneration of skeletal muscle fibers following injury: a review. Med Sci Sports Exerc. 1983;15(3):187-98.

[50] Charge SBP, Rudnicki MA. Cellular and molecular regulation of muscle regeneration. Physiol Rev. 2004 Jan;84(1):209-38.

[51] Jarvinen TAH, Jarvinen TLN, Kaariainen M, Aarimaa V, Vaittinen S, Kalimo H, et al. Muscle injuries: optimising recovery. Best Pract Res Cl Rh. 2007 Apr;21(2):317-31.

[52] Mauro A. Satellite cell of skeletal muscle fibers. J Biophys Biochem Cytol. 1961 Feb; 9:493-5.

[53] Tripathi AK, Ramani UV, Rank DN, Joshi CG. In vitro expression profiling of myostatin, follistatin, decorin and muscle-specific transcription factors in adult caprine contractile myotubes. J Muscle Res Cell M. 2011 Aug;32(1):23-30.

[54] Megeney LA, Kablar B, Garrett K, Anderson JE, Rudnicki MA. MyoD is required for myogenic stem cell function in adult skeletal muscle. Gene Dev. 1996 May 15;10(10): 1173-83.

[55] Liu YB, Chu A, Chakroun I, Islam U, Blais A. Cooperation between myogenic regulatory factors and SIX family transcription factors is important for myoblast differentiation. Nucleic Acids Res. 2010 Nov;38(20):6857-71.

[56] Bates SJ, Morrow E, Zhang AY, Pham H, Longaker MT, Chang J. Mannose-6-phosphate, an inhibitor of transforming growth factor-beta, improves range of motion after flexor tendon repair. The Journal of Bone and Joint Surgery American Volume. 2006;88(11):2465-72.

[57] Border WA, Noble NA. Transforming growth factor beta in tissue fibrosis. N Engl J Med. 1994 Nov 10;331(19):1286-92.

[58] Lijnen PJ, Petrov VV, Fagard RH. Induction of cardiac fibrosis by transforming growth factor-beta(1). Mol Genet Metab. 2000 Sep-Oct;71(1-2):418-35.

[59] Waltenberger J, Lundin L, Oberg K, Wilander E, Miyazono K, Heldin CH, et al. Involvement of transforming growth factor-beta in the formation of fibrotic lesions in carcinoid heart disease. Am J Pathol. 1993 Jan;142(1):71-8.

[60] Wagner KR, McPherron AC, Winik N, Lee SJ. Loss of myostatin attenuates severity of muscular dystrophy in mdx mice. Ann Neurol. 2002 Dec;52(6):832-6.

[61] Zhu J, Li Y, Shen W, Qiao C, Ambrosio F, Lavasani M, et al. Relationships between transforming growth factor-beta1, myostatin, and decorin: implications for skeletal muscle fibrosis. The Journal of Biological Chemistry. 2007;282(35):25852-63.

[62] McPherron AC, Lawler AM, Lee SJ. Regulation of skeletal muscle mass in mice by a new TGF-beta superfamily member. Nature. 1997 May 1;387(6628):83-90.

[63] McCroskery S, Thomas M, Platt L, Hennebry A, Nishimura T, McLeay L, et al. Improved muscle healing through enhanced regeneration and reduced fibrosis in myostatin-null mice. J Cell Sci. 2005 Aug 1;118(Pt 15):3531-41.

[64] Thomas M, Langley B, Berry C, Sharma M, Kirk S, Bass J, et al. Myostatin, a negative regulator of muscle growth, functions by inhibiting myoblast proliferation. J Biol Chem. 2000 Dec 22;275(51):40235-43.

[65] Langley B, Thomas M, Bishop A, Sharma M, Gilmour S, Kambadur R. Myostatin inhibits myoblast differentiation by down-regulating MyoD expression. J Biol Chem. 2002 Dec 20;277(51):49831-40.

[66] McPherron AC, Lee SJ. Double muscling in cattle due to mutations in the myostatin gene. Proc Natl Acad Sci U S A. 1997 Nov 11;94(23):12457-61.

[67] Mosher DS, Quignon P, Bustamante CD, Sutter NB, Mellersh CS, Parker HG, et al. A mutation in the myostatin gene increases muscle mass and enhances racing performance in heterozygote dogs. PLoS Genet. 2007 May 25;3(5):e79.

[68] Schuelke M, Wagner KR, Stolz LE, Hubner C, Riebel T, Komen W, et al. Myostatin mutation associated with gross muscle hypertrophy in a child. N Engl J Med. 2004 Jun 24;350(26):2682-8.

[69] Wagner KR, Fleckenstein JL, Amato AA, Barohn RJ, Bushby K, Escolar DM, et al. A phase I/IItrial of MYO-029 in adult subjects with muscular dystrophy. Ann Neurol. 2008 May;63(5):561-71.

[70] Bogdanovich S, Krag TO, Barton ER, Morris LD, Whittemore LA, Ahima RS, et al. Functional improvement of dystrophic muscle by myostatin blockade. Nature. 2002 Nov 28;420(6914):418-21.

[71] Diel P, Schiffer T, Geisler S, Hertrampf T, Mosler S, Schulz S, et al. Analysis of the effects of androgens and training on myostatin propeptide and follistatin concentrations in blood and skeletal muscle using highly sensitive immuno PCR. Molecular and Cellular Endocrinology. 2010;330(1-2):1-9.

[72] Bleakley C, McDonough S, MacAuley D. The use of ice in the treatment of acute soft-tissue injury - A systematic review of randomized controlled trials. Am J Sport Med. 2004 Jan-Feb;32(1):251-61.

[73] Järvinen M, Lehto, MU. The effects of early mobilisation and immobilisation on the healing process following muscle injuries. Sports Med. 1993;15(2):78-89.

[74] Schaser KD, Disch AC, Stover JF, Lauffer A, Bail HJ, Mittlmeier T. Prolonged superficial local cryotherapy attenuates microcirculatory impairment, regional inflammation, and muscle necrosis after closed soft tissue injury in rats. Am J Sports Med. 2007 Jan;35(1):93-102.

[75] Markert CD, Merrick MA, Kirby TE, Devor ST. Nonthermal ultrasound and exercise in skeletal muscle regeneration. Arch Phys Med Rehabil. 2005 Jul;86(7):1304-10.

[76] Rantanen J, Thorsson O, Wollmer P, Hurme T, Kalimo H. Effects of therapeutic ultrasound on the regeneration of skeletal myofibers after experimental muscle injury. Am J Sports Med. 1999 Jan-Feb;27(1):54-9.

[77] Wilkin LD, Merrick MA, Kirby TE, Devor ST. Influence of therapeutic ultrasound on skeletal muscle regeneration following blunt contusion. Int J Sports Med. 2004 Jan; 25(1):73-7.

[78] Jarvinen T, Jarvinen, TLN., Kaariainen, M. Biology of muscle trauma. Am J Sport Med. 2005;33:745-66.

[79] Jarvinen M. Healing of a crush injury in rat striated muscle. 2. a histological study of the effect of early mobilization and immobilization on the repair processes. Acta Pathol Microbiol Scand A. 1975 May;83(3):269-82.

[80] Mackey AL, Kjaer M, Dandanell S, Mikkelsen KH, Holm L, Dossing S, et al. The influence of anti-inflammatory medication on exercise-induced myogenic precursor cell responses in humans. J Appl Physiol. 2007 Aug;103(2):425-31.

[81] Woods C, Hawkins RD, Maltby S, Hulse M, Thomas A, Hodson A. The Football Association Medical Research Programme: an audit of injuries in professional football--analysis of hamstring injuries. Br J Sports Med. 2004 Feb;38(1):36-41.

[82] De Smet AA, Best TM. MR imaging of the distribution and location of acute hamstring injuries in athletes. AJR Am J Roentgenol. 2000 Feb;174(2):393-9.

[83] Bruckner P, van der Rest M. Structure and function of cartilage collagens. Microsc Res Tech. 1994 Aug 1;28(5):378-84.

[84] Schulz RM, Bader A. Cartilage tissue engineering and bioreactor systems for the cultivation and stimulation of chondrocytes. Eur Biophys J. 2007 Apr;36(4-5):539-68.

[85] Aigner T, Sachse A, Gebhard PM, Roach HI. Osteoarthritis: pathobiology-targets and ways for therapeutic intervention. Adv Drug Deliv Rev. 2006 May 20;58(2):128-49.

[86] Goldring MB, Tsuchimochi K, Ijiri K. The control of chondrogenesis. J Cell Biochem. 2006 Jan 1;97(1):33-44.

[87] Fan Z, Chubinskaya S, Rueger DC, Bau B, Haag J, Aigner T. Regulation of anabolic and catabolic gene expression in normal and osteoarthritic adult human articular chondrocytes by osteogenic protein-1. Clin Exp Rheumatol. 2004 Jan-Feb;22(1):103-6.

[88] Curl WW, Krome J, Gordon ES, Rushing J, Smith BP, Poehling GG. Cartilage injuries: a review of 31,516 knee arthroscopies. Arthroscopy. 1997 Aug;13(4):456-60.

[89] Hjelle K, Solheim E, Strand T, Muri R, Brittberg M. Articular cartilage defects in 1,000 knee arthroscopies. Arthroscopy. 2002 Sep;18(7):730-4.

[90] Aroen A, Loken S, Heir S, Alvik E, Ekeland A, Granlund OG, et al. Articular cartilage lesions in 993 consecutive knee arthroscopies. Am J Sports Med. 2004 Jan-Feb;32(1): 211-5.

[91] Woolf AD, Pfleger B. Burden of major musculoskeletal conditions. Bulletin of the World Health Organization. 2003;81(9):646-56.

[92] Mithoefer K, Hambly K, Logerstedt D, Ricci M, Silvers H, Della Villa S. Current concepts for rehabilitation and return to sport after knee articular cartilage repair in the athlete. J Orthop Sports Phys Ther. 2012 Mar;42(3):254-73.

[93] Kiviranta I, Tammi M, Jurvelin J, Arokoski J, Saamanen AM, Helminen HJ. Articular cartilage thickness and glycosaminoglycan distribution in the canine knee joint after strenuous running exercise. Clin Orthop Relat Res. 1992 Oct(283):302-8.

[94] Khan IM, Gilbert SJ, Singhrao SK, Duance VC, Archer CW. Cartilage integration: evaluation of the reasons for failure of integration during cartilage repair. A review. Eur Cell Mater. 2008;16:26-39.

[95] Uchio Y, Ochi M. [Biology of articular cartilage repair--present status and prospects]. Clinical calcium. 2004 Jul;14(7):22-7.

[96] Hayes DW, Jr., Brower RL, John KJ. Articular cartilage. Anatomy, injury, and repair. Clinics in podiatric medicine and surgery. 2001 Jan;18(1):35-53.

[97] Shapiro F, Koide S, Glimcher MJ. Cell origin and differentiation in the repair of full-thickness defects of articular cartilage. J Bone Joint Surg Am. 1993 Apr;75(4):532-53.

[98] Redman SN, Oldfield SF, Archer CW. Current strategies for articular cartilage repair. Eur Cell Mater. 2005;9:23-32; discussion 23-32.

[99] Hunziker EB. Growth-factor-induced healing of partial-thickness defects in adult articular cartilage. Osteoarthritis Cartilage. 2001 Jan;9(1):22-32.

[100] Radosavljevič D DM, Gorenšek M, Koritnik B, Kregar-Velikovanja N. Operativno zdravljenje okvar sklepnega hrustanca v sklepu. Med Razgl. 2003, 47–57.

[101] Detterline AJ, Goldberg S, Bach BR, Jr., Cole BJ. Treatment options for articular cartilage defects of the knee. Orthop Nurs. 2005 Sep-Oct;24(5):361-6; quiz 7-8.

[102] Lewis PB, McCarty LP, 3rd, Kang RW, Cole BJ. Basic science and treatment options for articular cartilage injuries. J Orthop Sports Phys Ther. 2006 Oct;36(10):717-27.

[103] Steadman JR, Rodkey WG, Rodrigo JJ. Microfracture: surgical technique and rehabilitation to treat chondral defects. Clin Orthop Relat Res. 2001 Oct(391 Suppl):S362-9.

[104] Mow VC, Ratcliffe A, Rosenwasser MP, Buckwalter JA. Experimental studies on repair of large osteochondral defects at a high weight bearing area of the knee joint: a tissue engineering study. Journal of biomechanical engineering. 1991 May;113(2): 198-207.

[105] Steadman JR, Briggs KK, Rodrigo JJ, Kocher MS, Gill TJ, Rodkey WG. Outcomes of microfracture for traumatic chondral defects of the knee: average 11-year follow-up. Arthroscopy. 2003 May-Jun;19(5):477-84.

[106] Zaslav K, Cole B, Brewster R, DeBerardino T, Farr J, Fowler P, et al. A prospective study of autologous chondrocyte implantation in patients with failed prior treatment

for articular cartilage defect of the knee: results of the Study of the Treatment of Articular Repair (STAR) clinical trial. Am J Sports Med. 2009 Jan;37(1):42-55.

[107] Minas T, Gomoll AH, Rosenberger R, Royce RO, Bryant T. Increased failure rate of autologous chondrocyte implantation after previous treatment with marrow stimulation techniques. Am J Sports Med. 2009 May;37(5):902-8.

[108] Brittberg M, Lindahl A, Nilsson A, Ohlsson C, Isaksson O, Peterson L. Treatment of deep cartilage defects in the knee with autologous chondrocyte transplantation. The New England journal of medicine. 1994 Oct 6;331(14):889-95.

[109] Nazem K, Safdarian A, Fesharaki M, Moulavi F, Motififard M, Zarezadeh A, et al. Treatment of full thickness cartilage defects in human knees with Autologous Chondrocyte Transplantation. J Res Med Sci. 2011 Jul;16(7):855-61.

[110] Harris JD, Siston RA, Pan X, Flanigan DC. Autologous chondrocyte implantation: a systematic review. J Bone Joint Surg Am. 2010 Sep 15;92(12):2220-33.

[111] Knutsen G, Engebretsen L, Ludvigsen TC, Drogset JO, Grontvedt T, Solheim E, et al. Autologous chondrocyte implantation compared with microfracture in the knee. A randomized trial. J Bone Joint Surg Am. 2004 Mar;86-A(3):455-64.

[112] Knutsen G, Drogset JO, Engebretsen L, Grontvedt T, Isaksen V, Ludvigsen TC, et al. A randomized trial comparing autologous chondrocyte implantation with microfracture. Findings at five years. J Bone Joint Surg Am. 2007 Oct;89(10):2105-12.

[113] Bentley G, Biant LC, Carrington RW, Akmal M, Goldberg A, Williams AM, et al. A prospective, randomised comparison of autologous chondrocyte implantation versus mosaicplasty for osteochondral defects in the knee. J Bone Joint Surg Br. 2003 Mar; 85(2):223-30.

[114] Horas U, Pelinkovic D, Herr G, Aigner T, Schnettler R. Autologous chondrocyte implantation and osteochondral cylinder transplantation in cartilage repair of the knee joint. A prospective, comparative trial. J Bone Joint Surg Am. 2003 Feb;85-A(2): 185-92.

[115] Minas T. Autologous chondrocyte implantation for focal chondral defects of the knee. Clin Orthop Relat Res. 2001 Oct(391 Suppl):S349-61.

[116] Micheli LJ, Browne JE, Erggelet C, Fu F, Mandelbaum B, Moseley JB, et al. Autologous chondrocyte implantation of the knee: multicenter experience and minimum 3-year follow-up. Clinical journal of sport medicine : official journal of the Canadian Academy of Sport Medicine. 2001 Oct;11(4):223-8.

[117] Harris JD, Siston RA, Brophy RH, Lattermann C, Carey JL, Flanigan DC. Failures, re-operations, and complications after autologous chondrocyte implantation--a systematic review. Osteoarthritis Cartilage. 2011 Jul;19(7):779-91.

[118] Kock L, van Donkelaar CC, Ito K. Tissue engineering of functional articular cartilage: the current status. Cell and tissue research. 2012 Mar;347(3):613-27.

[119] Hutmacher DW, Goh JC, Teoh SH. An introduction to biodegradable materials for tissue engineering applications. Ann Acad Med Singapore. 2001 Mar;30(2):183-91.

[120] Moutos FT, Guilak F. Composite scaffolds for cartilage tissue engineering. Biorheology. 2008;45(3-4):501-12.

[121] Giza E, Sullivan M, Ocel D, Lundeen G, Mitchell ME, Veris L, et al. Matrix-induced autologous chondrocyte implantation of talus articular defects. Foot Ankle Int. 2010 Sep;31(9):747-53.

[122] Fortier LA, Barker JU, Strauss EJ, McCarrel TM, Cole BJ. The role of growth factors in cartilage repair. Clin Orthop Relat Res. [Review]. 2011 Oct;469(10):2706-15.

[123] Elder BD, Athanasiou KA. Synergistic and additive effects of hydrostatic pressure and growth factors on tissue formation. PLoS One. 2008;3(6):e2341.

Chapter 2

Novel Therapies for the Management of Sports Injuries

Robi Kelc, Jakob Naranda, Matevz Kuhta and
Matjaz Vogrin

Additional information is available at the end of the chapter

1. Introduction

With the contemporary active lifestyle and widespread professionalism in sport, the need for high-end injury therapies is growing. Conservative principles in managing various sports injuries usually do not meet the need of athletes and their coaches. In order to achieve better and faster recovery after injuries, significant effort has been made in the recent decade among researchers. Local growth factor application, targeted therapies using recombinant proteins and tissue engineering represent promising groups of future therapeutic options with promising results.

Healthy tendons and ligaments get injured either by a single application of force or by a repeated or sustained action that alters their mechanical characteristics. Genetic disorders, aging, decreased vascularity, endocrine influences, nutritional status, inactivity, immobilization, and exercise may cause tendon degeneration, thus rendering the tendon or ligament more susceptible to injury when force is applied. Hypovascularity is hypothesized to play the major role in this degeneration, both directly by causing an ischaemic environment for the fibroblast and indirectly both by contributing to the production of free radicals and by allowing for tissue hyperthermia to occur. Conservative management, such as rest, corticosteroid injection, orthotics, ultrasound, laser treatment, or shockwave treatment provide pain relief but, when they fail, surgery is required. Local growth factor application and tissue-engineering strategies, such as the development of scaffold microenvironments, responding cells, and signalling biofactors are currently generating potential areas for additional prospective investigation in tendon or ligament regeneration.

Cartilage tissue also comprises of limited intrinsic potential for healing due to the lack of blood supply and subsequent incomplete repair by local chondrocytes with inferior fibrocartilage formation. Surgical intervention is often the only option, but the repair of damaged cartilage is often less than satisfactory, and rarely restores full function or returns the tissue to its native normal state. The new concept of cartilage tissue preservation uses tissue engineering technologies, combining new biomaterials as a scaffold, applying growth factors and using stem cells and mechanical stimulation.

Skeletal muscle, on the other hand, has a great regenerative capacity; however, this process if often incomplete because of partial fibrous scar formation. Conservative therapies including cryotherapy, resting, physical therapy and pain relief medications don't often give satisfactory results and can even be controversial. While surgery is reserved for bigger tissue defects, the need for antifibrotic agents to improve muscle repair after injury is obvious. These and platelet-derived growth factors represent the future of biological therapies for this common type of sports injury.

Novel tissue-specific therapies are mainly molecular, based on pathophysiological processes after injury. Although they seem to significantly accelerate healing and shorten the recovery time, their true goal is to achieve better and more functional repair.

2. Biological therapy for better muscle regeneration

While spontaneous muscle fibre regeneration usually occurs after muscle injury, this process can often be slow and incomplete and accompanied by fibrotic infiltration, which compromises the restoration of contractile function [1]. Scar formation is the result of excessive wound healing leading to a poor functional outcome after trauma and surgery [2]. Successful muscle repair after injury is important for restoring mobility and patients' quality of life. We therefore have an important medical need for drugs that can promote or hasten muscle fibre regeneration, reduce fibrosis, and enhance muscle function [1].

Despite the clinical significance of muscle injuries, current treatment principles for injured skeletal muscle lack a firm scientific basis, and are based on performing RICE (Rest, Ice, Compression, Elevation) and sometimes prescribing non-steroidal anti-inflammatory drugs (NSAIDs). However, increasing evidence indicates that the administration of NSAIDs decreases regeneration and increases fibrosis by inhibiting inflammation [3, 4].

Incomplete muscle fibre regeneration and fibrotic infiltration can lead to long-term functional deficits and physical incapacitation [1]. In recent years of muscle regeneration research, many agents have been described to have a significant antifibrotic effect in patients with heart or kidney disease and systemic sclerosis. Consequently, researchers are testing these for muscle healing, as therapeutic targets are the same. Although these agents play a life-saving role in the previously mentioned diseases, their importance for muscle injuries could be substantial and for athletes specifically, vital.

Transforming growth factor-Beta (TGF-β) and myostatin have been identified as the main factors that stimulate fibrotic differentiation. It has been shown in *In vitro* and *In vivo* studies that drugs with anti-fibrotic properties that can prevent or minimize scar formation have the potential of standalone or adjuvant therapies (Table 1). Although the World Anti-Doping

Agency (WADA) prohibits any use of myostatin inhibitors in athletes, their potential to act only therapeutically at the site of injury without any performance enhancement may play an important role in muscle injury therapy in the future. In the following chapters, various agents are described that reportedly have beneficial effects on muscle healing after injury.

Class	Agent
Recombinant proteins	Follistatin
	Decorin
	Interferon-γ
	Suramin
	Relaxin
Autologous growth factors	Platelet-rich plasma (PrP)
Other bioactive agents	Mannose-6-phosphate (M6P)
	N-acetylcysteine (NAC)
	Angiotensin receptor blockers (ARBs)

Table 1. Agents with proven anti-fibrotic effects in *In vitro* or *In vivo* studies of skeletal muscle regeneration after injury

2.1. Recombinant proteins in muscle regeneration

Follistatin is an autocrine glycoprotein expressed in nearly all tissues of higher animals, with multiple effects on skeletal muscles as well as other tissues [5]. It is a functional antagonist of several members of the TGF-β family of secreted signalling factors, including myostatin - the most powerful inhibitor of muscle growth characterized to date [6, 7]. Follistatin was previously known as FSH-suppressing protein (FSP) as it was found to have inhibitory effect on pituitary secretion of follicle-stimulating hormone (FSH) [8]. Research into the development of therapies to antagonize myostatin has led to the discovery of several new functions exhibited by follistatin [9]. Several *In vivo* studies on follistatin have shown that it directly inhibits myostatin and also reduces myostatin-induced muscle wasting after systemic administration [5, 10]. In recent research, Zhu et al. reported on the stimulative effect of follistatin on MyoD, MyF5, and myogenin expression, which are myogenic transcription factors that promote muscle differentiation. They also showed its inhibitory effect on myostatin, activin A, and TGF-β, all of which are negative regulators of muscle cell differentiation [9]. Although various myostatin inhibitors have been described, follistatin can modulate other regulators of muscle mass in addition to myostatin [11]. For example, follistatin administration to MSTN-1- mice caused muscle mass increases beyond that stimulated by myostatin depletion [12, 13], suggesting that this may be a more potent approach than targeting myostatin alone. Intramuscular administration of gene therapy vectors expressing follistatin has increased muscle mass and strength in both young and aged mdx mice, as well as in nonhuman primates [14]. In order to investigate the mechanisms of the follistatin-induced muscle hypertrophy, Gilson et al. used irradiation to destroy the proliferative capacity of satellite cells. They found that not only inhibition of MSTN, but also of activin (ACT) and proliferation of satellite cells are involved in follistatin-induced muscle hypertrophy [12]. Follistatin thus might offer a novel therapeutic strategy for muscular injuries and dystrophy by suppressing the progression of muscle degeneration and permitting skeletal muscle mass restoration [15]. However, before translating follistatin-based therapies from the bench to the bedside, clear mechanisms of how follistatin promotes muscle regeneration require extensive investigation.

Decorin is a component of the extracellular matrix in all collagen-containing tissues [16] and is expressed at high levels in skeletal muscle during early development [17]. It is a small leucine-rich proteoglycan that can modulate the bioactivity of growth factors and act as a direct signalling molecule to various cells [18]. It was found to neutralize the effects of myostatin in both fibroblasts and myoblasts. It has been implicated in cell proliferation and differentiation due to its ability to bind growth factors and has been found to interact with collagen, fibronectin and thrombospondin, hence influencing processes such as fibrillogenesis, cell adhesion, and migration [19]. Fukushima et al. proved that decorin also inactivates the stimulating effect of TGF-β in myofibroblasts *In vitro*, which has a beneficial effect in muscle fibrosis and leads to enhancement of muscle regeneration and strength [20]. Recent reports showed that the injection of decorin into lacerated muscle improves both muscle structure and function, enabling nearly complete recovery of muscle strength [20-22]. Besides reducing fibrosis, decorin promotes muscle cell differentiation by upregulating follistatin, PGC-1α, and myogenic genes, including MyoD [23]. Thus, decorin appears to be a new molecule in the myostatin-signalling pathway [24-26]. It has been reported that muscle cells produce decorin and myostatin proteins at the same time, and that prenatal and postnatal expression of myostatin is similar [17].

Interferon (IFN)-γ is an inflammatory cytokine that was first identified as an antiviral factor [27]. A primary function of IFN-γ is activation of macrophages through the classical pathway, which promotes pathogen killing [28]. Later, IFN-γ was recognized as a pleiotropic cytokine that also plays a role in regulating different immune responses as well as influencing many physiological processes [29]. It has also been shown by Foster et al. in 2003 to not only down-regulate endogenous collagen expression, but also to effectively block TGFβ -mediated increases in collagen protein levels [30]. INF-γ also inhibits TGFβ signalling by inducing expression of SMAD 7, which participates in a negative feedback loop in the TGFβ signal transduction pathway [31]. Therefore, IFN-γ is thought to be an antifibrotic factor during tissue repair that can reduce synthesis of the extracellular matrix by disrupting signalling by the profibrotic cytokine TGF-β [31, 32]. IFN-γ has been found to influence skeletal muscle homeostasis and repair. In 1999 Shelton et al. reported age-dependent necrotizing myopathy in a transgenic mouse that constitutively overexpresses IFN-γ at the neuromuscular junction [33]. On the other hand, the administration of IFN-γ appears to improve the healing of skeletal muscle, limit fibrosis and therefore limit the function of a regenerating muscle [30]. In 2008, Cheng et al. showed that IFN-γ is expressed at both mRNA and protein levels in skeletal muscle following injury, and that the time course of IFN-γ expression correlated with the accumulation of macrophages, T-cells, and natural killer cells, as well as myoblasts, in damaged muscle. The administration of an IFN-γ receptor-blocking antibody to wild-type mice impaired induction of interferon response factor-1, reduced cell proliferation and decreased the formation of regenerating fibres [29]. In 2008, Chen et al. reported a synergistic effect of IFN-γ and IGF-1, which is known to have beneficial effects on muscle regeneration after injury. They showed that IFN-γ injected into injured muscle has the effect of anti-fibrosis, which is more significant than that of IGF-1. They concluded that a combined injection could improve muscle regeneration, while inhibiting fibrosis simultaneously, and promote the healing of injured muscle [34]. *Suramin*, an antiparasitic and antitumor drug, acts as a TGF-β inhibitor by competitively binding to the growth factor's receptor [35, 36]. It has been evaluated for potential clinical applications and has shown antifibrotic effects in chronic kidney diseases, wound healing of rabbit conjunctiva and glaucoma after trabeculotomy [37, 38]. Chan et al. showed that suramin effectively inhibits fibroblast proliferation and neutralizes the stimulating effect of TGF-β on the proliferation of fibroblasts *In vitro*. In vivo, they showed that the injection of suramin two weeks after strain injury reduces muscle fibrosis and enhances muscle regeneration, and thereby leads to improved muscle strength recovery [39]. Although suramin can lead to side effects when administered intravenously, local intramuscular injection may not elicit the same deleterious effects and could be very useful in improving muscle healing [39]. Taniguti et al. evaluated the effect of suramin on fibrosis in mdx mice, where TGF-β is highly unregulated in the diaphragm and the quadriceps muscle. Mice received suramin for seven weeks while performing exercise on a treadmill to worsen disease progression. Suramin protected limb muscles against damage and reduced the exercise-induced loss of strength over time. These findings support the role of TGF-β in fibrogenesis and myonecrosis during the later stages of disease in mdx mice [40].

Relaxin, a polypeptide cytokine/growth factor, is a member of the insulin-like growth factor (IGF) family. The historical role of relaxin has been in reproduction, in which it functions to inhibit uterine contraction and induce growth and softening of the cervix. It can reduce type I and type III collagen deposition, increase procollagenase synthesis, and, by doing so, reduce fibrous scar tissue formation in many tissues [41, 42]. In an *In vivo* model of pulmonary fibrosis, relaxin treatment dramatically decreased bleomycin-induced collagen content in the lung, alveolar thickening, and improved the overall fibrosis score [43]. Recent studies using the relaxin-null mouse model have demonstrated age-associated pulmonary fibrosis in these animals that can be reversed by relaxin treatment [42]. In an innovative study, adenoviral-mediated delivery of relaxin was used to treat cardiac fibrosis caused by transgenic overexpression of the β2-adrenergic receptor, resulting in a dramatic decrease in interstitial collagen content in the left ventricle, but not other (nonfibrotic) chambers of the heart [44]. In a recent study, Mu et al. injected relaxin intramuscularly into the injured site of the mouse to observe its function *In vivo*. Results showed that relaxin promoted myogenic differentiation, migration, and activation of matrix metalloproteinases (MMPs) of cultured myoblasts *In vitro*. Relaxin also promoted activation of muscle satellite cells and increased its local population compared with non-treated control muscles. Meanwhile, both angiogenesis and revascularization were increased, while the extended inflammatory reaction was repressed in the relaxin-treated injured muscle. [45]

2.2. Platelet-rich plasma in muscle injury therapy

Among new therapeutic options for achieving more efficient healing, autologous thrombo-cytes have a very important place. Although there is no randomized prospective study confirming its value, platelet-rich plasma as a source of autologous growth factors is thought to be used by many sports physicians for treating muscle injuries. The use of platelet-derived preparations was prohibited by WADA until 2011 but was removed from the list after considering the lack of current evidence concerning the use of the method for the purposes of performance enhancement as current studies did not reveal a potential for performance enhancement beyond the therapeutic effect [46].

PrP (or platelet-rich plasma) may be defined as a volume of the plasma fraction of autologous blood having a platelet concentration above the baseline [47]. Normal platelet counts in blood range from 150000/µL to 350000/µL. Platelet-rich plasma contains a 3 to 5-fold increase in growth factor (GF) concentrations, sometimes more [47,48]. Platelet-rich plasma can only be made from anticoagulated blood [47]. The process begins by adding citrate to whole blood to bind the ionized calcium and inhibit the clotting cascade, followed by one or two centrifugation steps to separate red and white blood cells from platelets. When using anticoagulated PrP, activation is critical, as clotting results in the release of GF from the platelet α-granules (degranulation). PrP may be activated immediately before application, or it can occur *In vivo*. There is no consensus on the timing of PrP activation, or even whether activation is necessary at all [47]. Approximately 70% of the stored GF is released within 10 minutes, and more than 95% of the GF is released within 1 hour. Some GF is produced by the platelets during the next 8 to 10 days. Originally, bovine thrombin was used as an activating agent; however, a rare but major risk of coagulopathy from antibody formation has restricted its use for activation. Calcium chloride ($CaCl_2$) and autologous prepared thrombin are now used for activation instead. The $CaCl_2$ is added during the second centrifugation step to form a dense fibrin matrix in which platelets are trapped and release GF. Soluble collagen type I may also be used for activation. It is important to note that the composition of commercially derived PrP products differ qualitatively and quantitatively [49]. The most important difference is in the concentration of platelets as well as in the concentration of leukocytes in the preparation. Whether leukocytes have a positive or negative role is not clear yet. The paradigm suggests that neutrophils infiltrate injured tissue and in the process of assisting the removal of disrupted tissue, exacerbate or increase the original damage [49].

Platelet-rich plasma can potentially enhance healing by the delivery of various GF and cytokines from the α-granules contained in platelets. Platelets also contain subpopulations of α-granules that undergo differential release during activation, a potentially important point in understanding how PrP is activated and acts [47, 48]. Platelets contain, synthesize and release large amounts of biologically active proteins that promote tissue regeneration. Researchers have identified more than 1100 types of proteins inside platelets or on their surface [47-49]. The most commonly studied platelet proteins include platelet-derived growth factor (PDGF), transforming growth factor (TGF-β), platelet-derived epidermal growth factor (PD-EGF), vascular endothelial growth factor (VEGF), insulin-like growth factor I and II (IGF-I, IGF-II), fibroblastic growth factor (FGF), and cytokines, including proteins such as platelet factor 4 (PF4) and CD40L. The roles of the above listed growth factors are listed in Table 2 [47, 48, 50].

Growth Factor	Target tissue/cell	Function
FGF	Blood vessels, smooth muscle, skin fibroblasts and other cells	Proliferative and angiogenic action Stimulates collagen production
VEGF	Blood vessels	Stimulates vascularisation by stimulating vascular endothelial cells
TGF-β	Blood vessels, skin cells, fibroblasts, monocytes	Stimulates fibroblast production Stimulates production of collagen type-I and fibronectin
PDGF A+B	Fibroblasts, smooth muscle cells, chondrocytes, osteoblasts, mesenchymal stem cells	One of the first growth factors to be expressed after injury
		Stimulates other growth factor secretion Stimulates angiogenesis and macrophage activation
		Chemotaxic and proliferative action on fibroblasts, stimulates collagen synthesis
PD-EGF	Blood vessel, skin cells fibroblasts and other cells	Stimulates epidermal regeneration and wound healing by stimulating keratinocytes and dermal fibroblasts Promotes cell growth, recruitment, differentiation
		Stimulates cytokine secretion
IGF-I, II	Bone, blood vessel, skin, other tissue fibroblasts	Chemotactic for fibroblasts
		Stimulates protein synthesis
		Enhances bone formation
PF-4	Neutrophils, fibroblasts	Stimulates influx of neutrophils Chemotactic for fibroblasts
Myostatin,		
Leukaemia inhibitory factor (LIF),		Mainly function on bone/skeletal muscle adaptation and repair
mechano growth factor (MGF), Bone morphogenetic protein (BMP)		
(a member of TGF-β superfamily)		

Table 2. Growth factors released from platelets and their function

In vitro studies showed that the application of PrP enhances gene expression of the ECM proteins, has mitogenic activity, promotes tenocyte proliferation and induces secretion of other growth factors [47]. Importantly, animal studies showed that all positive effects of PrP are neglected when no mechanical stimuli are applied to the tendon during the healing peri-od, e.g. if the tendon is immobilised. Besides increased expression of growth factors, PrP was found to increase the expression of matrix degrading enzymes. PrP may also promote antibacterial effects. In addition to opsonophagocytosis, chemotaxis, and oxidative microbi-cidal activity, platelets and leukocytes can release a variety of small cationic peptides (anti-bacterial peptides) that have bactericidal activity [47].

When treating ligament injuries with PrP, animal studies suggest that use of PDGF-BB may improve the quality of healing medial collateral ligaments, and in a similar way PrP may influence the healing of other ligaments [51]. The effect of PrP may be dose and time-related [52]. However, extra-articular ligaments showed better wound site filling and increased the presence of finbrinogen and GF when healing as compared to intra-articular ligaments (like ACL), but the application of PRP can improve the results after ACL injury [53].

To date, no major adverse effects of PrP have been noted in humans. No adverse effects were observed when PrP was infiltrated in 808 patients, mainly with osteoarthritis [54]. The use of bovine thrombin for activation may cause a hypersensitivity reaction and is therefore avoided in modern preparation techniques [47]. To date, there is no evidence of a systemic effect of local PrP injection or carcinogenesis. The latter may be mainly due to the short *In vivo* half-lives and local bioavailability of GF produced by PrP [47]. At the moment, PrP is permitted by WADA (The World Anti-Doping Agency) by all routes of administration since 2011 [47].

The International Olympic Committee Consensus Statement expresses that current evidence suggests the use of PrP to be safe. They proposed that what type of PrP product is used and how it has been prepared, validated and tested should be made clear [47].

Suggested techniques for the application of PrP and post-injection recommendations of the International Olympic Committee Consensus Statement are [47]:

1. PrP is considered to act best when placed at the site of injured tissue; therefore ultra-sound guidance is advisable for accurate needle placement to the injured site.

2. With respect to tendon administration, there is no agreement on whether the needle should be placed inside the tendon or in the surrounding tendon sheath. In the pres-ence of exudates around the tendon, it is suggested that it be evacuated before PrP is injected.

3. If PrP is administered at arthroscopy, it is suggested that the injection be administered after emptying the joint of arthroscopic fluid. In the case of open surgery, the applica-tion of PrP can be undertaken using one of the gel or semi-solid forms.

4. Patients should follow general recommendations after an injection with rest, ice, and limb elevation for 48 hours. Depending on the site of treatment and extent and duration of the condition, patients may follow an accelerated rehabilitation protocol under ap-propriate supervision.

In the XX *(number needed for chapter: physiology of sports injuries)* chapter of this book, all phas-es of healing in an injured tissue are described. They are influenced by a number of growth factors that control cell functions through direct interactions with extracellular parts of the transmembrane receptors. Because thrombocytes represent a major source of growth factors in blood clots, the idea to concentrate them at the site of injury is well accepted. The effects of several individual growth factors have been studied in muscle regeneration. Results from *In vitro* studies are variable; however, their obvious role in regeneration is not to be neglected. Growth factors together with macrophages and products of the cyclooxygenase 2 (COX-2) regulatory pathway regulate the inflammatory phase during regeneration in skeletal muscle [55]. IGF-1 and FGF have been shown to have positive effects on healing and fast-twitch tetanic strength in a murine model of muscle laceration [56]. In case of gastrocnemius contusion, the local application of both GFs lead to higher satellite cell activation in bigger muscle fibre development [57]. Despite the promising potential of PrP for treatment of muscle injuries, some doubts have arisen concerning their use. Due to application of exogenous TGF-β into the tissue, which has been proven to be highly responsible for tissue scarring, some experts are not defenders of this particular therapeutic option. However, in a recent *In vitro* study using human myoblast cell lines it was shown that PrP-derived growth factors promote satellite and muscle cell proliferation as well as inhibiting fibrotic differentiation, mainly due to down-expression of TGF-β [58].

To date there are no randomized control studies confirming the real role of PrP in treating muscle injuries [59], nor was any sample in clinical studies large enough to represent relevant statistical data [48]. However, the preclinical data seems to be promising enough for clinical studies to take place.

2.3. Other bioactive agents to improve muscle healing

Manose-6-Phosphate (M6P) is a natural inhibitor of TGF-β, a carbohydrate molecule with structural similarity to TGF-β and has been shown to reduce its activity [2, 60]. In an experiment by Roberts et al., M6P reduced scarring in incision wounds in rats [61]. In another recent study M6P significantly reduced TGF-β1-mediated transformation of human corneal fibroblasts into myofibroblasts and is therefore a potential modulator of corneal wound healing that may reduce haze after refractive surgery [62]. Regarding the musculoskeletal system, only a few studies on tendons had been performed to date. In an experiment by Bates et al. the antifibrotic effect of M6P was under observation *In vitro* and *In vivo*, where primary cell cultures from the rabbit flexor tendon sheath, epitenon, and endotenon were established and supplemented with TGF-β along with increasing doses of M6P. They also transected and immediately repaired rabbit flexor tendons. M6P solution was added to the repair sites and compared to a placebo group. They found that M6P is effective in reducing TGF-β upregulated collagen production, which correlated with the finding that a single intraoperative dose of M6P improved the postoperative range of motion. Because of its nonimmunogenic property and because it is easily produced, M6P could be an ideal candidate for clinical application in muscle injuries [2]. Yang et al. studied the effects of M6P on TGF-β peptide and receptor expression in order to provide the experimental basis for preventing tendon-healing adhesion by M6P. They found that M6P can significantly decrease the expressions of TGF-β peptide, TGF-β receptor, TGF-β mRNA and may therefore provide a means of modulating the effects of TGF-β on adhesion formation in flexor tendon wound healing [63].

Although *N-acetylcysteine (NAC)* is a non-toxic aminothiol widely known as an antidote to acetaminophen overdose, it has multiple other uses supported by varying levels of evidence, like chronic obstructive pulmonary disease exacerbation, prevention of contrast-induced kidney damage during imaging procedures, and treatment of infertility in patients with clomiphene-resistant polycystic ovary syndrome [64]. Recent studies have emphasized the role of oxidative stress as the molecular basis of lung fibrosis. NAC has a strong reductive capacity that inhibits the TGF-β-stimulated collagen production in cultured fibroblasts [65]. Moreover, it has been shown by Hagiwara et al. that the aerosolized administration of NAC attenuates the lung fibrosis induced by bleomycin in mice [66] suggesting the suppressing effects of antioxidant TGF-b1 signalling *In vitro* and *In vivo*. A recent study demonstrated that NAC reduces the disulfide bonds of TGF-b1 and changes the bioactive form to the inactive form [67]. It also changes the binding activity of TGF-b1 to its receptor in hepatic stellate cells, suggesting that the effect of antioxidant NAC is based on a direct blockade of TGF-b1 function and signalling. However, whether NAC can modulate the TGF-b1-induced tissue repair, mediator production, and differentiation in human lung fibroblasts has not been fully elucidated [68]. Sugiura et al. recently reported that NAC affects the production of fibronectin and vascular endothelial growth factor (VEGF), which are believed to be important mediators of repair and remodelling. The effect of NAC on the TGF-β induces differentiation to myofibroblasts by assessing a smooth muscle actin (a-SMA) expression [68]. Although treatment with NAC has been shown to attenuate interstitial fibrosis in mouse models of hypertrophic cardiomyopathy mutation and several other pathological states [69], no studies have been performed on the effects of NAC in muscle regeneration after injury. However, since it has been shown to have beneficial effects on diseases that share the same pathophysiological core with the process of muscle fibrosis, the effects of NAC could potentially be beneficial in this pathology as well. Because it is a safe, inexpensive, and well-tolerated antioxidant with a well-defined mechanism of action, a highly favourable risk/benefit ratio and low rate of adverse events [64], researchers will probably study the effects of NAC in muscle repair in the future.

Angiotensin-converting enzyme (ACE) inhibitors and angiotensin receptor blockers (ARBs) have also shown beneficial effects in studies of muscle healing. ACE is a circulating enzyme that participates in the body's renin-angiotensin-aldosterone system (RAAS), which modulates extracellular volume and arterial vasoconstriction. Its inhibitors reduce morbidity, mortality, hospital admissions, and decline in physical function and exercise capacity in congestive heart failure patients. These therapeutic effects are attributed primarily to beneficial cardiovascular actions of these drugs [70]. Observations have linked pathologic fibrosis in various organ systems to the local effects of angiotensin II. The modulation of angiotensin II with angiotensin-converting enzyme inhibitors or angiotensin II receptor blockers has demonstrated decreased fibrosis and improved function in liver, kidney, and lung tissue [71-74]. Injured cardiac muscle also demonstrates dysfunction related to fibrosis. Myocardium exposed to decreased levels of angiotensin II, either through the use of ACE inhibitors or ARBs, has also demonstrated a measurably improved function [75, 76]. However, it has been suggested that ACE inhibitor-induced positive effects may also be mediated by direct action on the skeletal muscle [70]. Recent studies reported on the beneficial side effects of ACE inhibitors in hypertensive patients free of chronic heart failure [70]. Treatment with ACE inhibitors was associated with better performance and muscular outcomes, and genetic studies also support the hypothesis that the ACE system may be involved in physical performance and skeletal muscle function [77, 78]. Moreover, elite athletes, particularly those in endurance sports, have also demonstrated findings consistent with inherent differences in their body's metabolism of angiotensin II, with decreased exposure resulting in improved skeletal muscle function [70, 79, 80]. In an *In vitro* and *In vivo* study by Bedair et al. angiotensin receptor blocker therapy significantly reduced fibrosis and led to an increase in the number of regenerating myofibres in acutely injured skeletal muscle and may therefore provide a safe, clinically available treatment for improving healing after skeletal muscle injury [81].

3. Future perspectives of cartilage tissue repair

Damage to articular cartilage is of great clinical consequence since the cartilage tissue comprises of limited intrinsic potential for healing due to the lack of blood supply and subsequent incomplete repair by local chondrocytes with inferior fibrocartilage formation. Surgical intervention is often the only option, but the repair of damaged cartilage is often less than satisfactory, and rarely restores full function or returns the tissue to its native normal state.

Tissue engineering of articular cartilage still remains challenging due to the special structure of cartilage tissue consisting of multiphasic cellular architecture and great weight-bearing characteristics. Good knowledge and understanding of cartilage structure, its metabolism, and the process of chondrogenesis enables *In vitro* cartilage production in terms of tissue engineering. The new concept of cartilage tissue preservation uses tissue-engineering technologies, combining new biomaterials as a scaffold, the application of growth factors, the use of stem cells, and mechanical stimulation. Scaffolds enable 3-dimensional environmental conditions to promote hyaline-like cartilage production. Additionally, various types of growth factors, which are the endogenous regulators of chondrogenesis, can be applied locally or in culture condition to promote cartilage development. Further studies are attempting to create the ideal scaffold and explore the synergistic effect of concomitant application of growth factors and mechanical loading. In clinical practice, new generations of autologous chondrocyte implantation (ACI) are based on the use of biodegradable materials that serve as temporary cell-carriers for the *In vitro* growth and subsequent implantation into the cartilage defect. Moreover, single stage procedures appear attractive, as they consist of natural chondral tissue inserted on the carrier and can reduce cost and patient morbidity since they avoid second operation and cell culturing procedures.

3.1. Tissue engineering of articular cartilage

The field of tissue engineering uses the principles of cell biology, engineering, and medicine in order to produce such a construct that can successfully replace damaged tissue. Engineered tissue should comprise of the characteristics of the native intact tissue in terms of histological structure, morphology, function, and mechanical properties. The challenges of tissue engineering of articular cartilage include isolating and culturing cells to gain relevant and reproducible constructs with good durability *In vivo*. A demanding and crucial role in the process of *In vitro* culturing represents phenotype regulation, *In vitro* expansion, scaffold design, the use of bioreactor, etc. All of these components should be optimized to advance cartilage tissue engineering from culturing to clinical application. In particular, there is still a need to develop suitable scaffolds that can provide a 3-dimensional environment for the cell to adhere to and adequately proliferate. Additionally, scaffolds should be mechanically strong and biocompatible. Cartilage tissue engineering usually uses bioactive molecules (growth factors) and mechanical loading to promote differentiation towards a cartilage phenotype [82].

3.1.1. Biomaterials and scaffolds

Scaffolds are engineered extracellular matrices that serve as an artificial structure capable of supporting 3-dimensional tissue formation. Cells are often implanted or seeded into these scaffolds and different biomaterials are used that allow cell attachment, growth, differentiation, and regeneration of functional cartilage tissue. Scaffolds were developed with the aim to improve the biological performance of chondrocytes as well as render the surgical technique easier. In cartilage tissue engineering, scaffolds should comprise of the following characteristics; they should be biocompatible (not triggering inflammatory response and not toxic), offering temporary support to cells, mechanically strong to protect cells and withstand *In vivo* forces during joint movement, and bioactive to provide cellular attachment and migration. Additionally, scaffolds should be biodegradable, serving as a temporary construct that is later replaced by a newly synthesized extracellular matrix (ECM) [83]. With time, the transplanted chondrocytes take over the function of the cell carrier; therefore they should be degraded once they have served their purpose. The ideal biodegradable scaffold should also enable uniform cell spreading possible [84-87].

In general, scaffolds are divided into natural material, synthetic polymers, and new materials. Natural materials include collagen, hyaluronic acid, fibrin glue, chitosan, agarose, and alginate. Their advantage is excellent biocompatibility since they are natural bodily constituents, thus degradation is physiological and non-toxic. On the other hand, their use includes sourcing, processing, and the risk of disease transmission. Synthetic polymers, especially PLA (poly alfa-hydroxil acid polymers) and PLGA (*poly lactic-co-glycolic acid*) are also widely used due to the approval of the FDA. Their major advantage is the design flexibility (highly porous 3-dimensional structure) and no risk of disease transmission. The disadvantages are acid degradation products, inflammatory response, and chronic inflammation due to high molecular weight proteins. Novel materials have been introduced recently, such as silk, cellulose, and other synthetic materials (biodegradable elastomer, polycaprolactone, poly (ether ester) copolymer scaffolds). Additionally, the combination of different materials is applied [88], e.g. gelatin and hyaluronic acid have been combined with a fibrin glue and chondroitin-6-suplphate. Furthermore, scaffolds to support bone formation (hydroxiapatite) were combined with the chitosan to enable the regeneration of osteochondral lesions.

The new approach represents the development of smart matrices that actively support cartilage formation and not only provide mechanical function but also allow control over cell metabolism, tissue formation, enable adjustment of the physical properties, inclusion of ECM motifs and active substances such as GF incorporated in microspheres to allow temporally and spatially controlled delivery of GF in scaffolds [87].

Although most of these developments seem to be promising for future clinical application, they are mainly used *In vitro* and in animal models [84-87]. Chondrocytes previously expanded and seeded onto scaffold produce a characteristic ECM rich in proteoglycans, collagen type II and aggrecan. After implantation in the full thickness femoral defect in rabbits, it promoted healing and regenerated a cartilage-like tissue [89]. The future prospective for cartilage repair is also based on the quality of integration between the newly formed tissue and the native tissue for achieving stable healing.

3.1.2. Growth factors

Growth factors and their signaling pathways are the essential regulators of chondrogenesis during tissue engineering and thus are the prime candidates for engineering of cartilage tissue. Chondrogenesis is a multistep process that comprises of several steps: precursor cell condensation, differentiation towards chondrogenic phenotype, secretion of cartilage specific ECM components (collagen type II, aggrecan and others), chondrocytes proliferation in the area of growth plate, further differentiation towards hypertrophy, and replacement of cartilage with the bone tissue. All of the steps are regulated by different and overlapping signals (Figure 1).

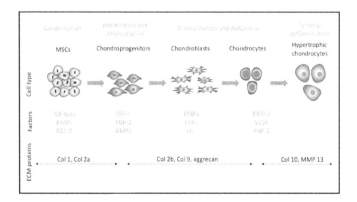

Figure 1. Schematic diagram of different stages of chondrogenesis (including main growth factors and alterations in ECM)

In general, GFs are endogenous regulators of chondrogenesis and their logical choice of use appears to be promising to stimulate anabolic responses and the repair of articular cartilage. For example, in *In vitro* cartilage formation it is essential to promote early chondrocytes differentiation and proliferation while trying to prevent further differentiation towards hypertrophy. However, the design and optimization of all GF's for a particular tissue engineering and/or local application is complex and has to consider the combination of different factors, their timing, concentrations, etc.

The most important factors currently used in tissue engineering are the members of transforming growth factor β (TGF-β) family, Bone Morphogenetic Protein (BMP), Insulin-like growth factors (IGF), Fibroblast Growth Factors (FGF), especially FGF-2 and FGF-18, Epidermal Growth Factor (EGF) and Vascular-Endothelial Growth Factors (VEGFs). The summary of the effect of different GFs on chondrocytes/cartilage is presented in Table 4. It is becoming increasingly apparent that GFs work synergistically and simultaneously to induce and promote cartilage formation; e.g.: TGF-β1 and FGF-2 [90] together with IGF-1 [91], BMP-7 and IGF-1 [91], TGFβ3 and BMP [92], etc. Based on the concept that several different GFs work in combination during cartilage repair, the use of PrP, autologous conditioned serum (ACS), and bone marrow concentrate were used in cartilage repair techniques [93].

	Growth factors	Effect on chondrocytes/cartilage
TGF-β	Transforming Growth Factor β	Stimulates synthesis of ECM Decreases catabolic activity
BMP-2	Bone Morphogenetic Protein - 2	Stimulates synthesis of ECM Increased ECM turnover (increased aggrecan degradation)
BMP-7	Bone Morphogenetic Protein - 7	Stimulates ECM synthesis Decrease cartilage degradation
IGF-1	Insulin-like growth factors	Stimulates ECM synthesis Decreases matrix catabolism
FGF-2	Fibroblast Growth Factors-2	Decreases aggrecanase activity Antagonizes PG synthesis
FGF-18	Fibroblast Growth Factors-18	Increases chondrocyte proliferation and stimulates ECM

Table 3. Proven effects of various growth factors on cartilage

3.1.3. Mesenchymal stem cells

Mesenchymal stem cells (MSCs) are pluripotent cells found in multiple human adult tissues including bone marrow, synovial tissues, and adipose tissues. They are of great interest for scientists involved in cell therapy and tissue engineering since they have self-renewal capacity and multilineage differentiation potential. Depending on the cultivation conditions, they can differentiate into adipogenic, ostegenic or chondrogenic cells as well as form bone, cartilage, and fat. Currently, researchers are exploring the possibilities of manipulating the stem cells under laboratory conditions into mature chondrocytes that can then be integrated into scaffolds for later application [94,95]. There are many studies reporting the isolation and characterization of MSCs from adult human synovium and periosteum and providing evidence about their multipotency at the single cell level [96, 97]. It was also demonstrated that human MSCs from different tissues possess distinctive biological properties [98]. Additionally, there is still the issue of whether MSCs are capable of forming stable hyaline-like cartilage as opposed to that formed during the process of endochondral ossification, which is later replaced with bone. The variability in biological responses of MSCs and no standardized MSC bioprocessing to obtain MSC preparations with consistent, reproducible, and quality-controlled biological potency for therapeutic applications limit the use of MSCs in clinical practice. On the other hand, the use of MSCs as chondrocyte substitutes in an ACI-equivalent procedure has become highly attractive since MCSs are easily accessible, easy to isolate and capable of expanding into culture as opposed to articular chondrocytes with limited proliferative capacity and rapid de-differentiation *In vitro*.

Furthermore, MCSs appear to be immune privileged under certain conditions [94-97]. Altogether, these properties would allow the generation of large batches of quality controlled MCSs preparations ready for allogenic use. In addition, limitations in patient-to-patient variability would be circumvented [93]. In animal models, MSCs have already shown significant potential for cartilage repair and novel approaches using MSCs as an alternative cell source to patient-derived chondrocytes are being tested [89, 99]. However, preclinical and clinical studies should be conducted in order to evaluate whether the implantation of MCSs results in a cartilage formation that is as durable as the one following the implantation of articular chondrocytes. Additionally, the application of MCSs can be further expanded to non-localized chronic lesions in osteoarthritis patients [100].

3.1.4. Mechanical load

A potential strategy in cartilage functional tissue engineering comprises of the effect of mechanical stimuli applied during *In vitro* tissue formation. Several studies demonstrated that mechanical forces stimulate the synthesis of ECM and may even enhance the mechanical properties of the developing tissue [101, 102]. After physical stimuli are applied to the tissue, the intracellular mechanisms convert mechanical signals into biochemical events responsible for regulating the transcription of genes governing cell growth and differentiation. This effect proved to be further intensified with concomitant application of growth factors and mechanical load in a synergistic manner [103, 104]. Various bioreactor systems have been developed in order to form cartilaginous grafts with similar biomechanical characteristics compared to native intact cartilage tissue [105-107]. Due to the complexity of the load and motion patterns within an articular joint, new bioreactors with multi-axial loading patterns are designed to recreate the *In vivo* situation [106, 107]. The interesting aspect of cartilage repair in clinical practice represents cell-based strategies that are not culture-intensive and allow single surgical procedure. Hence, a natural environment is the most suitable for tissue development therefore cell culture and bioreactors may not be required [108].

3.2. Clinical application of tissue engineering in cartilage repair

Cartilage repair has gained great interest since autologous cartilage implantation (ACI) has become an established treatment. The first line of treatment options remains microfracturing, due to low cost, arthroscopic procedure, and ease of performance.

Bone marrow stimulation techniques as well as ACI represent the cell-based approach for tissue regeneration in which the attendance of specific cells with the ability of proliferation and differentiation in desired cell phenotype plays a crucial role. In the case of bone marrow stimulating techniques, these cells are recruited from the bone marrow either by drilling or microfracturing; as such they are released from the medullar canal and subsequently form the blot clot on the side of the lesion. However, the final result is fibrous cartilage with inferior biomechanical properties compared to native hyaline cartilage. On the other hand, the histological analysis of random biopsy specimens after ACI procedure indicated the presence of type-II collagen and hyaline-like cartilage within the healing tissue.

ACI is both technically demanding and associated with a high percentage of reoperations. The modification of this cell therapy was designed to reduce complications such as periosteal hypertrophy, the need for second look arthroscopy, the development of fibrocartilage tissue with variable amount of hyaline cartilage, etc. The next generation of ACI was developed by replacing the periosteal patch with a biocompatible matrix and selecting cells of potentially improved chondrogenic potential. For example, second generation ACI uses collagen-covered autologous cultured chondrocyte implantation and in third-generation ACI, special cell carriers or cell-seeded scaffolds were created. Fourth generation cartilage repair focuses on growth factors and gene therapy, the use of stem cells and tissue engineering [109, 110]. In general, arthrotomy and a two-stage procedure are the most commonly used, but all-arthroscopic techniques and one-stage procedures (e.g. technique with minced articular cartilage) have become highly attractive treatment techniques. Additionally, preimplantation chondrocyte phenotype manipulation has also shown excellent outcomes.

3.2.1. Second generation ACI

Second generation ACI is still a two-step procedure, but in contrast to classical ACI it involves culturing in 3-dimensional conditions, which favours the maintenance of phenotypic stability of chondrocytes. In particular, chondrocytes are cultured on the scaffold that is biocompatible, enables cellular growth, and as such represents the graft to be transplanted. These scaffolds/matrices containing the chondrocytes are implanted on the chondral lesion and attached with fibrin glue. In this manner, periosteal grafts and their suturing onto healthy cartilage are not necessary. These techniques were developed in an attempt to resolve some of the most common problems indicated by the standard ACI technique such as periosteal hypertrophy, which is a source of complaints about localized pain among some patients.

The scaffolds used in second generation ACI should comprise all of the following futures: biocompatibility (no inflammatory response), biodegradability (controlled rate of degradation), bioactivity (promote maintenance of phenotype and proliferation), and permeability (to ensure nutrition). Natural and synthetic scaffolds can be used. The concern about the synthetic scaffolds is the risk of the harmful effect of degradation products on surrounding tissue. A comparison of the first and second-generation ACI has shown rather equivalent short-term clinical outcomes, with similar complications and a similar rate of reoperation [110]. A variety of scaffolds have been introduced, implanted either through a small arthrotomy or arthroscopically and will be presented briefly: collagen-covered ACI (CACI or ACI-C), Hyalograft C based on hyaluronic acid and membrane/matrix induced ACI (MACI) and others.

The main innovation in CACI is the use of bioresorable collagen membrane cover instead of the periosteal cover. Initial reports showed clinical improvements of this second generation ACI with fewer complications compared to classical ACI. The clinical and functional assessment after two years showed that 74% of patients had good or excellent results following CACI compared to 67% after classical ACI (ACI-P or PACI – periosteal ACI). Revision arthroscopy was required in 36.4% in the PACI group one year after surgery due to shaving for hypertrophy compared to none in the CACI group [111]. In the systemic review of ACI procedures including 82 studies they reported that the failure rate was highest in PACI (7.7%) compared to CACI (1.5%). Similarly, the highest rate of unplanned re-operation was in the PACI group (27%) compared to CACI (5%) [112].

Matrix-induced ACI (MACI) was first introduced in 1998. In this technique, cells are seeded directly onto the surface of a biodegradable type I/III collagen membrane and as such overcome the shortcomings of the original periosteum-covered technique. The membrane is a bi-layer structure, smooth on one side and rough and more porous on the inner side, with incorporated cells to stimulate cartilage matrix specific molecules. It was shown that chondrocytes can adhere and maintain their phenotypic characteristics while seeded onto a type I/III collagen membrane [113]. The procedure requires limited exposure of the joint ensuring shorter operation time and less morbidity. The rate of failure was low (0-6.3%) and mainly due to symptomatic graft hypertrophy or detachment. However, clinical, arthroscopic, and histological outcomes are comparable for CACI and MACI [114]. Additionally, MACI was also significantly more effective after two years compared to microfracturing [115]. Although significantly improved results after 5 years were reported, MACI still remains the cost-intensive alternative [116].

Hyalograft C implants autologous cells onto an esterified hyaluronic acid scaffold. It was reported that 76% of patients had no pain and 88% had no mobility problems. Additionally, 96% of patients' treated knee was assessed to be normal by the surgeon and cartilage repair was graded arthroscopically as normal or nearly normal in 96%. The majority of second-look biopsies showed hyaline-like cartilage and a very low rate of complications were recorded [117]. Several other studies also reported positive clinical results with Hyalograft C [118, 119]. Similarly, in two comparative studies, researchers found superiority over hyaluronic-acid based chondrocytes transplantation at five years follow up in respect to microfracture in young, active patients [120, 121].

3.2.2. Third and fourth generation ACI

Recently, further technological advances have led to a third-generation ACI, where chondrocytes are embedded into three-dimensionally constructed scaffolds (i.e. 3-dimensional environment) for cell growth [122]. This novel approach uses: chondro-inductive or chondro-conductive matrix; autogenous or alogenous cells treated *In vitro* in order to induce cell proliferation, differentiation and production of ECM; a single-stage surgical approach; and mechanical stimulation to improve the material properties and maturation of the implant [123]. Such mature tissue might ensure shorter rehabilitation and shorten the time to achieve clinical efficiency. For example, the DeNovo Engineered Tissue (ET) graft (Zimmer, Warsaw) is generated from juvenile cartilage cells under special laboratory conditions and is hyaline-like. It is engineered by ISTO Technologies and the FDA approved ISTO's Investigational New Drug (IND) application for Neocartilage in 2006, which allowed them to pursue clinical trials of the product in humans.

Likewise, Neocart (Histogenics, Waltham, MA), a bioengineered tissue patch containing an autologous chondrocyte population matured in a biodegradable collagen matrix, uses bioreactor technology (hydrostatic pressure with modified flow rates and low oxygen) to stimulate ECM accumulation and suppress long-term degradation. A recent randomized study suggests that the safety of autologous cartilage tissue implantation, with the use of the NeoCart technique is similar to that of microfracture and associated with greater clinical efficacy at two years after treatment [124]. However, there are still technical problems remaining regarding the initial fixation technique, subchondral and edge integration, long-term durability, etc. [125].

A number of new generation ACI methods for implanting cultured autologous chondrocytes in a biodegradable matrix are currently in development or testing. These include Chondroselect (characterized chondrocyte implantation, TiGenex, Phase III trial), BioCart II (ProChon Biotech, Phase II trial), Cartilix (polymer hydrogel, Cartilix), MACI® (matrix-induced ACI, Verigen, available outside of the U.S.), Cartipatch (solid scaffold with an agarose-alginate matrix, TBF Tissue Engineering, Phase III trial), NeoCart (ACI with a 3-dimensional chondromatrix, Histogenics, Phase II trial) and Hyalograft C (ACI with a hyaluronic acid-based scaffold, Fidia Advanced Polymers). Although the clinical use of these second-generation ACI products has been reported in Europe, none are approved for use in the U.S. at this time [126].

The future of fourth generation cartilage repair focuses on gene therapy, the use of stem cells (bone marrow, adipose, or muscle derived) and tissue engineering. MSCs are an attractive cell source due to their differentiation capacities. To expand and deliver MSCs to the site of defect, the cells should be seeded into an appropriate scaffold that is biocompatible, mechanically stable, permeable, and biodegradable. A variety of biomaterials were introduced, e.g. carbohydrate polymers (hyaluronan, agarose, alginate, PLA/PLGA) that are protein-based (collagen, fibrin, gelatin) in order to obtain homogenous distribution within a 3-dimensional matrix.

Future generations of cartilage tissue engineering will also include methods to control the genome to direct chondrogenic differentiation towards a hyaline-like pathway. In this manner, the local cellular environment can be coordinated by a tightly regulated GFs that signal molecules to regulate cellular maturation and proliferation. Additionally, with the use of gene therapy, either viral or non-viral vectors can be applied into cells, which then express chondrogenic GF. Gene transfer enables localized exposure of bioactive proteins or gene products to the site of tissue lesions. There have been numerous cDNAs cloned and used for biological stimulation of cartilage healing in terms of mitosis induction, synthesis of ECM components, induction of chondrogenesis by progenitor cells, inhibiting inflammatory response, etc. Researching involves identification and specific gene combinations that could be incorporated into vectors and delivered to target cells [127]. Current data indicates that efficient delivery and expression of certain genes may have an effect on overall healing response in cartilage tissue and is capable of turning the repair response towards the synthesis of a more hyaline cartilage tissue [128]. The novel approach in cartilage tissue engineering is the use of cell population certification (screening of gene markers, positive and negative factors, gene expression score - ChondroCelect), which enables prediction of whether cells are capable of making stable hyaline-like cartilage *In vitro*. By selecting those characterized cells with a high probability of maintaining a chondrogenic phenotype, the effectiveness of transplanted chondrocytes would be maximized.

3.2.3. One-step surgery

Recent directions in cartilage repair are moving towards the possibility of performing one-step surgery, including the use of MCS and GF, and to avoid the first surgery, harvesting cell material, and subsequent cell cultivation. Numerous studies reported that bone marrow stem cells are a useful source for restoring cartilage defects. Additionally, by the concomitant use of PRP and MCS it is possible to develop a single step procedure.

Single stage procedures can be divided into two categories: cell free implants (scaffolds) and cell-based implants (further subdivided according to the cell type utilized; auto- and allografts). One of the most common cell-free procedures is AMIC (autologous matrix-induced chondrogenesis). The technique requires a cell free implant that is "smart" enough to provide the appropriate stimuli to induce orderly and durable tissue regeneration. Moreover, it should be capable of inducing in situ cartilage formation. The AMIC procedure comprises of microfracturing combined with the implant of a porcine collagen type I/III bilayer matrix to stabilize blood clot formation.

The first reports on the AMIC technique were promising and the results were comparable to standard ACI with the advantage of a single stage technique and no donor site morbidity [129]. In a study with the mean follow up rate of 37 months, they reported highly satisfactory results in 87% with MRI showing moderate to complete filling and normal to hyperdense signal [130]. Another possibility is to use bone marrow concentrate (BMC) for MCS in treating cartilage defects. The technique consists of harvesting 40-60ml of bone marrow aspirate from the iliac crest, centrifugation, and the use of special enzymes to activate the BMC and produce the sticky clot material that is placed on the side of the lesion; finally the defect is covered with a collagen membrane.

An attractive option in terms of cell-based technologies is represented by minced articular cartilage procedures for repairing articular cartilage, as they are one-staged, autologous and inserted on scaffold carriers that provide chondro-milieu, mechanical protection and even distribution of the cells within the defect. The principle of the minced cartilage procedure is to obtain hyaline-like "minced" cartilage pieces supplemented with the scaffold delivery system. Minced cartilage represents the source of cells and even relatively large defects can be treated with a small amount of cells; specifically, one-tenth of the cartilage that originally covered a defect is required. The proposed advantages of this procedure over conventional treatment are the elimination of the need for in-vitro cell expansion and a second surgical procedure. Several technologies are being investigated and are in current late stage trials [131]. The autograft cell-based procedure CAIC (Mitek, USA) is currently under phase III evaluation. During the procedure, autologous cartilage is harvested with the special shaver device, then morcellized and secured on resorbable polymer mesh with fibrin glue. DeNovo NT Graft ("Natural Tissue Graft", Zimmer, Warsaw) is a similar application used for treatment of the cartilage lesions limited to an articular surface with intact subchondral bone. It utilizes morcelized juvenile cartilage, which is secured with the fibrin glue. As there is no use of chemicals and minimal manipulation, a DeNovo NT Graft does not require FDA approval and is currently available in the United States. Both CAIS and DeNovo NT techniques rely on chondrocytes migration out of the cartilage tissue with subsequent matrix production to fill the defect [130-132]. Early animal and preclinical models have demonstrated hyaline-like cartilage. Clinical experience is limited, with short-term studies demonstrating both procedures to be safe, feasible, and effective, with improvements in subjective patient scores, and with magnetic resonance imaging [133].

4. Strategies to improve ligament and tendon repair

Tendons and ligaments are avascular and hypocellular with distinct mechanical features that make them difficult for currently available treatments to reach a complete functional repair of the damaged tissue. Tendon injuries, whether acute or chronic, are commonly managed either conservatively or surgically. Conservative management, such as rest, corticosteroid injection, orthotics, ultrasound, laser treatment, or shockwave provide pain relief but, when they fail, surgery is required [134].

Surgical repair may be indicated in acute injuries. In chronic lesions, excision of the involved area might be performed. However, repaired tendons have inferior properties when compared to healthy ones. The loss of mechanical features is mainly due to a distorted extra cellular matrix (ECM) composition and a misalignment of collagen fibrils of the scar tissue [134]. Another option is to use tendon or ligament grafts, but graft-augmentation devices and artificial prostheses have also been developed [135]. Because current treatment is suboptimal, alternative therapies have been developed, such as the delivery of growth factors, the development of engineered scaffolds or the application of stem cells.

4.1. Grafts and graft-augmentation devices

Autografts are used widely to repair the affected tendon and prevent instability due to the damaged ligament. The most commonly used autografts include hamstring tendons (semitendinosus and gracilis) and bone-patellar ligament (middle third)-bone. Several factors are important in the selection of the graft tissue reconstruction, such as the initial mechanical properties of the graft tissue, morbidity resulting from graft harvesting, graft healing, and the initial mechanical properties of the graft fixation, [134].

Allografts represent an alternative option to autografts for tendon and ligament repair. Because of high cost, limited accessibility, associated risk of disease transmission and tissue rejection with the use of allografts, autografts are preferred.

Immediately after a reconstruction with autograft or allograft, the fixation site, not the graft midsubstance, is considered to be the weakest point; following that period, the process of ligamentization influences the mechanical properties of the graft, making it more vulnerable.

To prevent injuries of the graft until integration into the bone and the process of ligamentization is complete, graft augmentation devices were developed to provide immediate post-surgical protection. They share mechanical loads with the biological graft until the graft itself is capable of withstanding local tensile and compressive forces [134]. Graft augmentation devices should be resorbable, but the rate of resorption should be limited by gradual transfer of mechanical loads to the biological graft [134, 135].

4.2. Tissue engineering

Tissue engineering (TE) combines biological materials and cells into a construct that is eventually able to replace the regenerated tissue [136], through the merging of three areas: scaffold microenvironment, stem cells, and signalling biofactors. The goal is to reconstruct a ligament/tendon by providing a scaffold seeded with cell-inducing neotissue formation that adequately meets the required biological and mechanical properties [136,137]. Engineering fibrous tissues, such as tendons and ligaments, requires the use of fibre-based scaffolds, because they should possess appropriate mechanical properties to withstand high stresses, but also high porosity and surface area to allow the seeded cells to proliferate and regenerate the tissue [137].

4.2.1. Stem cells and scaffolds

The purpose of TE with responding cells is to induce a regenerative response instead of scarring. Tissue engineering can be divided into two subtypes: the *In vivo* approach and the *ex vivo-de novo*. The *In vivo* approach permits the self-regeneration of small tissue lesions [138]. The *ex vivo-de novo* approach is designed to produce functional tissue that can be implanted in the body. Several cells have been used: tenocytes, fibroblasts and stem cells. The latter can be derived from bone marrow, human tendons (ACL, PCL), adipose tissue or embryonic derived stem cells [138].

Upon injury, elongated fibroblast cells resident in the tendon are activated by the inflammatory response for collagen deposition. To conduct this function, tenocytes are assisted by tendon-derived stem cells (TDSCs) [139].

MSCs do not differentiate spontaneously during *In vitro* culture, which permits a controlled microenvironment, such as to dictate the differentiation of MSCs after implantation. Because they are more easily isolated and banked from bone marrow compared to TDSCs, they represent a more optimal source of stem cells suitable for therapeutic use. MSCs have been induced to differentiate to tenocytes through the Wnt signalling pathway and cyclic mechanical stimulation that mimics normal processes [140]. It was also found that platelet-rich plasma (PrP) stimulates both MSCs and TDSCs [139].

Adipose-derived stem cell (ASC) use for tendon regeneration and repair has recently been taken into consideration. In a recent study, the role of these stem cells in primary tendon healing has been investigated by a local autologous ASC-mixed platelet-rich plasma (PrP) application at the site of tendon injury in a control to PrP application only [141]. The tensile strengths experimental groups were found to be significantly higher in comparison to the control group and, along with higher expression of collagen type I, FGF and VEGF levels in the experimental group, ASCs seems to enhance primary tendon healing.

It is now well accepted that seeded grafts vastly improve outcomes over un-seeded grafts. Recently, collagen matrices cultured with MSCs have appeared on the horizon for tendon repair [142-144]. The isoelectric focusing technique aligns collagen fibres to the parameters of the target tissue, adjusting the density, alignment, and strength of dense connective tissue (Gurkan: Comparison of morphology, orientation, and migration of tendon derived fibroblasts and bone marrow stromal cells on electrochemically aligned collagen constructs 2010). These matrices support a higher proliferation rate of MSCs compared to randomly oriented collagen. Currently, the versatility of synthetic polymers shows great promise in tissue engineering. Poly (1.8 octanediol-co-citrate) scaffold (POC) is a highly reproducible elastomeric material capable of being used as a synthetic scaffold to support cell growth. Instead of attaching tendinous grafts to bone via screws, the optimal approach is reconstruction using the collaboration of synthetic materials with MSCs. Paradoxically, the very complexity of the fibrocartilage interface makes it a perfect candidate for POC utilization. A scaffold with three distinct regions would allow formation of a collagenous tendon along one edge, osseous material along the other, and a middle zone representing the transition from tendon to bone. Given the capacity of MSCs to differentiate into osteogenic and tenogenic lineages, a single cell population seeded onto the scaffold could regenerate the complex fibrocartilage interface. Additionally, POC scaffolds could be crafted according to the target tendon interface, relying on Wolff's Law to govern the dynamics and load of the tendon aimed for reconstruction [139].

4.2.2. Bioreactors

A bioreactor in TE is a device that simulates a physiological environment in order to promote cell or tissue growth In vivo. Tendons respond to mechanical forces by changing the metabolism as well as their structural and mechanical properties. Without the appropriate biomechanical stimulation, newly formed tissue will lack appropriate collagenous organization and alignment for sufficient load-bearing capacity [134, 145, 146]. When subjected to mechanical stimulation In vitro, embryonic stem cells exhibited tenocyte-like morphology and positively expressed tendon-related gene markers, as well as other mechanosensory structures and molecules (cilia, integrins and myosin). In ectopic transplantation, the TE tendon under In vivo mechanical stimulus displayed more regularly aligned cells and larger collagen fibres that enabled enhanced tendon regeneration in situ, as evidenced by better histological scores and superior mechanical performance characteristics [145]. In a recent study, rabbit flexor tendons were deprived of cells and exposed to cyclic strain in a bioreactor, in comparison to a control, which was kept unloaded in a medium for 5 days [147]. The tendons were then implanted to bridge a zone II defect in the rabbit, followed by determination of ultimate tensile strength and elastic modulus after 4 weeks. Both were significantly improved in tendon constructs that were exposed to cyclic strain, and the histology showed an increased cellularity in the bioreactor tendons. In another study, it was showed that the material properties of human allograft tissue-engineered constructs can be enhanced by re-seeding and dynamic conditioning [148]. It was found that while conditioning duration has a significant effect on material properties, the load magnitude does not. The issue of attrition in biomechanical properties with time following cycle completion must be addressed before bioreactor preconditioning can be successfully introduced as a step in the processing of these constructs for clinical application.

4.2.3. Growth factors

Following acute tendon injury, circulation-derived cells play a crucial role in the healing processes of tissue. It was shown, that locally injected PrP is useful as an activator of circulation-derived cells for the enhancement of the initial tendon healing process [149]. PrP also improves the mechanical properties of tendons in the early phase following acute injury, in terms of increase in the force at failure, ultimate stress, and stiffness; but the effect seems to vanish in the long-term follow up [150]. To date, there is still a debate regarding the positive effect of PrP following acute tendon injury. There are studies that confirm the positive effect of PrP on tendon healing, since an earlier return to sports, decreased cross-sectional area of tendon, and improved earlier range of ankle motion, following Achilles tendon reconstruction was noted [151]. It is speculated that In vivo use of PrP, as well as platelet-poor plasma to a certain extent, in tendon injuries might accelerate the catabolic demarcation of traumatically injured tendon matrices and promote angiogenesis and formation of a fibrovascular callus [152]. A study showed that platelets influence only the early phases of regeneration, but this allows for mechanical stimulation to start driving neo-tendon development at an earlier time point, which kept it constantly ahead of the controls [153]. However, all studies do not confirm the positive effect of PrP; in fact a possible negative effect of PrP on the functional results after the reconstruction of an Achilles tendon during a long-term follow up was observed [154].

In chronic tendon lesions, especially tendinopathy, the use of PrP is focused on restoring normal tissue composition while avoiding further degeneration. Ultrasound-guided injections of PrP were effective in reducing pain in elbow tendinosis, medial epicondylitis [155] and jumper's knee [156]. Until now, few high-quality studies on the use of autologous GF injections for the management of chronic tendinopathy showed no significant improvement compared to a control group, but in those studies, autologous blood was injected and not PrP [157-159]. Currently, there is level 3 (limited) evidence that PrP injections improve pain or function in chronic tendinopathy [160]. More research on basic science and the clinical application of PrP needs to be undertaken before a final recommendation for PrP administration for the treatment of tendinosis can be made [47, 160].

A study performed at our department showed that the administration of PrP when reconstructing ACL with a hamstring autograft enhances early graft revascularization in the interface zone between graft and bone in the tibial tunnel; furthermore, PrP stimulates the formation of a sclerotic bony ring around the graft [161]. Platelet-leukocyte gel, applied locally, can also improve knee stability in the first three-month period and especially in the second three-month period [162]. Studies indicate that the delivery of PrP mimics and accelerates physiological healing and reparative tissue processes in graft healing and graft ligamentization process. Therefore, such therapy could improve knee stability and shorten the period of rehabilitation after reconstructive knee surgery. However, not all studies on humans confirm the positive effect of PrP. In one study after ACL reconstruction using patellar tendon graft with the application of PrP, researchers did not find any statistically important difference in inflammatory parameters, appearance of the graft on MRI, or clinical evaluation using validated scores [163]. Still others did not find any differences in graft fixation after ACL reconstruction with hamstring allograft and application of PrP [164].

4.3. Extracorporeal shock wave therapy

Extracorporeal shock wave therapy (ESWT) is a technique used in the treatment of tendon disorders, particularly calcific tendinopathy. The treatment is an extension of renal lithotripsy. It is a non-invasive modality used to stimulate healing, particularly in ligament, tendon, or bone structures. A high-energy sound wave rapidly increases pressure as it travels through the tissue, which results in cavitation that causes microtrauma. This stimulates an increase in blood flow and new blood vessel formation in the target area. Studies showed an increase in inflammatory cytokines and growth factors, as well as the regulation of tumour necrosis factor, interleukin, and bone morphogenetic protein following ESWT. Studies indicate that differentiated tenocytes are metabolically "activated" by ESWT and significantly induced proliferation and production of collagen (mainly type I) compared with untreated cells [165, 166]. Not all studies were able to show a positive effect of ESWT, but this was later argued to be a possible consequence of topical anaesthetics that interfere with ESWT treatment [167].

Numerous other substances have been used in the treatment of tendon disorders, including sclerosants, calcium gluconate, heparin, dextrose, and aprotinin; however, more studies have to be performed to prove their efficiency [168]. To date, no optimal treatment modalities for injured tendons or ligaments have been proposed. In fact, sheathed tendons may heal differently from those not enclosed in sheaths and the process of healing of an intra-articular ligament may differ from an extra-articular ligament. Recent studies support the idea that scaffolds can provide an alternative for tendon augmentation and that tissue engineering has an enormous therapeutic potential. In recent years studies revealed that tendon healing and regeneration may be improved by the application of several growth factors and the use of PrP expanded widely. Today, many different producers provide PrP of different composition that makes studies hard to compare. Future studies will have to explain which concentrations of PrP works the best, where it is effective and what the role of accompanying leucocytes is.

5. Conclusion

Regenerative medicine holds great promise for sports medicine with aim to develop novel therapies that will replace, repair, or promote tissue regeneration. It is an increasingly expanding area of research with hopes of providing therapeutic treatments for diseases and/or injuries that conventional medicines cannot effectively treat. Skeletal muscle has a great self-regenerative capacity, but it is unfortunately limited by fibrotic infiltration. Although none of the antifibrotic agents to improve skeletal muscle regeneration have been tested on humans to date, its clinical implications are potentially far-reaching and include not only sports-related injuries, but also diseases such as muscular dystrophies and trauma- and surgery-related injury. With emerging novel therapeutic targets this is an important area of research and presents a basis for further possibilities to study different mechanisms of action and effects drug combinations for improving muscle regeneration.

Biomaterials play an important role in directing tissue growth and may provide another tool to manipulate and control stem cell behaviour. Growth factors and therapies using mesenchymal stem cells, scaffolds, and tissue engineering using bioreactors represent promising strategies for tendon, ligament and cartilage repair. While therapies using growth factors seem to be well established in case of the first two, lack of scientific evidence still makes them questionable. In the future of cartilage repair, the modification of cellular differentiation following microfracture could be alternated with the use of exogenous growth factors and scaffolds in order to retain chongrogenic phenotype and to improve the quality of repair tissue generated in the defect. The important future prospective of cartilage repair is also focused on the quality of the bonding and integration of the newly engineered tissue to native cartilage to achieve stable healing. This holds potential for tissue-engineered strategies that would enable repairing complex cartilage lesions together with the subchondral bone and other structures. However, as with all innovations, carefully conducted studies should be carried out to access the efficiency for cartilage regeneration. Furthermore, long term prospective randomized studies are needed to confirm the encouraging preliminary results.

Author details

Robi Kelc, Jakob Naranda, Matevz Kuhta and Matjaz Vogrin

Department of Orthopaedic Surgery, University Medical Centre Maribor, Slovenia

References

[1] Gehrig SM, Lynch GS. Emerging drugs for treating skeletal muscle injury and promoting muscle repair. Expert Opin Emerg Dr. 2011 Mar;16(1):163-82.

[2] Bates SJ, Morrow E, Zhang AY, Pham H, Longaker MT, Chang J. Mannose-6-phosphate, an inhibitor of transforming growth factor-beta, improves range of motion after flexor tendon repair. J Bone Joint Surg Am. 2006 Nov;88A(11):2465-72.

[3] Mishra DK, Friden J, Schmitz MC, Lieber RL. Anti-inflammatory medication after muscle injury. A treatment resulting in short-term improvement but subsequent loss of muscle function. J Bone Joint Surg Am. 1995 Oct;77(10):1510-9.

[4] Shen W, Li Y, Tang Y, Cummins J, Huard J. NS-398, a cyclooxygenase-2-specific inhibitor, delays skeletal muscle healing by decreasing regeneration and promoting fibrosis. Am J Pathol. 2005 Oct;167(4):1105-17.

[5] Nakatani M, Takehara Y, Sugino H, Matsumoto M, Hashimoto O, Hasegawa Y, et al. Transgenic expression of a myostatin inhibitor derived from follistatin increases skeletal muscle mass and ameliorates dystrophic pathology in mdx mice. Faseb Journal. 2008 Feb;22(2):477-87.

[6] Amthor H, Connolly D, Patel K, Brand-Saberi B, Wilkinson DG, Cooke J, et al. The expression and regulation of follistatin and a follistatin-like gene during avian somite compartmentalization and myogenesis. Dev Biol. 1996 Sep 15;178(2):343-62.

[7] McPherron AC, Lawler AM, Lee SJ. Regulation of skeletal muscle mass in mice by a new TGF-beta superfamily member. Nature. 1997 May 1;387(6628):83-90.

[8] Findlay JK. An update on the roles of inhibin, activin, and follistatin as local regulators of folliculogenesis. Biol Reprod. 1993 Jan;48(1):15-23.

[9] Zhu J, Li Y, Lu A, Gharaibeh B, Ma J, Kobayashi T, et al. Follistatin Improves Skeletal Muscle Healing after Injury and Disease through an Interaction with Muscle Regeneration, Angiogenesis, and Fibrosis. Am J Pathol. 2011 May 31.

[10] Amthor H, Nicholas G, McKinnell I, Kemp CF, Sharma M, Kambadur R, et al. Follistatin complexes Myostatin and antagonises Myostatin-mediated inhibition of myogenesis. Dev Biol. 2004 Jun 1;270(1):19-30.

[11] Foley JW, Bercury SD, Finn P, Cheng SH, Scheule RK, Ziegler RJ. Evaluation of systemic follistatin as an adjuvant to stimulate muscle repair and improve motor function in Pompe mice. Mol Ther. 2010 Sep;18(9):1584-91.

[12] Gilson H, Schakman O, Kalista S, Lause P, Tsuchida K, Thissen JP. Follistatin induces muscle hypertrophy through satellite cell proliferation and inhibition of both myostatin and activin. Am J Physiol Endocrinol Metab. 2009 Jul;297(1):E157-64.

[13] Lee SJ, McPherron AC. Regulation of myostatin activity and muscle growth. P Natl Acad Sci USA. 2001 Jul 31;98(16):9306-11.

[14] Kota J, Handy CR, Haidet AM, Montgomery CL, Eagle A, Rodino-Klapac LR, et al. Follistatin gene delivery enhances muscle growth and strength in nonhuman primates. Sci Transl Med. 2009 Nov 11;1(6):6ra15.

[15] Hiroki E, Abe S, Iwanuma O, Sakiyama K, Yanagisawa N, Shiozaki K, et al. A comparative study of myostatin, follistatin and decorin expression in muscle of different origin. Anat Sci Int. 2011 Mar 18.

[16] Hocking AM, Shinomura T, McQuillan DJ. Leucine-rich repeat glycoproteins of the extracellular matrix. Matrix Biol. 1998 Apr;17(1):1-19.

[17] Nishimura T, Futami E, Taneichi A, Mori T, Hattori A. Decorin expression during development of bovine skeletal muscle and its role in morphogenesis of the intramuscular connective tissue. Cells Tissues Organs. 2002;171(2-3):199-214.

[18] Stander M, Naumann U, Dumitrescu L, Heneka M, Loschmann P, Gulbins E, et al. Decorin gene transfer-mediated suppression of TGF-beta synthesis abrogates experimental malignant glioma growth in vivo. Gene Ther. 1998 Sep;5(9):1187-94.

[19] Ungefroren H, Ergun S, Krull NB, Holstein AF. Expression of the Small Proteoglycans Biglycan and Decorin in the Adult Human Testis. Biol Reprod. 1995 May;52(5): 1095-105.

[20] Fukushima K, Badlani N, Usas A, Riano F, Fu FH, Huard J. The use of an antifibrosis agent to improve muscle recovery after laceration. Am J Sport Med. 2001 Jul-Aug; 29(4):394-402.

[21] Li Y, Foster W, Deasy BM, Chan Y, Prisk V, Tang Y, et al. Transforming growth factor-beta1 induces the differentiation of myogenic cells into fibrotic cells in injured skeletal muscle: a key event in muscle fibrogenesis. Am J Pathol. 2004 Mar;164(3): 1007-19.

[22] Sato K, Li Y, Foster W, Fukushima K, Badlani N, Adachi N, et al. Improvement of muscle healing through enhancement of muscle regeneration and prevention of fibrosis. Muscle Nerve. 2003 Sep;28(3):365-72.

[23] Li Y, Li J, Zhu J, Sun B, Branca M, Tang Y, et al. Decorin gene transfer promotes muscle cell differentiation and muscle regeneration. Mol Ther. 2007 Sep;15(9):1616-22.

[24] Kishioka Y, Thomas M, Wakamatsu JI, Hattori A, Sharma M, Kambadur R, et al. Decorin enhances the proliferation and differentiation of myogenic cells through suppressing myostatin activity. J Cell Physiol. 2008 Jun;215(3):856-67.

[25] Miura T, Kishioka Y, Wakamatsu J, Hattori A, Hennebry A, Berry CJ, et al. Decorin binds myostatin and modulates its activity to muscle cells. Biochem Biophys Res Commun. 2006 Feb 10;340(2):675-80.

[26] Zhu J, Li Y, Shen W, Qiao C, Ambrosio F, Lavasani M, et al. Relationships between transforming growth factor-beta 1, myostatin, and decorin - Implications for skeletal muscle fibrosis. J Biol Chem. 2007 Aug 31;282(35):25852-63.

[27] Wheelock EF. Interferon-Like Virus-Inhibitor Induced in Human Leukocytes by Phytohemagglutinin. Science. 1965 Jul 16;149(3681):310-1.

[28] Farrar MA, Schreiber RD. The molecular cell biology of interferon-gamma and its receptor. Annu Rev Immunol. 1993;11:571-611.

[29] Cheng M, Nguyen MH, Fantuzzi G, Koh TJ. Endogenous interferon-gamma is required for efficient skeletal muscle regeneration. Am J Physiol Cell Physiol. 2008 May;294(5):C1183-91.

[30] Foster W, Li Y, Usas A, Somogyi G, Huard J. Gamma interferon as an antifibrosis agent in skeletal muscle. J Orthop Res. 2003 Sep;21(5):798-804.

[31] Ulloa L, Doody J, Massague J. Inhibition of transforming growth factor-beta/SMAD signalling by the interferon-gamma/STAT pathway. Nature. 1999 Feb 25;397(6721): 710-3.

[32] Leask A, Abraham DJ. TGF-beta signaling and the fibrotic response. FASEB J. 2004 May;18(7):816-27.

[33] Shelton GD, Calcutt NA, Garrett RS, Gu D, Sarvetnick N, Campana WM, et al. Necrotizing myopathy induced by overexpression of interferon-gamma in transgenic mice. Muscle Nerve. 1999 Feb;22(2):156-65.

[34] Chen JW, Chen SY, Li HY, Shang XL, Wu ZY. [Effect of exogenous interferon gamma on the healing of injured skeletal muscle following injury]. Zhongguo Gu Shang. 2008 Jun;21(6):434-7.

[35] Schrell UM, Gauer S, Kiesewetter F, Bickel A, Hren J, Adams EF, et al. Inhibition of proliferation of human cerebral meningioma cells by suramin: effects on cell growth, cell cycle phases, extracellular growth factors, and PDGF-BB autocrine growth loop. J Neurosurg. 1995 Apr;82(4):600-7.

[36] Zumkeller W, Schofield PN. Growth factors, cytokines and soluble forms of receptor molecules in cancer patients. Anticancer Res. 1995 Mar-Apr;15(2):343-8.

[37] Liu N, Tolbert E, Ponnusamy M, Yan H, Zhuang S. Delayed administration of suramin attenuates the progression of renal fibrosis in obstructive nephropathy. J Pharmacol Exp Ther. 2011 May 27.

[38] Mietz H, Krieglstein GK. Suramin to enhance glaucoma filtering procedures: a clinical comparison with mitomycin. Ophthalmic Surg Lasers. 2001 Sep-Oct;32(5):358-69.

[39] Chan YS, Li Y, Foster W, Fu FH, Huard J. The use of suramin, an antifibrotic agent, to improve muscle recovery after strain injury. Am J Sport Med. 2005 Jan;33(1):43-51.

[40] Taniguti AP, Pertille A, Matsumura CY, Santo Neto H, Marques MJ. Prevention of muscle fibrosis and myonecrosis in mdx mice by suramin, a TGF-beta1 blocker. Muscle Nerve. 2011 Jan;43(1):82-7.

[41] Masterson R, Hewitson TD, Kelynack K, Martic M, Parry L, Bathgate R, et al. Relaxin down-regulates renal fibroblast function and promotes matrix remodelling in vitro. Nephrol Dial Transpl. 2004 Mar;19(3):544-52.

[42] Samuel CS, Unemori EN, Mookerjee I, Bathgate RAD, Layfield SL, Mak J, et al. Relaxin modulates cardiac fibroblast proliferation, differentiation and collagen production and reverses cardiac fibrosis in vivo. Endocrinology. 2004 Sep;145(9):4125-33.

[43] Unemori EN, Pickford LB, Salles AL, Piercy CE, Grove BH, Erikson ME, et al. Relaxin induces an extracellular matrix-degrading phenotype in human lung fibroblasts in vitro and inhibits lung fibrosis in a murine model in vivo. J Clin Invest. 1996 Dec 15;98(12):2739-45.

[44] Bathgate RA, Lekgabe ED, McGuane JT, Su Y, Pham T, Ferraro T, et al. Adenovirus-mediated delivery of relaxin reverses cardiac fibrosis. Mol Cell Endocrinol. 2008 Jan 2;280(1-2):30-8.

[45] Mu X, Urso ML, Murray K, Fu F, Li Y. Relaxin regulates MMP expression and promotes satellite cell mobilization during muscle healing in both young and aged mice. Am J Pathol. 2010 Nov;177(5):2399-410.

[46] Official WADA Website. 2012; Available from: http://www.wada-ama.org/en/Media-Center/Archives/Articles/WADA-2011-Prohibited-List-Now-Published/.

[47] International Olympic Commitee: IOC Consensus Statement on the use of platelet-rich plasma (PRP) in sports medicine. http://www.olympic.org/Documents/Reports/EN/IOC_PRP_Consensus_Statement-ENG.pdf.

[48] Foster TE, Puskas BL, Mandelbaum BR, Gerhardt MB, Rodeo SA. Platelet-rich plasma: from basic science to clinical applications. Am J Sports Med. 2009 Nov;37(11): 2259-72.

[49] Sanchez M, Anitua E, Orive G, Mujika I, Andia I. Platelet-rich therapies in the treatment of orthopaedic sport injuries. Sports medicine. 2009;39(5):345-54.

[50] Bachl N, Derman W, Engebretsen L, Goldspink G, Kinzlbauer M, Tschan H, et al. Therapeutic use of growth factors in the musculoskeletal system in sports-related injuries. The Journal of sports medicine and physical fitness. 2009 Dec;49(4):346-57.

[51] Hildebrand KA, Woo SL, Smith DW, Allen CR, Deie M, Taylor BJ, et al. The effects of platelet-derived growth factor-BB on healing of the rabbit medial collateral ligament. An in vivo study. The American journal of sports medicine. 1998 Jul-Aug;26(4): 549-54.

[52] Batten ML, Hansen JC, Dahners LE. Influence of dosage and timing of application of platelet-derived growth factor on early healing of the rat medial collateral ligament. Journal of orthopaedic research: official publication of the Orthopaedic Research Society. 1996 Sep;14(5):736-41.

[53] Murray MM, Spindler KP, Abreu E, Muller JA, Nedder A, Kelly M, et al. Collagen-platelet rich plasma hydrogel enhances primary repair of the porcine anterior cruci-

ate ligament. Journal of orthopaedic research: official publication of the Orthopaedic Research Society. 2007 Jan;25(1):81-91.

[54] Wang-Saegusa A, Cugat R, Ares O, Seijas R, Cusco X, Garcia-Balletbo M. Infiltration of plasma rich in growth factors for osteoarthritis of the knee; short-term effects on function and quality of life. Archives of orthopaedic and trauma surgery. 2011 Mar; 131(3):311-7.

[55] Shen W, Li Y, Zhu JH, Schwendener R, Huard J. Interaction between macrophages, TGF-beta 1, and the COX-2 pathway during the inflammatory phase of skeletal muscle healing after injury. J Cell Physiol. 2008 Feb;214(2):405-12.

[56] Menetrey J, Kasemkijwattana C, Day CS, Bosch P, Vogt M, Fu FH, et al. Growth factors improve muscle healing in vivo. J Bone Joint Surg Br. 2000 Jan;82B(1):131-7.

[57] Wright-Carpenter T, Klein P, Schaferhoff P, Appell HJ, Mir LM, Wehling P. Treatment of muscle injuries by local administration of autologous conditioned serum: A pilot study on sportsmen with muscle strains. Int J Sports Med. 2004 Nov;25(8): 588-93.

[58] Kelc R, Trapecar, M., Gradisnik, L., Mlakar, R., Rupnik, MS., Cencic, A., Vogrin, M. New therapeutic strategy for muscle repair after injury: platelet-rich plasma and TGF-ß antagonists. Poster presentation. Development, function and repair of the muscle cell: Frontiers in myogenesis; New York, USA2011.

[59] Mishra A, Woodall J, Vieira A. Treatment of Tendon and Muscle Using Platelet-Rich Plasma. Clin Sport Med. 2009 Jan;28(1):113-+.

[60] Dennis PA, Rifkin DB. Cellular activation of latent transforming growth factor beta requires binding to the cation-independent mannose 6-phosphate/insulin-like growth factor type II receptor. Proc Natl Acad Sci U S A. 1991 Jan 15;88(2):580-4.

[61] Roberts A, Sporn, MB. Transforming growth factor-beta. Clark R, editor. New York: Plenum; 1996.

[62] Angunawela RI, Marshall J. Inhibition of transforming growth factor-beta1 and its effects on human corneal fibroblasts by mannose-6-phosphate. Potential for preventing haze after refractive surgery. J Cataract Refract Surg. 2010 Jan;36(1):121-6.

[63] Yang R, Xia C, Wang X, Sun K, Yang X, Tian S, et al. [Effects of mannose-6-phosphate on transforming growth factor beta and transforming growth factor beta receptor expression of flexor tendon cells]. Zhongguo Xiu Fu Chong Jian Wai Ke Za Zhi. 2010 Jan;24(1):64-8.

[64] Millea PJ. N-acetylcysteine: multiple clinical applications. Am Fam Physician. 2009 Aug 1;80(3):265-9.

[65] Liu RM, Liu Y, Forman HJ, Olman M, Tarpey MM. Glutathione regulates transforming growth factor-beta-stimulated collagen production in fibroblasts. Am J Physiol Lung Cell Mol Physiol. 2004 Jan;286(1):L121-8.

[66] Hagiwara SI, Ishii Y, Kitamura S. Aerosolized administration of N-acetylcysteine attenuates lung fibrosis induced by bleomycin in mice. Am J Respir Crit Care Med. 2000 Jul;162(1):225-31.

[67] Meurer SK, Lahme B, Tihaa L, Weiskirchen R, Gressner AM. N-acetyl-L-cysteine suppresses TGF-beta signaling at distinct molecular steps: the biochemical and biological efficacy of a multifunctional, antifibrotic drug. Biochem Pharmacol. 2005 Oct 1;70(7): 1026-34.

[68] Sugiura H, Ichikawa T, Liu X, Kobayashi T, Wang XQ, Kawasaki S, et al. N-acetyl-L-cysteine inhibits TGF-beta1-induced profibrotic responses in fibroblasts. Pulm Pharmacol Ther. 2009 Dec;22(6):487-91.

[69] Marian AJ, Senthil V, Chen SN, Lombardi R. Antifibrotic effects of antioxidant N-acetylcysteine in a mouse model of human hypertrophic cardiomyopathy mutation. J Am Coll Cardiol. 2006 Feb 21;47(4):827-34.

[70] Onder G, Vedova CD, Pahor M. Effects of ACE inhibitors on skeletal muscle. Curr Pharm Des. 2006;12(16):2057-64.

[71] Lim DS, Lutucuta S, Bachireddy P, Youker K, Evans A, Entman M, et al. Angiotensin II blockade reverses myocardial fibrosis in a transgenic mouse model of human hypertrophic cardiomyopathy. Circulation. 2001 Feb 13;103(6):789-91.

[72] Otsuka M, Takahashi H, Shiratori M, Chiba H, Abe S. Reduction of bleomycin induced lung fibrosis by candesartan cilexetil, an angiotensin II type 1 receptor antagonist. Thorax. 2004 Jan;59(1):31-8.

[73] Paizis G, Gilbert RE, Cooper ME, Murthi P, Schembri JM, Wu LL, et al. Effect of angiotensin II type 1 receptor blockade on experimental hepatic fibrogenesis. J Hepatol. 2001 Sep;35(3):376-85.

[74] Suga S, Mazzali M, Ray PE, Kang DH, Johnson RJ. Angiotensin II type 1 receptor blockade ameliorates tubulointerstitial injury induced by chronic potassium deficiency. Kidney Int. 2002 Mar;61(3):951-8.

[75] Gremmler B, Kunert M, Schleiting H, Ulbricht LJ. Improvement of cardiac output in patients with severe heart failure by use of ACE-inhibitors combined with the AT1-antagonist eprosartan. Eur J Heart Fail. 2000 Jun;2(2):183-7.

[76] Swedberg K, Kjekshus J. Effects of enalapril on mortality in severe congestive heart failure: results of the Cooperative North Scandinavian Enalapril Survival Study (CONSENSUS). Am J Cardiol. 1988 Jul 11;62(2):60A-6A.

[77] Savo A, Maiorano PM, Onder G, Bernabei R. Pharmacoepidemiology and disability in older adults: can medications slow the age-related decline in physical function? Expert Opin Pharmacother. 2004 Feb;5(2):407-13.

[78] Jones A, Woods DR. Skeletal muscle RAS and exercise performance. Int J Biochem Cell Biol. 2003 Jun;35(6):855-66.

[79] Frederiksen H, Bathum L, Worm C, Christensen K, Puggaard L. ACE genotype and physical training effects: a randomized study among elderly Danes. Aging Clin Exp Res. 2003 Aug;15(4):284-91.

[80] Frederiksen H, Gaist D, Bathum L, Andersen K, McGue M, Vaupel JW, et al. Angiotensin I-converting enzyme (ACE) gene polymorphism in relation to physical performance, cognition and survival--a follow-up study of elderly Danish twins. Ann Epidemiol. 2003 Jan;13(1):57-65.

[81] Bedair HS, Karthikeyan T, Quintero A, Li Y, Huard J. Angiotensin II receptor blockade administered after injury improves muscle regeneration and decreases fibrosis in normal skeletal muscle. Am J Sports Med. 2008 Aug;36(8):1548-54.

[82] Hildner F, Albrecht C, Gabriel C, Redl H, van Griensven M. State of the art and future perspectives of articular cartilage regeneration: a focus on adipose-derived stem cells and platelet-derived products. J Tissue Eng Regen Med. 2011 Apr;5(4):e36-51.

[83] Tuli R, Li WJ, Tuan RS. Current state of cartilage tissue engineering. Arthritis research & therapy. [Review]. 2003;5(5):235-8.

[84] Taboas JM, Maddox RD, Krebsbach PH, Hollister SJ. Indirect solid free form fabrication of local and global porous, biomimetic and composite 3D polymer-ceramic scaffolds. Biomaterials. 2003 Jan;24(1):181-94.

[85] Stoop R. Smart biomaterials for tissue engineering of cartilage. Injury. 2008 Apr;39 Suppl 1:S77-87.

[86] Moutos FT, Guilak F. Composite scaffolds for cartilage tissue engineering. Biorheology. 2008;45(3-4):501-12.

[87] Wang X, Wenk E, Zhang X, Meinel L, Vunjak-Novakovic G, Kaplan DL. Growth factor gradients via microsphere delivery in biopolymer scaffolds for osteochondral tissue engineering. J Control Release. 2009 Mar 4;134(2):81-90.

[88] Ameer GA, Mahmood TA, Langer R. A biodegradable composite scaffold for cell transplantation. J Orthop Res. 2002 Jan;20(1):16-9.

[89] Grigolo B, Lisignoli G, Desando G, Cavallo C, Marconi E, Tschon M, et al. Osteoarthritis treated with mesenchymal stem cells on hyaluronan-based scaffold in rabbit. Tissue engineering Part C, Methods. [Research Support, Non-U.S. Gov't]. 2009 Dec; 15(4):647-58.

[90] Pei M, He F, Vunjak-Novakovic G. Synovium-derived stem cell-based chondrogenesis. Differentiation. 2008 Dec;76(10):1044-56.

[91] Cals FL, Hellingman CA, Koevoet W, Baatenburg de Jong RJ, van Osch GJ. Effects of transforming growth factor-beta subtypes on in vitro cartilage production and mineralization of human bone marrow stromal-derived mesenchymal stem cells. J Tissue Eng Regen Med. 2012 Jan;6(1):68-76.

[92] Rui YF, Du L, Wang Y, Lui PP, Tang TT, Chan KM, et al. Bone morphogenetic pro-
      tein 2 promotes transforming growth factor beta3-induced chondrogenesis of human
      osteoarthritic synovium-derived stem cells. Chin Med J (Engl). 2010 Nov;123(21):
      3040-8.

[93] Fortier LA, Barker JU, Strauss EJ, McCarrel TM, Cole BJ. The role of growth factors in
      cartilage repair. Clin Orthop Relat Res. [Review]. 2011 Oct;469(10):2706-15.

[94] Kramer J, Hegert C, Guan K, Wobus AM, Muller PK, Rohwedel J. Embryonic stem
      cell-derived chondrogenic differentiation in vitro: activation by BMP-2 and BMP-4.
      Mech Dev. 2000 Apr;92(2):193-205.

[95] Richardson SM, Hoyland JA, Mobasheri R, Csaki C, Shakibaei M, Mobasheri A. Mes-
      enchymal stem cells in regenerative medicine: opportunities and challenges for artic-
      ular cartilage and intervertebral disc tissue engineering. J Cell Physiol. 2010 Jan;
      222(1):23-32.

[96] Ronziere MC, Perrier E, Mallein-Gerin F, Freyria AM. Chondrogenic potential of
      bone marrow- and adipose tissue-derived adult human mesenchymal stem cells. Bi-
      omed Mater Eng. 2010;20(3):145-58.

[97] Hildner F, Albrecht C, Gabriel C, Redl H, van Griensven M. State of the art and fu-
      ture perspectives of articular cartilage regeneration: a focus on adipose-derived stem
      cells and platelet-derived products. J Tissue Eng Regen Med. 2011 Jan 10.

[98] Sakaguchi Y, Sekiya I, Yagishita K, Muneta T. Comparison of human stem cells de-
      rived from various mesenchymal tissues: superiority of synovium as a cell source.
      Arthritis and rheumatism. 2005 Aug;52(8):2521-9.

[99] Yan H, Yu C. Repair of full-thickness cartilage defects with cells of different origin in
      a rabbit model. Arthroscopy. [Research Support, Non-U.S. Gov't]. 2007 Feb;23(2):
      178-87.

[100] Csaki C, Schneider PR, Shakibaei M. Mesenchymal stem cells as a potential pool for
      cartilage tissue engineering. Annals of anatomy = Anatomischer Anzeiger: official or-
      gan of the Anatomische Gesellschaft. 2008 Nov 20;190(5):395-412.

[101] Mahmoudifar N, Doran PM. Chondrogenesis and cartilage tissue engineering: the
      longer road to technology development. Trends in biotechnology. 2012 Mar;30(3):
      166-76.

[102] Schulz RM, Bader A. Cartilage tissue engineering and bioreactor systems for the cul-
      tivation and stimulation of chondrocytes. Eur Biophys J. 2007 Apr;36(4-5):539-68.

[103] Elder BD, Athanasiou KA. Synergistic and additive effects of hydrostatic pressure
      and growth factors on tissue formation. PLoS One. [Research Support, N.I.H., Extra-
      mural]. 2008;3(6):e2341.

[104] Mauck RL, Nicoll SB, Seyhan SL, Ateshian GA, Hung CT. Synergistic action of growth factors and dynamic loading for articular cartilage tissue engineering. Tissue Eng. 2003 Aug;9(4):597-611.

[105] Shieh AC, Athanasiou KA. Principles of cell mechanics for cartilage tissue engineering. Ann Biomed Eng. [Review]. 2003 Jan;31(1):1-11.

[106] Waldman SD, Couto DC, Grynpas MD, Pilliar RM, Kandel RA. Multi-axial mechanical stimulation of tissue engineered cartilage: review. Eur Cell Mater. [Research Support, Non-U.S. Gov't]. 2007;13:66-73; discussion -4.

[107] Elder BD, Athanasiou KA. Hydrostatic pressure in articular cartilage tissue engineering: from chondrocytes to tissue regeneration. Tissue Eng Part B Rev. [Review]. 2009 Mar;15(1):43-53.

[108] Grad S, Eglin D, Alini M, Stoddart MJ. Physical stimulation of chondrogenic cells in vitro: a review. Clin Orthop Relat Res. [Review]. 2011 Oct;469(10):2764-72.

[109] Marlovits S, Zeller P, Singer P, Resinger C, Vecsei V. Cartilage repair: generations of autologous chondrocyte transplantation. European journal of radiology. 2006 Jan; 57(1):24-31.

[110] Harris JD, Siston RA, Pan X, Flanigan DC. Autologous chondrocyte implantation: a systematic review. J Bone Joint Surg Am. [Review]. 2010 Sep 15;92(12):2220-33.

[111] Bentley G, Biant LC, Carrington RW, Akmal M, Goldberg A, Williams AM, et al. A prospective, randomised comparison of autologous chondrocyte implantation versus mosaicplasty for osteochondral defects in the knee. J Bone Joint Surg Br. 2003 Mar; 85(2):223-30.

[112] Harris JD, Siston RA, Brophy RH, Lattermann C, Carey JL, Flanigan DC. Failures, re-operations, and complications after autologous chondrocyte implantation--a systematic review. Osteoarthritis Cartilage. [Review]. 2011 Jul;19(7):779-91.

[113] Gigante A, Bevilacqua C, Ricevuto A, Mattioli-Belmonte M, Greco F. Membrane-seeded autologous chondrocytes: cell viability and characterization at surgery. Knee Surg Sports Traumatol Arthrosc. 2007 Jan;15(1):88-92.

[114] Bartlett W, Skinner JA, Gooding CR, Carrington RW, Flanagan AM, Briggs TW, et al. Autologous chondrocyte implantation versus matrix-induced autologous chondrocyte implantation for osteochondral defects of the knee: a prospective, randomised study. J Bone Joint Surg Br. 2005 May;87(5):640-5.

[115] Basad E, Ishaque B, Bachmann G, Sturz H, Steinmeyer J. Matrix-induced autologous chondrocyte implantation versus microfracture in the treatment of cartilage defects of the knee: a 2-year randomised study. Knee Surg Sports Traumatol Arthrosc. [Randomized Controlled Trial]. 2010 Apr;18(4):519-27.

[116] Behrens P, Bitter T, Kurz B, Russlies M. Matrix-associated autologous chondrocyte transplantation/implantation (MACT/MACI)--5-year follow-up. The Knee. [Clinical Trial]. 2006 Jun;13(3):194-202.

[117] Marcacci M, Berruto M, Brocchetta D, Delcogliano A, Ghinelli D, Gobbi A, et al. Articular cartilage engineering with Hyalograft C: 3-year clinical results. Clin Orthop Relat Res. 2005 Jun(435):96-105.

[118] Pavesio A, Abatangelo G, Borrione A, Brocchetta D, Hollander AP, Kon E, et al. Hyaluronan-based scaffolds (Hyalograft C) in the treatment of knee cartilage defects: preliminary clinical findings. Novartis Foundation symposium. [Review]. 2003;249:203-17; discussion 29-33, 34-8, 39-41.

[119] Podskubka A, Povysil C, Kubes R, Sprindrich J, Sedlacek R. [Treatment of deep cartilage defects of the knee with autologous chondrocyte transplantation on a hyaluronic Acid ester scaffold (Hyalograft C)]. Acta chirurgiae orthopaedicae et traumatologiae Cechoslovaca. 2006 Aug;73(4):251-63.

[120] Kon E, Gobbi A, Filardo G, Delcogliano M, Zaffagnini S, Marcacci M. Arthroscopic second-generation autologous chondrocyte implantation compared with microfracture for chondral lesions of the knee: prospective nonrandomized study at 5 years. Am J Sports Med. [Comparative Study]. 2009 Jan;37(1):33-41.

[121] Kon E, Filardo G, Berruto M, Benazzo F, Zanon G, Della Villa S, et al. Articular cartilage treatment in high-level male soccer players: a prospective comparative study of arthroscopic second-generation autologous chondrocyte implantation versus microfracture. Am J Sports Med. 2011 Dec;39(12):2549-57.

[122] Kuroda T, Matsumoto T, Mifune Y, Fukui T, Kubo S, Matsushita T, et al. Therapeutic strategy of third-generation autologous chondrocyte implantation for osteoarthritis. Upsala journal of medical sciences. [Research Support, Non-U.S. Gov't]. 2011 May; 116(2):107-14.

[123] Hettrich CM, Crawford D, Rodeo SA. Cartilage repair: third-generation cell-based technologies--basic science, surgical techniques, clinical outcomes. Sports Med Arthrosc. [Review]. 2008 Dec;16(4):230-5.

[124] Crawford DC, DeBerardino TM, Williams RJ, 3rd. NeoCart, an autologous cartilage tissue implant, compared with microfracture for treatment of distal femoral cartilage lesions: an FDA phase-II prospective, randomized clinical trial after two years. J Bone Joint Surg Am. 2012 Jun 6;94(11):979-89.

[125] McNickle AG, Provencher MT, Cole BJ. Overview of existing cartilage repair technology. Sports Med Arthrosc. [Review]. 2008 Dec;16(4):196-201.

[126] AHCCS AsMA. AHCCCS Medical Policy Manual: Medical and Behavioral Health Policy Manual. Arizona2012.

[127] Kessler MW, Ackerman G, Dines JS, Grande D. Emerging technologies and fourth generation issues in cartilage repair. Sports Med Arthrosc. [Review]. 2008 Dec;16(4): 246-54.

[128] Steinert AF, Noth U, Tuan RS. Concepts in gene therapy for cartilage repair. Injury. 2008 Apr;39 Suppl 1:S97-113.

[129] Schiavone Panni A, Cerciello S, Vasso M. The manangement of knee cartilage defects with modified amic technique: preliminary results. Int J Immunopathol Pharmacol. 2011 Jan-Mar;24(1 Suppl 2):149-52.

[130] Gille J, Schuseil E, Wimmer J, Gellissen J, Schulz AP, Behrens P. Mid-term results of Autologous Matrix-Induced Chondrogenesis for treatment of focal cartilage defects in the knee. Knee Surg Sports Traumatol Arthrosc. 2010 Nov;18(11):1456-64.

[131] McCormick F, Yanke A, Provencher MT, Cole BJ. Minced articular cartilage--basic science, surgical technique, and clinical application. Sports Med Arthrosc. [Review]. 2008 Dec;16(4):217-20.

[132] Farr J, Cole BJ, Sherman S, Karas V. Particulated articular cartilage: CAIS and DeNovo NT. The journal of knee surgery. 2012 Mar;25(1):23-9.

[133] Cole BJ, Farr J, Winalski CS, Hosea T, Richmond J, Mandelbaum B, et al. Outcomes after a single-stage procedure for cell-based cartilage repair: a prospective clinical safety trial with 2-year follow-up. Am J Sports Med. 2011 Jun;39(6):1170-9.

[134] Rodrigues MT, Reis RL, Gomes ME. Engineering tendon and ligament tissues: present developments towards successful clinical products. Journal of tissue engineering and regenerative medicine. 2012 Apr 12.

[135] Mascarenhas R, MacDonald PB. Anterior cruciate ligament reconstruction: a look at prosthetics--past, present and possible future. McGill journal of medicine: MJM: an international forum for the advancement of medical sciences by students. 2008 Jan; 11(1):29-37.

[136] Hoffmann A, Gross G. Tendon and ligament engineering: from cell biology to in vivo application. Regenerative medicine. 2006 Jul;1(4):563-74.

[137] Sahoo S, Cho-Hong JG, Siew-Lok T. Development of hybrid polymer scaffolds for potential applications in ligament and tendon tissue engineering. Biomedical materials. 2007 Sep;2(3):169-73.

[138] Longo UG, Lamberti A, Petrillo S, Maffulli N, Denaro V. Scaffolds in tendon tissue engineering. Stem cells international. 2012;2012:517165.

[139] Thaker H, Sharma AK. Engaging stem cells for customized tendon regeneration. Stem Cells Int. 2012;2012:309187.

[140] Kuo CK, Tuan RS. Mechanoactive tenogenic differentiation of human mesenchymal stem cells. Tissue Eng Part A. 2008 Oct;14(10):1615-27.

[141] Uysal CA, Tobita M, Hyakusoku H, Mizuno H. Adipose-derived stem cells enhance primary tendon repair: Biomechanical and immunohistochemical evaluation. J Plast Reconstr Aesthet Surg. 2012 Jul 6.

[142] Kishore V, Bullock W, Sun X, Van Dyke WS, Akkus O. Tenogenic differentiation of human MSCs induced by the topography of electrochemically aligned collagen threads. Biomaterials. 2012 Mar;33(7):2137-44.

[143] Butler DL, Juncosa-Melvin N, Boivin GP, Galloway MT, Shearn JT, Gooch C, et al. Functional tissue engineering for tendon repair: A multidisciplinary strategy using mesenchymal stem cells, bioscaffolds, and mechanical stimulation. J Orthop Res. 2008 Jan;26(1):1-9.

[144] Awad HA, Boivin GP, Dressler MR, Smith FN, Young RG, Butler DL. Repair of patellar tendon injuries using a cell-collagen composite. J Orthop Res. 2003 May;21(3): 420-31.

[145] Chen JL, Yin Z, Shen WL, Chen X, Heng BC, Zou XH, et al. Efficacy of HESC-MSCs in knitted silk-collagen scaffold for tendon tissue engineering and their roles. Biomaterials. 2010 Dec;31(36):9438-51.

[146] Doroski DM, Levenston ME, Temenoff JS. Cyclic tensile culture promotes fibroblastic differentiation of marrow stromal cells encapsulated in poly(ethylene glycol)-based hydrogels. Tissue engineering Part A. 2010 Nov;16(11):3457-66.

[147] Thorfinn J, Angelidis IK, Gigliello L, Pham HM, Lindsey D, Chang J. Bioreactor optimization of tissue engineered rabbit flexor tendons in vivo. J Hand Surg Eur Vol. 2012 Feb;37(2):109-14.

[148] Woon CY, Kraus A, Raghavan SS, Pridgen BC, Megerle K, Pham H, et al. Three-dimensional-construct bioreactor conditioning in human tendon tissue engineering. Tissue Eng Part A. 2011 Oct;17(19-20):2561-72.

[149] Kajikawa Y, Morihara T, Sakamoto H, Matsuda K, Oshima Y, Yoshida A, et al. Platelet-rich plasma enhances the initial mobilization of circulation-derived cells for tendon healing. Journal of cellular physiology. 2008 Jun;215(3):837-45.

[150] Lyras DN, Kazakos K, Verettas D, Botaitis S, Agrogiannis G, Kokka A, et al. The effect of platelet-rich plasma gel in the early phase of patellar tendon healing. Archives of orthopaedic and trauma surgery. 2009 Nov;129(11):1577-82.

[151] Sanchez M, Anitua E, Azofra J, Andia I, Padilla S, Mujika I. Comparison of surgically repaired Achilles tendon tears using platelet-rich fibrin matrices. The American journal of sports medicine. 2007 Feb;35(2):245-51.

[152] de Mos M, van der Windt AE, Jahr H, van Schie HT, Weinans H, Verhaar JA, et al. Can platelet-rich plasma enhance tendon repair? A cell culture study. The American journal of sports medicine. 2008 Jun;36(6):1171-8.

[153] Virchenko O, Aspenberg P. How can one platelet injection after tendon injury lead to a stronger tendon after 4 weeks? Interplay between early regeneration and mechanical stimulation. Acta orthopaedica. 2006 Oct;77(5):806-12.

[154] Schepull T, Kvist J, Norrman H, Trinks M, Berlin G, Aspenberg P. Autologous platelets have no effect on the healing of human Achilles tendon ruptures: a randomized single-blind study. The American journal of sports medicine. 2011 Jan;39(1):38-47.

[155] Mishra A, Pavelko T. Treatment of chronic elbow tendinosis with buffered platelet-rich plasma. The American journal of sports medicine. 2006 Nov;34(11):1774-8.

[156] Kon E, Filardo G, Delcogliano M, Presti ML, Russo A, Bondi A, et al. Platelet-rich plasma: new clinical application: a pilot study for treatment of jumper's knee. Injury. 2009 Jun;40(6):598-603.

[157] Kalaci A, Cakici H, Hapa O, Yanat AN, Dogramaci Y, Sevinc TT. Treatment of plantar fasciitis using four different local injection modalities: a randomized prospective clinical trial. Journal of the American Podiatric Medical Association. 2009 Mar-Apr; 99(2):108-13.

[158] Kiter E, Celikbas E, Akkaya S, Demirkan F, Kilic BA. Comparison of injection modalities in the treatment of plantar heel pain: a randomized controlled trial. Journal of the American Podiatric Medical Association. 2006 Jul-Aug;96(4):293-6.

[159] Lee TG, Ahmad TS. Intralesional autologous blood injection compared to corticosteroid injection for treatment of chronic plantar fasciitis. A prospective, randomized, controlled trial. Foot & ankle international/American Orthopaedic Foot and Ankle Society [and] Swiss Foot and Ankle Society. 2007 Sep;28(9):984-90.

[160] de Vos RJ, van Veldhoven PL, Moen MH, Weir A, Tol JL, Maffulli N. Autologous growth factor injections in chronic tendinopathy: a systematic review. British medical bulletin. 2010;95:63-77.

[161] Vogrin M, Rupreht M, Dinevski D, Haspl M, Kuhta M, Jevsek M, et al. Effects of a platelet gel on early graft revascularization after anterior cruciate ligament reconstruction: a prospective, randomized, double-blind, clinical trial. European surgical research Europaische chirurgische Forschung Recherches chirurgicales europeennes. 2010;45(2):77-85.

[162] Vogrin M, Rupreht M, Crnjac A, Dinevski D, Krajnc Z, Recnik G. The effect of platelet-derived growth factors on knee stability after anterior cruciate ligament reconstruction: a prospective randomized clinical study. Wiener klinische Wochenschrift. 2010 May;122 Suppl 2:91-5.

[163] Nin JR, Gasque GM, Azcarate AV, Beola JD, Gonzalez MH. Has platelet-rich plasma any role in anterior cruciate ligament allograft healing? Arthroscopy: the journal of arthroscopic & related surgery: official publication of the Arthroscopy Association of North America and the International Arthroscopy Association. 2009 Nov;25(11): 1206-13.

[164] Silva A, Sampaio R. Anatomic ACL reconstruction: does the platelet-rich plasma ac-
       celerate tendon healing? Knee surgery, sports traumatology, arthroscopy: official
       journal of the ESSKA. 2009 Jun;17(6):676-82.

[165] Vetrano M, d'Alessandro F, Torrisi MR, Ferretti A, Vulpiani MC, Visco V. Extracor-
       poreal shock wave therapy promotes cell proliferation and collagen synthesis of pri-
       mary cultured human tenocytes. Knee surgery, sports traumatology, arthroscopy:
       official journal of the ESSKA. 2011 Dec;19(12):2159-68.

[166] Furia JP. High-energy extracorporeal shock wave therapy as a treatment for inser-
       tional Achilles tendinopathy. The American journal of sports medicine. 2006 May;
       34(5):733-40.

[167] Costa ML, Shepstone L, Donell ST, Thomas TL. Shock wave therapy for chronic
       Achilles tendon pain: a randomized placebo-controlled trial. Clinical orthopaedics
       and related research. 2005 Nov;440:199-204.

[168] Rees JD, Maffulli N, Cook J. Management of tendinopathy. The American journal of
       sports medicine. 2009 Sep;37(9):1855-67.

Chapter 3

Patellofemoral Instability: Diagnosis and Management

Alexander Golant, Tony Quach and Jeffrey Rosen

Additional information is available at the end of the chapter

1. Introduction

Patellofemoral articulation plays a major role in locomotion and other activities that involve knee flexion and extension. Problems of patellofemoral tracking are very common, ranging from mild lateral maltracking and tilt, to frank instability and dislocation of the patella. Patellofemoral instability can be defined as movement of the patella out of its normal position, and can be divided into dislocation and subluxation. Natural history of this condition is that of a relatively high recurrence. Even in the absence of recurrent instability, patients who sustain patella dislocation or subluxation may develop a number of significant problems, including persistent knee pain, functional limitations, decreased athletic performance, and arthritic degeneration of the patellofemoral articulation. Especially for the recurrent dislocator, surgical treatment plays an important role in management, since the natural history of this condition is that of relatively poor return to normal function.

Direction of patellofemoral instability is almost always lateral (rare cases of medial dislocation have been reported to occur secondary to iatrogenic causes). Overall incidence of this injury has been shown to be around 6 per 100,000, with the highest incidence occurring in the 2nd decade of life (around 30 per 100,000), and becoming significantly lower after 30 years of age (around 2 per 100,000).[1,2]Traditionally, this injury was thought to occur in sedentary, overweight, adolescent females, but most recent data has shown this stereotype to be inaccurate, with most injuries actually occurring in young athletic individuals, often males, during sports participation and other intense physical activity. [3]

Proper articulation and movement of the patella within the femoral trochlear groove requires complex interplay between a number of important static and dynamic soft-tissue stabilizers, the bony architecture of the patellofemoral joint, and the overall alignment of the lower extremity. Abnormalities in one or more of these factors can result in or predispose to clinically relevant patellofemoral instability, and are described below.

2. Anatomy of the patellofemoral joint and factors contributing to instability

2.1. Osseous anatomy of the patellofemoral articulation

Instability of the patellofemoral articulation can occur when the bony anatomy of the patella, the femoral trochlea, or both is abnormal, i.e. dysplastic. In order to understand how dysplasia contributes to instability, normal anatomy and biomechanics of this joint have to first be described.

The patella is the largest sesamoid bone in the body, i.e. it is a bone that is imbedded within a tendon – in this case the extensor mechanism of the knee. It has a multifaceted articular surface, with lateral and medial facets separated by a central ridge, and a much smaller odd facet located far medially. The articular cartilage of the patella is the thickest in the body, designed to withstand significant joint reactive forces that occur at the patellofemoral joint, which range from 0.5 to 9.7 x body weight with daily activities, and may approach values of 20 x body weight with certain sporting activities. [4]

The patella's most important function is as a fulcrum for the extensor mechanism. It increases the distance of the line of action of the extensor mechanism from the center of rotation of the knee, thereby increasing the force that can be generated by contraction of the quadriceps. Total patellectomy has been shown to decrease the maximum force generated by the quadriceps by 50%. [5]

Anatomy of the femoral trochlea typically closely matches the articular shape of the patella, with a longer and higher lateral wall that serves as the most important bony restraint to lateral translation. In full extension the patella sits on the non-articular anterior surface of the distal femur, and typically enters the trochlea at 20-30 degrees of knee flexion, depending on the length of the patella tendon. The contact area increases and moves proximally with greater flexion; the lateral facet engages the trochlea first, while the medial facet engages it last.

Since the flexion angle at which the patella engages the trochlea depends on the length of the patella tendon, patella alta – the condition in which the length of the patella tendon is abnormally increased and the patella position is abnormally high - contributes to instability by increasing the range at which there is no bony contribution to stability. Patella alta has been shown to be associated with recurrent patellofemoral instability. [6,7]

Once the patella enters the trochlea, dysplasia of the patella, the trochlea, or both, can contribute to instability by decreasing the bony restraint and consequently the amount of energy required to dislocate. Patellofemoral dysplasia has been classified by Dejour et al. [8] (Figure 1) Dysplasia typically occurs on both sides of the joint, with congruous articulation between the two bones, although incongruous articulation can also occur, and leads to some of the worst instability.

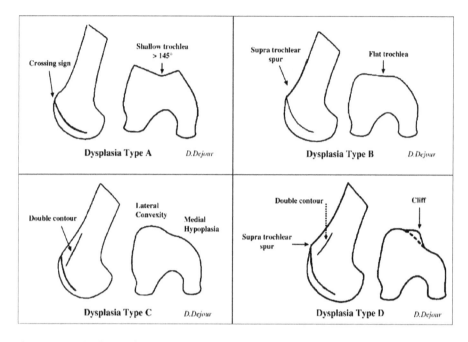

Figure 1. Dejour classification of trochlea dysplasia

2.2. Soft-tissue stabilizers

Soft-tissue structures important to the patellofemoral joint include the lateral retinaculum, the iliotibial band, and vastus lateralis muscle on the lateral side, and the medial retinaculum, medial patellofemoral ligament, and the vastus medialis oblique muscle on the medial side. Normally, these all work in concert to provide proper stability and tracking of the patellofemoral articulation. When medial stabilizers are weakened or disrupted, the typical lateral instability may occur. Tightness or excessive force by the lateral stabilizers typically does not cause actual instability, as long as the medial structures are normal, but may cause symptomatic abnormalities in patella tilt and tracking, as described below.

The lateral retinaculum tightness is commonly implicated in abnormal lateral tilt of the patella. However, it is not considered to be a major factor contributing to lateral instability of the patella. Lateral release alone in the setting of instability has been shown to result in 100% rate of recurrence [9], indicating the very limited, if any, contribution of the lateral retinaculum to development of lateral instability. Moreover, biomechanically the lateral retinaculum may even contribute up to 10% to medial stability [10], and addition of a lateral release to medial soft-tissue repairs has been shown to actually decrease the force required to dislocate the patella, compared to medial repair alone. [11]

Iliotibial band (ITB) is a continuation of tensor fascia lata, which originates on the anterior superior iliac spine, and inserts on the Gerdy's tubercle of the anterolateral proximal tibia. It exerts its effect on the patellofemoral joint via fibers attaching to the lateral retinaculum. Abnormal tightness of the ITB can result in lateral patellar maltracking with pain, and is a common finding in patellofemoral tracking abnormalities and patellofemoral pain syndrome (which is one of the most common causes of anterior knee pain). Non-operative treatment with stretching and therapeutic modalities can be quite successful in decreasing ITB tightness and alleviating symptoms.

The other dynamic stabilizer on the lateral side is the vastus lateralis muscle, which has a force vector 30-40 degrees lateral to anatomic femoral axis. Disruption of the attachment of the vastus lateralis to the patella from overly aggressive and excessively proximal lateral retinacular release can result in iatrogenic instability of the patella in the medial direction. [12]

The main dynamic stabilizer on the medial side, counteracting the pull of the vastus lateralis and the ITB, is the vastus medialis oblique (VMO) muscle, which has a 60 degree force vector to the anatomic femoral axis, and is most active at 0-30 degrees of knee flexion. In addition to its role as a dynamic stabilizer [13], the VMO also serves as a static stabilizer, and its sectioning has been shown to produce increased lateral translation of the patella. [14] After an injury to the quadriceps muscle group, the VMO is the typically the first to weaken and last to recover.

The most important of the static medial soft-tissue stabilizers is the medial patellofemoral ligament (MPFL), which provides 53-60% of the check-rein to lateral displacement of the patella at 0-30 degrees of knee flexion. [10, 15] Because of its importance for stability, MPFL's anatomy and function have been extensively studied. This ligament is located in the second layer of the medial knee - deep to the crural fascia, superficial to the knee joint capsule - in the same layer as the superficial medial collateral ligament (MCL). It is a very thin ligament, measuring 0.44mm in thickness, withan average length of 58mm, an hourglass shape, measuring approximately 13mm width at its midpoint, 17mm on the patella side, and 15mm on the femoral side. [16-18]MPFL attaches to the proximal half of the medial border of the patella and to the medial femoral condyle. Its femoral attachment is located anterior and distal to the adductor tubercle, and posterior and proximal to the medial femoral epicondyle and the origin of the MCL. [17,18]

Sectioning of the MPFL in cadaveric studies has been shown to increase lateral patella subluxation by 50% [19], and decrease the force required to translate the patella laterally by 10mm by 50%. [20] MPFL functions isometrically (meaning its length is unchanged) during early flexion, mostly between 0-30 degrees of flexion, where it is the most important static stabilizer; it becomes progressively lax after 70 degrees of flexion. Isometry of the MPFL has been found to be most sensitive to the femoral insertion. Therefore, it is crucial to locate the anatomic femoral insertion site of the MPFL during surgical repair or reconstruction of this ligament.

2.3. Lower extremity malalignment/Q-angle

In addition to abnormalities of bones and soft-tissues around the patellofemoral joint, instability of this joint can also result from abnormalities in the overall alignment of the lower extremity, especially those abnormalities that increase laterally-directed forces on the patella. Clinically, this can be measured by assessing the Q-angle.

The Q-angle is defined as the complement of the angle between the force vectors of the quadriceps and patella tendons. The Q-angle typically measures 12 degrees in males and 16 degrees in females, is highest in extension, and represents the laterally directed force acting on the patella. Malalignment that increases the Q-angle increases the laterally-directed forces and thus predisposes to patellofemoral instability. The Q-angle is increased by genu valgum, femoral anteversion, external tibial torsion, and pes planus.

To summarize contributions of various anatomic structures to patellofemoral stability, stability in extension and early flexion (up to 30 degrees) is primarily dependent on integrity and function of the medial soft-tissue stabilizers, both static (MPFL) and dynamic (VMO), while stability in greater degrees of flexion is dependent to a greater degree on bony architecture and congruity of the femoral trochlea and the patella. Factors contributing to instability include 1) inadequate bony restraints, such as patella alta and patellofemoral dysplasia; 2) inadequate medial soft-tissue restraints, such as VMO weakness or MPFL disruption/attenuation; and 3) excessive laterally-directed forces, typically resulting from lower extremity malalignment producing a high Q-angle. (Table 1)

Inadequate Bony Restraints of the Patellofemoral Joint	Femoral trochlea dysplasia (excessively shallow)
	Patella dysplasia
	Combined patellofemoral dysplasia
	Patella alta
Inadequate Medial Soft-tissue Restraints	MPFL tear or elongation
	VMO disruption
	VMO weakness
Lower extremity malalignment	Abnormally high Q-angle
	Excessive femoral anteversion
	Excessive external tibial torsion
	Genu valgum
	Proximal tibia vara
	Pes planus

Table 1. Factors Predisposing to Patellofemoral Instability

3. Clinical presentation of patellofemoral instability

The two most common types of clinical presentation of patella instability are 1) acute dislocation from an injury, and 2) recurrent instability (either dislocation or subluxation), typically occurring with minor or no injury, with a history of previous dislocation. Another common presenting complaint related to patellofemoral tracking is painful maltracking without sensation of instability, with or without history of previous dislocation.

3.1. Acute dislocation

Acute dislocation may occur from a direct or an indirect mechanism of injury. Indirect mechanism accounts for the majority of acute dislocations, and occurs most commonly with cutting, pivoting, and squatting movements with sports and other strenuous physical activities. Typically the foot is planted, the femur is rotated internally and/or the tibia is rotated externally, and there is a valgus force at the knee joint; in this position, sudden contraction of the quadriceps produces a strong laterally directed force vector, resulting in dislocation of the patella. Dislocation from a direct injury mechanism, which is much less common, occurs when the patella is struck with a laterally directed blow.

Most cases of acute patella dislocation reduce spontaneously as the knee is brought into extension, and therefore evaluation in the emergency room or doctor's office may not readily provide the diagnosis. Patient may report feeling or hearing a "pop" or a "snap" and seeing/feeling their kneecap "move out of place", followed by spontaneous reduction with a "clunk" as the knee is extended. On presentation typical complaints are those of pain, swelling, limited motion, and difficulty bearing weight. Occasionally the reduction is not spontaneous and requires reduction in the emergency room (by gently extending the knee and manipulating the patella back into the trochlear groove).

Physical examination after acute dislocation may be significantly limited by guarding due to pain and hemarthrosis (bleeding) in the knee. If this is the case, arthrocentesis should be considered, with aspiration of the hemarthrosis and injection of a short-acting local anesthetic. This allows for a more accurate examination of the knee, as well as quicker restoration of knee motion and strength.

Examination should focus on ruling out fractures, injuries to major ligamentous stabilizers of the knee joint, and finally assessing patellar stability. Combination of hemarthrosis and a sports-related mechanism of injury may initially suggest a diagnosis of ananterior cruciate ligament (ACL) tear, and careful examination of anterior, posterior, varus, valgus, and rotational stability of the knee should be performed.

Patients may exhibit medial knee tenderness and ecchymosis (bruising) at the femoral origin of the MPFL, near the medial epicondyle and adductor tubercle, and injury to the MCL (which also originates in this area) should be ruled out. There is often tenderness over the medial facet and lateral femoral condyle. Less commonly there is a palpable soft-tissue defect adjacent to the medial facet, especially if there is a complete tear at the VMO insertion. Range of motion of the knee is usually very limited due to pain and apprehension; crepitus during motion (in a knee without preexisting arthritis) is concerning for osteochondral fracture and presence of intraarticular fragments. Examination of patellar medial-lateral translation with the knee extended and at 30 degrees of flexion should be attempted, but may not be possible due to patient guarding. Apprehension with attempted lateral translation at 30 degrees of knee flexion is suggestive of patella instability and is known as the "patella apprehension" test.

3.2. Recurrent instability

Patients with this problem sometimes report a clear history of recurrent dislocations or subluxations, but in other cases the presentation is more vague, and may include such complaints as sensation of the whole knee giving out, weakness of the knee, anterior and anterolateral pain, difficulty navigating stairs, and inability to participate in sports. A thorough history and careful physical examination are essential to arrive at the correct diagnosis. Important history points include previous injuries and dislocations, provoking activities and positions of the knee, family history of instability or laxity of other joints, and childhood problems of the lower extremity (including those of the hip and foot).

Physical examination must include evaluation of lower extremity alignment, including measurement of the Q-angle, as well as a comparison to the contralateral knee. The Q-angle is typically measured in a supine position, and is formed by the intersection of a line drawn from the ASIS (anterior superior iliac spine) to the patella and from the patella to the tibial tubercle.

Examination of patients with patella instability should also assess genu varum ("bowlegs") or genu valgum ("knock-knees"), external tibial torsion, femoral anteversion (best assessed by abnormally increased femoral internal rotation with the patient prone), pes planus ("flat feet"), and generalized ligamentous laxity. Strength of the quadriceps, hip flexors, abductors, and rotators must be assessed, as weakness in these muscle groups can contribute to patellofemoral maltracking and instability.

The patella itself can be evaluated for resting position, tilt, passive translation, apprehension, and dynamic tracking. In extension and 30 degrees of knee flexion the patella position should be central within the trochlear groove, and while it may rest laterally tilted, the examiner should be able to "lift it off" the lateral trochlea and bring it to at least a horizontal position. Inability to do this suggests excessive tightness of the lateral retinaculum. With the knee in flexion, the normal position of the patella should be pointing directly forward; a "grosshopper eyes" appearance may be noted in patients with recurrent instability or lateral maltracking, with both patellae pointing superiorly and laterally.

Passive lateral translation of the patella is measured with the knee flexed to 30 degrees and the quadriceps muscles relaxed, and must be compared to the contralateral side. Passive lateral translation should be no more than one half the patellar width, without sensation of apprehension or pain. Pain and/or crepitus with patellar compression into the groove ("patella grind") may indicate arthritis or osteochondral injury. Finally, patellofemoral tracking during active knee range of motion should be central. Abnormal tracking is classically manifested by a positive "J-sign", which is a sudden lateral movement of the patella as it exists the femoral trochlea during terminal extension.

4. Radiographic imaging of patellofemoral instability

Radiographic imaging is essential for proper evaluation of a patient suspected of having patellofemoral instability. The imaging modalities most commonly used for this condition include plain radiographs, magnetic resonance imaging (MRI), and ultrasound (US). The computed tomography (CT) scan is used less commonly. Initial evaluation should always begin with plain radiographs, while more advanced imaging is ordered as necessary, based on clinical examination and plain radiographic findings.

The plain radiographic evaluation should include a minimum of three views – anterior-posterior (AP), lateral, and axial, or "sunrise", views. The AP view allows assessment of coronal plan malalignment, such as genu varum or valgum, as well as presence of any tibiofemoral arthritis. The lateral view is used to assess patella alta or baja.Several signs of trochlear dysplasia can also be appreciated on the lateral view, including the crossing sign, supratrochlear spur, and the double contour. [8](Figure 2)

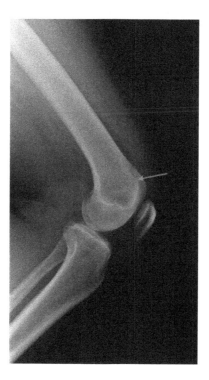

Figure 2. "Crossing sign" on a preoperative lateral radiograph in a 35 year old female with recurrent instability, significant malalignment and trochlea dysplasia. This sign represents abnormally elevated floor of the trochlear groove rising above the top of the wall of one of the femoral condyles (arrow).

The two most commonly used techniques for axial, or "sunrise", radiographs of the knee, are Merchant's and Laurin views. These views, especially in comparison to the contralateral knee (ideally on the same cassette) are invaluable in detecting such abnormalities as lateral patellar tilt, patellar subluxation, dysplasia, patellofemoral arthritis, vertical fractures of the patella (including avulsion fractures), and osteochondral fragments. A number of angles and indices measured on the axial views have been described to objectively characterize patellofemoral dysplasia, subluxation and tilt. The sulcus angle (normally 138 +/- 6 degrees) for example, as measured on the Merchant view, identifies trochlear dysplasia when it is greater than145 degrees, and has been noted to beabnormal in significant number of patients with patella instability. [21](Figure 3)

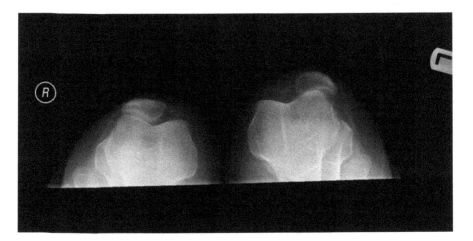

Figure 3. Example of a shallow trochlea, with a sulcus angle measuring 148 degrees, and lateral patella subluxation, in the same patient from Figure 2, on a preoperative Merchant's view

The more advanced imaging modalities used in evaluation of patellofemoral instability include ultrasound, CT, and MRI. Ultrasound was recently shown in one study to have a 90% accuracy and predictive value in identifying the location and severity of injury to the MPFL. [22]MRI also has high sensitivity and accuracy in detecting MPFL injuries [23], and additionally is very useful for indentifying articular cartilage damage and osteochondral fragments, over 40% of which may be missed on plain radiographs. [24,25]A relatively high number of associated injuries have been found on MR imaging of knees after patella dislocation, including as many as 21% with meniscal tears, 19% with MCL injury, 7% with patella fractures, 13% with loose bodies, and 49% with osteochondral injury. [25] Finally, in cases where the history, physical examination and plain radiographs are inconclusive, MRI can help arrive at the diagnosis of a recent acute patella dislocation by demonstrating a classic bone bruising pattern on the medial patella facet and the lateral femoral condyle.(Figure 4)

The most common location of MPFL injury from a patella dislocation has been debated. What is known for certain is that this ligament can tear anywhere along its course, including femoral avulsions, patella avulsions, and midsubstance ruptures. Moreover, a not insignificant number of patients may have combined injuries, and some studies suggest that these may be more common in children compared to adults. [25, 26]

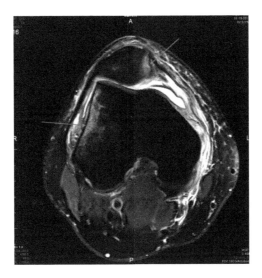

Figure 4. Classic bone bruise pattern of the lateral femoral condyle and medial patella facet after an acute first-time patella dislocation; other than a partial tear of the MPFL no other abnormalities were noted in this 45 year old male.

CT imaging during work-up of patellofemoral instability is most useful for assessing bony anatomy(dysplasia and incongruence) and malalignment. CT imaging is probably most useful in assessing the tibial tubercle to trochlear groove distance (TT-TG distance), which measures the lateral offset of the tibial tubercle from the deepest point of the trochlear groove, and is considered to be the true measure of the Q-angle. The normal TT-TG distance is a range of 7-17mm (average 13mm), whereas values of greater than 20mm have been found to be predictive of patellofemoral instability [27], and should prompt consideration of a distal (tibial tubercle) realignment procedure when surgical treatment is contemplated (discussed below).

In summary, radiographic imaging of patellofemoral instability should always begin with a series of plain radiographs, including an AP, lateral, and sunrise views. Acute dislocations should receive additional imaging with a MRI, to assess injury to the MPFL, and evaluate for intraarticular fragments and other associated injuries. An ultrasound can also be used to evaluate the MPFL, but is less helpful in assessing articular cartilage injuries. Finally, a CT scan is most commonly used for pre-operative assessment of trochlear dysplasia, tibial tubercle offset, and localization of bony fragments.

5. Non-operative treatment of patellofemoral instability

While it is reasonable to attempt non-operative treatment for most first-time acute patella dislocations, it is important to remember that "non-operative treatment" does not mean "no treatment". Initial management should be aimed at controlling pain and swelling, and protecting the knee from further injury.

There is no consensus on the type and duration of immobilization after an acute episode of patellar dislocation. Treatment protocols reported in the literature range from immediate range of motion and weightbearing to brace or cast immobilization in full extension for 6 weeks. Studies have shown that more rigid methods of knee immobilization (i.e. with a cast), result in lower risk of recurrent dislocations, but higher risk of knee stiffness. [28]

The authors' treatment protocol for acute first-time dislocation includes immobilization with a knee brace locked in extension for a minimum of 2 weeks, with weight-bearing allowed in the brace. Younger patients (who tend to be at a higher risk of recurrent dislocation) may be immobilized for a longer period of time, up to 4 weeks for documented complete tears of the MPFL.

Once the acute inflammation has subsided, physical therapy is helpful to reduce swelling, improve range of motion and muscle strength, stabilize patellofemoral tracking, regain proprioception of the knee, and normalize the gait pattern. Physical therapists often prefer to do patella taping during rehabilitation, as it has been shown in some studies to increase quadriceps muscle torque, control patellar motion, and activate VMO earlier than VL during stairs ascent/descent. [29,30] With regard to strengthening exercises, studies have shown that closed-chain exercises may be more efficacious in strengthening the vastus medialis,compared to open-chain exercises.[31,32]

Pre-requisites for allowing return to sportsinclude complete resolution of pain and swelling, no sensation of instability, full range of motion of the knee, and return of at least 80% of quadriceps muscle strength. This may be expected by approximately 3 months from initial injury. A patellar-stabilizing low-profile brace may be worn for athletic activities, although no studies have demonstrated efficacy of bracing in preventing recurrence of instability. [33]

6. Natural history of patellofemoral instability

Studies looking at the natural history of a first-time patella dislocation suggest an overall rate of recurrence of 15-44%, while persistence of instability after one episode of recurrence can be as high as 65%. [28,34,35]There is 7 times higher odds of recurrent instability in patients with a previous history of dislocation, compared to first-time dislocators, with the risk being higher for both knees. [2] The initial injury from a first time dislocation compromises the integrity of the MPFL. A torn or stretched out MPFL decreases the energy required to dislocate the patella laterally, and may predispose to recurrent instability even with less strenuous activities. Recurrent dislocations may produce further injury to the articular cartilage, ligaments and retinaculum, with irreversible articular cartilage damage being especially of concern, particularly in the young patients.(Figure 5)

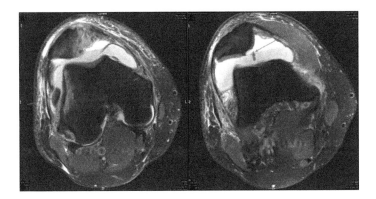

Figure 5. Axial MRI images of the same patient in Figure 4 after a 2nd dislocation, this time producing multiple osteochondral fragments with significant injury to both the patella and femoral articular surfaces

Even in the absence of recurrent instability, the natural history of a first-time patella dislocation may include other problems, such as persistent pain, mechanical symptoms, and knee-related dysfunction with inability to return to pre-injury functional status. Unsatisfactory results of non-surgically treated patella dislocators were as high at 63% and 75% in some studies. [28,35] Over half the patients with a first-time patella dislocation reported, at 6 months after the injury, being significantly limited in their ability to engage in strenuous physical activity, and unable to return to sports. [1]

Despite the relatively unsatisfactory outcomes of non-operative treatment for patellofemoral instability, the natural history of a first-time dislocation has not been significantly improved by an acute medial repair. A number of prospective trials (level 1 and 2) comparing medial repair versus non-operative treatment for first time dislocation showed no difference in recurrent instability or functional outcome scores. [36-40] Therefore, non-operative treatment is typically recommended after the initial episode of instability, with indications for acute surgery including presence of osteochondral fragments or persistent static patella subluxation. [24]

7. Surgical treatment of patellofemoral instability

The surgical procedures for patella instability can be divided into the general categories of proximal and distal realignment. (Table 2) Proximal realignment most commonly is done to the soft-tissue stabilizers, and includes procedures such as VMO advancement, medial retinaculum and MPFL imbrication, MPFL repair, and MPFL reconstruction. Distal realignment is typically done by changing the position of the tibial tubercle via one of several osteotomies (Elmslie-Trillat, Fulkerson AMZ, and Hughston). Patellofemoral instability which results from severe dysplasia of the femoral trochlea can also be treated with reshaping of the trochlea (trochleaplasty). The surgical procedures and their outcomes are discussed below.

	Proximal Realignment	Distal Realignment
Soft-tissue procedures	Medial retinaculum and MPFL imbrication	Procedures mostly of historic significance
	MPFL repair	–Rough-Goldthwait (lateral slip of patella
	MPFL reconstruction	tendon transferred medially)
	VMO advancement	–Galleazzi (semitendinosis tendon transferred
		to the patella)
Bony procedures	Femoral trochleaplasty	Tibial tubercle osteotomy/transfer
		–Hughston (for patella alta)
		–Elmslie-Trillat (for instability)
		–Fulkerson/AMZ (for instability and arthritis)

Table 2. Surgical Options for Treatment of Patellofemoral Instability

7.1. Lateral retinacular release

As previously mentioned, lateral retinacular is the one procedure that has definitively been shown to be ineffective as a stand-alone surgical option for treatment of patella instability. [33] Studies have demonstrated a very high instability recurrence rate (up to 100% in one study) and poor results in terms of patient satisfaction when lateral release was used as the main surgical treatment for patella instability. [9,41,42] Even as an add-on procedure to medial repair or reconstruction, the utility of the lateral release has been questioned [11], and therefore this procedure should be reserved for patients with significant static lateral tilt of the patella, lateral patellofemoral compression and pain. Lateral retinacular release can be performed with an arthroscopic or an open approach, and involves dividing the lateral retinacular layer from the level of the patella tendon up to the insertion of the vastus lateralis. Care must be taken to protect the lateral geniculate artery while performing the proximal portion of the release.

7.2. MPFL repair

Most proximal soft-tissue realignment procedures focus on restoring the integrity of the MPFL, as injury to this ligament is considered the "essential lesion" of patella instability. With its important to patellofemoral stability well demonstrated in multiple biomechanical studies, some argue that full dislocation is impossible without significant MPFL injury. [43] Clinical reports support this notion, showing a ruptured MPFL in as many as 90% of acute dislocations [44], and either rupture or attenuated MPFL in almost 100% of cases of recurrent instability. [45] After an acute injury the MPFL either fails to heal or heals in a non-anatomic position, losing its isometry and ability to work properly as a medial stabilizer. Restoration of MPFL integrity, including its anatomic insertion sites, has been shown to restore patellofemoral tracking to normal [15,19,46], and is an important component of any surgical plan for patella stabilization. Options for restoring MPFL integrity include imbrication/tightening of the elongated ligament, repair of the ligament, or reconstruction of the ligament.

Ideal situation for an MPFL repair is an acute injury with avulsion from the patella or femoral insertion site, in a patient without significant predisposing factors such as dysplasia or malalignment. Femoral avulsions may be especially important injuries to consider for acute repair study, since at least one study demonstrated much higher rate of recurrent instability in first-time dislocators with MPFL avulsion from the femur. [47] MFPL avulsions from the insertion sites can be repaired through bone tunnels or with suture anchors, and mid-substance ruptures can be repaired with a strong non-absorbable braided suture. The repair is typically performed open, but arthroscopic techniques for repairing avulsion from the patella have also been described. [48,49]

Imbrication of the medial stabilizing structures is sometimes used for cases of mild recurrent instability (subluxation, rather than frank dislocation), and an intact but elongated MPFL. It is a "non-anatomic" procedure, which cannot address problems at the insertion sites of the ligament. With inability to precisely quantify how much of the ligament and retinaculum should be imbricated, this procedure may either fail to restore appropriate tension to the MPFL and result in recurrent instability, or over-tension the medial stabilizers and result in excessive compressive forces of the medial side of the patellofemoral joint. [50] Medial imbrication can be done arthroscopically or open,[51-53]and is similar in its technique and goals to capsular plication in the shoulder.

Outcomes ofmedial repair and imbrication procedures have shown promise in some studies[49,51,54-59], including one prospective study that demonstrated a higher rate of return to pre-injury activity level after arthroscopic repair, when compared to non-operative treatment. [40] However, randomized controlled trials have not shown any significant benefit of surgical repaircompared to non-operative treatment for first-time dislocators, with similar rates of recurrent instability and similar functional outcomes scores. [36-39]

A 2007 systematic review of 70 level I-IV trials evaluating medial repair and non-operative treatment for first-time patella dislocators concluded that initial management of these injuries should be non-operative except in select cases, including: 1) presence of intraarticular osteochondral fragments (Figure 6); 2) what the authors describe as "significant disruption of medial patellar stabilizers"; 3) lateral subluxation of the patella on the injured side, when compared to otherwise normal contralateral alignment (Figure 7); 4) persistent symptoms despite non-operative treatment; and 5) recurrent instability event.[24] With regard to recurrent instability, MPFL repair has been shown to have a relatively high rate of failure (26-46%) [60,61], and is not recommended as a stand-alone procedure.

7.3. MPFL reconstruction

Given the relative failure of medial repair to decrease the risk of recurrent instability and improve functional outcomes, much attention over the past two decades has been directed to MPFL reconstruction. Historically, non-anatomic procedures (such as Roux-Goldthwait and Galleazzi transfers),were used to re-create the medial stabilizers, but in the long-term these procedures has shown relative high rates of recurrent instability (22%), osteoarthritis (78%), and patient dissatisfaction (54%). [62] Unlike these and other medial soft-tissue stabilization procedures, the recently popularized techniques of MPFL reconstruction have shown excellent outcomes in terms of recurrent instability and function, [63] as well as relatively low risk of development and progression of arthritis. [64]

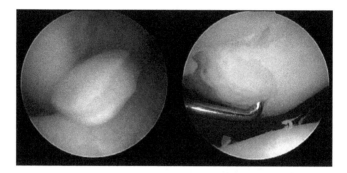

Figure 6. Arthroscopic picture of a large osteochondral fragment after a previous patella dislocation, and a donor site on the medial patellar facet from which it likely originated (overgrown with fibrocartilage)

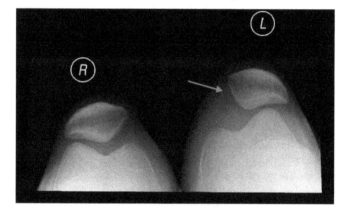

Figure 7. Axial radiograph showing static subluxation of the left patella in a 16 year old boy after an acute first-time dislocation. Note the small bony fleck adjacent to the medial patella facet, representing patellar avulsion of the MPFL.

The first report of anatomic MPFL reconstruction was described by Ellera Gomes in 1992 [65], and since then many variations on the procedure have been described. Variations in surgical techniques include different choices of surgical approach, graft material, and fixation method. Furthermore, there are options of associated procedures to be performed along with the MFPL reconstruction, such as the lateral retinacular release, VMO advancement, and tibial tubercle transfer. To the authors' knowledge, there have not been any comparative studies showing advantage of one technique or approach over the other.

The typical grafts used for MPFL reconstruction (most commonly the semitendinosus tendon) have biomechanical properties significantly superior to those of the native MPFL, with higher strength, stiffness, and load to failure. [17,66] The advantage of these superior biomechanical characteristics is the ability of the graft to withstand greater loads in cases of dysplasia and malalignment. Conversely, overtightening or malpositioning the graft can lead to maltracking and excessive medial compressive forces.

Multiple studies of MPFL reconstruction for acute and recurrent patella instability have shown excellent results, with low rates of recurrent instability, low complications rates, and good improvement in subjectively and objectively reported outcomes. [63,65,67-73] However, no consensus has been achieved with regard to the surgical approach, choice of graft, graft positioning, and fixation methods. [63,72] With this in mind, several important points of the surgical technique of MPFL reconstruction, with the relevant pearls and pitfalls, deserve mention.

7.4. MPFL reconstruction: Technical pearls and technical errors

A single or a double incision technique may be used, and the goal of both approaches should be to comfortably and safely access the femoral and patella insertion sites of the MPFL; visualization of the mid-substance of the ligament is less important. However, the layer where MPFL normally runs (2nd layer of the medial knee – same layer that contacts the superficial MCL and VMO aponeurosis) must be identified, so that the graft can be properly placed into this layer, and remain extraarticular.

Next, patella and femoral insertion sites of the MPFL are located and prepared for graft implantation. While patellar insertion site of the MPFL can be approximated to the proximal half of the medial facet, the femoral attachment site needs to be located more precisely, as isometry and function of this ligament are especially sensitive to its femoral insertion. Locating the femoral insertion site may be difficult with direct visualization, especially through a small incision, and intraoperative radiographic imaging (fluoroscopy) is typically used to localize this site via previously described landmarks. [74] Once both patella and femoral sites are indentified and prepared, the graft is secured to one of the sites (surgeon's choice), brought through the 2nd layer of the knee to the other site, tensioned, and secured. Multiple techniques for graft fixation on both the patella and femoral sides exist, including suture anchors, bone tunnels, interference screws, knotless anchors, and suspensory buttons. While no single technique has been shown to be superior to others in clinical studies, suture anchor fixation of the graft to the surface of the bone has been shown to be weaker than fixation of the graft within a tunnel. [43]

Technical errors of MPFL reconstruction typically result from improper graft position and/or graft tension. Recurrent instability can occur when the tension on the reconstructed ligament is inadequate. In biomechanical studies properly tensioned grafts have been shown to restore stability and normal tracking of the patellofemoral articulation without excessive contact pressures, while overtensioned grafts restricted motion and resulted in increased medial patellofemoral pressures. [75] Malpositioning the graft and making it too short may as much as double the graft tension in flexion [76], which is likely to lead to eventual development of patellofemoral arthrosis.

The authors' preferred technique for MPFL reconstruction is with a double-incision approach, using a semitendinosis autograft or allograft (based on patient preference). The medial facet of the patella is exposed first and burred down to bleeding bone, to encourage healing. Two tunnels are created in the medial facet by reaming over guidewires (Figure 8A), the position of which can be checked with fluoroscopy (Figure 8B). The graft is loaded onto an adjustable suspensory fixation device and its free ends aresecured into the patellar tunnels with interference screws. (Figure 8C) The femoral insertion site is identified with fluoroscopy using a radiographic template (Figure 8D) and a guidewire is drilled into this area, exiting on the lateral side of the knee. Once this guidewire is in place, a suture is passed from the patellar insertion to the femoral guidewire, and the knee is then taken through the range of motion to assess isometry of the suture at the early angles of flexion, which predicts the isometry of the reconstructed ligament. A femoral tunnel is then reamed to but not through the lateral cortex (Figure 8E). The graft is now brought through the appropriate layer to the entrance of the femoral tunnel (Figure 8F); the button of the suspensory deviceis passed through the tunnel and flipped on the lateral femoral cortex, and the graft is then drawn into the tunnel (Figure 8G and 8H). The graft tension is then adjusted, and once appropriate tension is obtained, interference screw is used to back-up graft fixation at the medial aperture of the femoral tunnel. Additional procedures are performed as necessary.

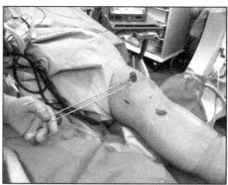

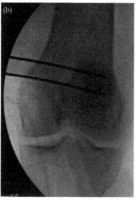

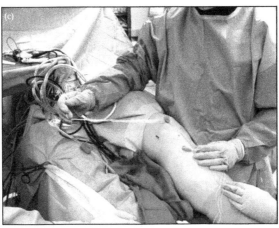

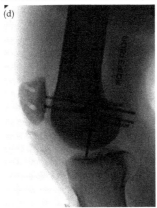

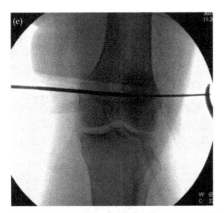

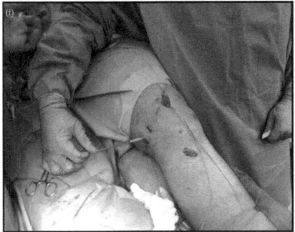

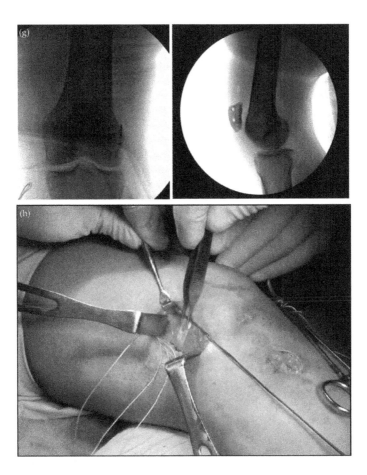

Figure 8. MPFL reconstruction with a double incision technique, using semitendinosus autograft, interference screws/ knotless anchors on the patella side, and interference screw + cortical suspensory button-loop device on the femoral side. a) guidewires drilled into the medial facet of the patella; note the incision for semitendinosus harvest; b) position of the guidewires confirmed radiographically; c) semitendinosus graft secured to the patella; d) intraoperative lateral image showing a radiographic template overlying the distal femur, allowing placement of the guidewire in the appropriate position for a femoral tunnel; e) femoral tunnel is reamed under fluoroscopic visualization; f) graft is passed to the femoral tunnel; g) intraoperative radiographs (AP and lateral) of the final reconstruction, demonstrating patella tunnels and the suspensory button-loop fixation device on the lateral femoral cortex; h) intraoperative photograph of the final reconstruction (different case – single incision technique, with gracilis autograft)

7.5. Distal realignment – Tibial tubercle osteotomies

A number of osteotomies and transfers of the tibial tubercle have been described, aiming to realign, offload or do both to the patellofemoral joint. These can address such problems as patella alta and excessively high Q-angle.

Hughston osteotomy transfers the tibial tubercle distally and medially. It improves the TT-TG distance and also inferiorizes the position of the patella, and is a useful surgical procedure for severe patella alta. However, there is a risk with this procedure of globally increased patellofemoral contact pressure.

In the absence of patella alta, the two osteotomies most commonly for patellofemoral instability are the Elmslie-Trillat osteotomy, otherwise known as Tibial Tubercle Medialization (TTM), and the Fulkerson osteotomy, otherwise known as tibial tubercle anteromedialization (AMZ). Elmslie Trillat is a single-plane osteotomy that translates the tibia tubercle straight medially, and has demonstrated relatively low rates of recurrent instability, good functional outcomes and return to activities, although patient satisfaction decreases over time. [77-79] The AMZ is an oblique-plane osteotomy, translating the tubercle anteriorly and medially, (Figure 9) allowing both improvement of the TT-TG distance and offloading of the lateral and distal patella facet and the lateral femoral trochlea, and is commonly used both for patellofemoral instability and lateral patellofemoral arthrosis. It does, however, increase the load on the medial trochlea and patella, and is contraindicated when there is preexisting arthritis in these areas. A number of studies evaluating outcomes of the AMZ have shown 74-95% good or excellent results, with better outcomes in males, patients with intact patellar cartilage, and in cases when osteotomy was done for instability (and not for painful maltracking/arthritis). [80-82]

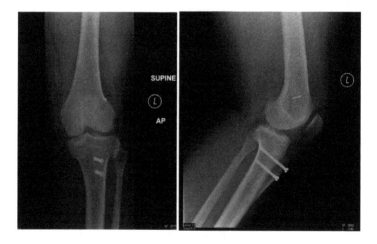

Figure 9. Postoperative radiographs after AMZ procedure (combined with MPFL reconstruction), in the same patient as in Figures 2 and 3 (AP and Lateral views).

7.6. Proximal Bony Realignment - Trochleaplasty

Femoral trochleaplasty is a relatively new procedure which seeks to address severe femoral trochlea dysplasia, such as with "dome-shaped" trochlea. The surgical technique involves removing a sulcus of cancellous bone from under the trochlear groove, and then impacting the cortical shell into this space. The procedure has been shown to improve stability of the patellofemoral joint, but does not prevent development of subsequent patellofemoral arthritis. [83]

7.7. Algorithm for Selecting Appropriate Treatment for a Patient with Patellofemoral Instability (Table 3)

Initial management of a first-time dislocator should include immobilization of the knee in extension and appropriate imaging, including plain radiographs (bilateral patellofemoral views for comparison) and an MRI. Patients without osteochondral injury, static subluxation, or predisposing factors can typically be treated nonoperatively, with a period of immobilization (2-4 weeks), followed by therapy to restore motion, strength, stability and proprioception. Consideration may be given to acute MPFL repair in cases of severe injury to the ligament, especially avulsions from bone. The authors prefer to perform such a repair with two suture anchors.

Patients with significant osteochondral injury typically require arthroscopic or open procedure to remove or repair the fragment, and consideration should be given to addressing the MPFL injury at the same time, with repair or reconstruction. Patients with significant predisposing factors such as dysplasia or malalignment are at particularly high risk for recurrent dislocation with non-operative treatment, and should be considered for MFPL reconstruction, even after a first-time dislocation. The goal of this seemingly aggressive approach is to prevent recurrent instability that may result in additional osteochondral injury, and thus predispose to patellofemoral arthrosis.

Recurrent dislocators who wish to remain active and athletic, as well as patients who experience instability with daily activities, typically require MPFL reconstruction, although arthroscopic or open plication of the MPFL and medial retinaculum can be done for patients with mild instability (subluxation, rather than dislocation) and no significant dysplasia or malalignment. In patients with recurrent instability and lower extremity malalignment consideration should be given to tibial tubercle transfer. Selection of appropriate osteotomy is as follows: Hughston osteotomy (distal and medial) for patella alta, Elmslie-Trillat (medial) for recurrent instability with increased TT-TG distance but normal patellar height, and Fulkerson/AMZ (anterior and medial) for recurrent instability and lateral patellofemoral arthrosis or compression. Patients with severe trochlear dysplasia, such as a "dome-shaped trochlea" should be considered for trochleaplasty.

8. Post-operative rehabilitation after patellofemoral stabilization

Immediate postoperative care is focused on multimodal pain management program, swelling control, and protecting the repair, reconstruction or osteotomy.Physical therapy protocols vary depending on the degree of preoperative instability, the type of surgery performed (bony versus soft-tissue, repair versus reconstruction, etc.), and patient-specific factors.

Presenting event	Associated factors	Recommended treatment
First-time dislocation	No dysplasia No malalignment No intraarticular fragments No static subluxation of the patella	Non-operative (initial immobilization, followed by rehabilitation therapy)
First-time dislocation	Intraaticular fragments	Arthroscopy or open procedure for fragment removal or repair
First-time dislocation	MPFL avulsion from bone (femur or patella) AND static subluxation of the patella (compared to contralateral side)	Acute MPFL repair (with suture anchors)
First-time dislocation	Patellofemoral dysplasia and/or malalignment	MFPL reconstruction +/- tibial tubercle osteotomy (TTO)
Recurrent dislocation	No significant dysplasia or malalignment	MPFL reconstruction
Recurrent dislocation	Significant malalignment (high Q-angle, TT-TG distance > 20mm)	MPFL reconstruction with TTO
Recurrent dislocation	Severe trochlear dysplasia	MPFL reconstruction with trochleaplasty
Recurrent subluxation	No dysplasia or malalignment, intact MPFL	Consider arthroscopic or open imbrication of the MFPL and medial retinaculum

Table 3. Algorithm for selecting appropriate treatment for a patient with patella instability

For soft-tissue procedures, the knee is initially immobilized in extension, and weight-bearing with the brace locked in extension is typically allowed. The brace is continued for 6-8 weeks or until quadriceps control is regained. Typically, after MPFL reconstruction, especially with secure graft fixation in bone tunnels, limited passive range of motion of the knee can be initiated immediately after surgery. In cases of MPFL avulsion repairs with suture anchors the authors prefer to immobilize the knee for 3-4 weeks prior to initiating any range of motion, to allow some healing of the repair.

The majority of bony procedures performed for patellofemoral instability are tibial tubercle osteotomies, and the goal of early rehabilitation after this type of surgery is to prevent excessive traction on the patella tendon. Therefore, an extension brace is worn, weight-bearing is typically protected for 4-6 weeks, while passive range of motion may be allowed to a limited degree, as long as fixation of the osteotomy is secure. Active knee extension is typically restricted for at least 6 weeks, or until the osteotomy is healed.

The postoperative physical therapy protocol after patellofemoral stabilization is typically divided into 3 phases. (Table 4) Phase I (0-6 weeks) focuses on controlling the inflammatory process, protecting the bony or soft tissue fixation, and regaining quadriceps and VMO control, typically with isometric strengthening. Phase II (6-12 weeks) involves exercises to regain full range of motion, patella mobilization and continued VMO strengthening to stabilize patellar tracking, and return to a normal gait pattern. Phase III (after 12 weeks) progresses with strengthening and endurance exercises to regain full quadriceps strength and proprioception. Return to sporting activity is allowed only when the patient has no pain, no sensation of instability, regains full range of motion, andhas normal or near normal quadriceps strength. For tibial tubercle transfers healing of the osteotomy on radiographs should be confirmed prior to allowing sports participation. Return to full athletic activity typically takes 4-6 months after surgery.

Phase I (0-6 weeks)	Decrease inflammation
	Protect surgical fixation
	Regain quadriceps/VMO control (isometric strengthening)
Phase II (6-12 weeks)	Regain full range of motion
	Mobilize the patella
	Continue quadriceps/VMO strengthening
	Normalize gait
Phase III (>12 weeks)	Achieve full strength
	Build up endurance
	Regain proprioception
Phase IV - Return to sports	No pain
	No sensation of instability
	Full range of motion
	Normal or near normal quadriceps strength
	Radiographic healing of osteotomy (if done)

Table 4. Postoperative Rehabilitation Protocol After Patellofemoral Stabilization Surgery

9. Conclusion

Patellofemoral instability typically affects the young and athletic patient population. Initial trial of non-operative treatment is warranted for patients after a first-time dislocation, and without intraarticular osteochondral fragments, severe injury to the medial stabilizers, significant malalignment or patellofemoral dysplasia. When surgical treatment is contemplated, the focus should be on restoring integrity of the MFPL and optimizing the alignment of the lower extremity and specifically of the patellofemoral articulation. MPFL reconstruction has produced the best results in patients with mild or no dysplasia and malalignment, while tibial tubercle osteotomies are indicated in patients with abnormally high Q-angle and increased TT-TG distance.

The natural history of acute patellofemoral instability is that of a relatively high rate of recurrence as well as long-term functional limitations and inability to return to baseline level of activity, and thus surgery often plays a role in management of these patients. Prospective randomized trials comparing different surgical techniques are needed to determine which treatment options provide optimal restoration of function, minimize recurrence, and decrease the risk of arthritic degeneration.

Author details

Alexander Golant*, Tony Quach and Jeffrey Rosen

*Address all correspondence to: alg9067@nyp.org

New York Hospital Queens, Flushing, NY and Weill Medical College of Cornell University, New York, USA

References

[1] Atkin DM, Fithian DC, Marangi KS, Stone ML, Dobson BE, Mendelsohn C.Character-istics of patients with primary acute lateral patellar dislocation and their recovery within the first 6 months of injury. Am J Sports Med. 2000;28(4):472-9.

[2] Fithian DC, Paxton EW, Stone ML, Silva P, Davis DK, Elias DA, White LM. Epidemi-ology and natural history of acute patellar dislocation. Am J Sports Med. 2004;32(5): 1114-21.

[3] Sillanpää P, Mattila VM, Iivonen T, Visuri T, Pihlajamäki H. Incidence and risk fac-tors of acute traumatic primary patellar dislocation. Med Sci Sports Exerc.2008;40(4): 606-11.

[4] Schindler OS, Scott WN. Basic kinematics and biomechanics of the patello-femoral joint. Part 1: The native patella. Acta Orthop Belg. 2011;77(4):421-31.

[5] Sutton FS Jr, Thompson CH, Lipke J, Kettelkamp DB. The effect of patellectomy on knee function. J Bone Joint Surg Am. 1976;58(4):537-40.

[6] Insall J, Goldberg V, Salvati E. Recurrent dislocation and the high-ridingpatella. Clin Orthop Relat Res. 1972;88:67-9.

[7] Kannus PA. Long patellar tendon: radiographic sign of patellofemoral painsyn-drome--a prospective study. Radiology. 1992;185(3):859-63

[8] Dejour H, Walch G, Neyret P, Adeleine P. [Dysplasia of the femoral trochlea]. [Arti-cle in French] Rev Chir Orthop Reparatrice Appar Mot. 1990;76(1):45-54.

[9] Kolowich PA, Paulos LE, Rosenberg TD, Farnsworth S. Lateral release of thepatella: indications and contraindications. Am J Sports Med. 1990;18(4):359-65

[10] Desio SM, Burks RT, Bachus KN. Soft tissue restraints to lateral patellartranslation in the human knee. Am J Sports Med. 1998;26(1):59-65.

[11] Bedi H, Marzo J. The biomechanics of medial patellofemoral ligament repairfollowed by lateral retinacular release. Am J Sports Med. 2010;38(7):1462-7.

[12] Pagenstert G, Wolf N, Bachmann M, Gravius S, Barg A, Hintermann B, Wirtz DC, Valderrabano V, Leumann AG. Open lateral patellar retinacular lengthening versus open retinacular release in lateral patellar hypercompression syndrome: a prospective double-blinded comparative study on complications and outcome. Arthroscopy. 2012;28(6):788-97.

[13] Sakai N, Luo ZP, Rand JA, An KN. The influence of weakness in the vastusmedialis oblique muscle on the patellofemoral joint: an in vitro biomechanicalstudy. Clin Biomech (Bristol, Avon). 2000;15(5):335-9.

[14] Goh JC, Lee PY, Bose K. A cadaver study of the function of the oblique part ofvastus medialis. J Bone Joint Surg Br. 1995;77(2):225-31.

[15] Conlan T, Garth WP Jr, Lemons JE. Evaluation of the medial soft-tissuerestraints of the extensor mechanism of the knee. J Bone Joint Surg Am. 1993;75(5):682-93

[16] Nomura E, Inoue M, Osada N. Anatomical analysis of the medial patellofemoralligament of the knee, especially the femoral attachment. Knee Surg SportsTraumatol Arthrosc. 2005;13(7):510-5.

[17] Amis AA, Firer P, Mountney J, Senavongse W, Thomas NP. Anatomy andbiomechanics of the medial patellofemoral ligament. Knee. 2003;10(3):215-20.

[18] LaPrade RF, Engebretsen AH, Ly TV, Johansen S, Wentorf FA, Engebretsen L.The anatomy of the medial part of the knee.J Bone Joint Surg Am. 2007;89(9):2000-10.

[19] Hautamaa PV, Fithian DC, Kaufman KR, Daniel DM, Pohlmeyer AM. Medial softtissue restraints in lateral patellar instability and repair. Clin Orthop Relat Res. 1998; (349):174-82.

[20] Senavongse W, Amis AA. The effects of articular, retinacular, or musculardeficiencies on patellofemoral joint stability: a biomechanical study in vitro. JBone Joint Surg Br. 2005;87(4):577-82

[21] Dejour D, Le Coultre B. Osteotomies in patello-femoral instabilities. SportsMed Arthrosc. 2007;15(1):39-46.

[22] Felus J, Kowalczyk B. Age-Related Differences in Medial PatellofemoralLigament Injury Patterns in Traumatic Patellar Dislocation: Case Series of 50Surgically Treated Children and Adolescents. Am J Sports Med. 2012 Sep 7; [Epub ahead of print] PMID: 22962292

[23] Sanders TG, Morrison WB, Singleton BA, Miller MD, Cornum KG. Medialpatellofemoral ligament injury following acute transient dislocation of thepatella: MR find-

ings with surgical correlation in 14 patients. J Comput AssistTomogr. 2001;25(6): 957-62.

[24] Stefancin JJ, Parker RD. First-time traumatic patellar dislocation: a systematic review. Clin Orthop Relat Res. 2007;455:93-101.

[25] Guerrero P, Li X, Patel K, Brown M, Busconi B. Medial patellofemoral ligament injury patterns and associated pathology in lateral patella dislocation: an MRIstudy. Sports Med Arthrosc Rehabil Ther Technol. 2009;1(1):17.

[26] Balcarek P, Walde TA, Frosch S, Schüttrumpf JP, Wachowski MM, Stürmer KM, Frosch KH. Patellar dislocations in children, adolescents and adults: a comparative MRI study of medial patellofemoral ligament injury patterns and trochlear groove anatomy.Eur J Radiol. 2011;79(3):415-20.

[27] Dejour H, Walch G, Nove-Josserand L, Guier C. Factors of patellar instability: an anatomic radiographic study.Knee Surg Sports Traumatol Arthrosc. 1994;2(1):19-26.

[28] Mäenpää H, Lehto MU. Patellar dislocation. The long-term results of nonoperative management in 100 patients. Am J Sports Med. 1997;25(2):213-7.

[29] Cowan SM, Bennell KL, Hodges PW. Therapeutic patellar taping changes the timing of vasti muscle activation in people with patellofemoral pain syndrome. Clin J Sport Med. 2002;12(6):339-47.

[30] McConnell J. Rehabilitation and nonoperative treatment of patellar instability. Sports Med Arthrosc. 2007;15(2):95-104.

[31] Stensdotter AK, Hodges PW, Mellor R, Sundelin G, Häger-Ross C. Quadriceps activation in closed and in open kinetic chain exercise. Med Sci Sports Exerc. 2003;35(12): 2043-7.

[32] Escamilla RF, Fleisig GS, Zheng N, Barrentine SW, Wilk KE, Andrews JR. Biomechanics of the knee during closed kinetic chain and open kinetic chain exercises. Med Sci Sports Exerc. 1998;30(4):556-69

[33] Colvin AC, West RV. Patellar instability. J Bone Joint Surg Am. 2008;90(12):2751-62.

[34] Cofield RH, Bryan RS. Acute dislocation of the patella: results of conservative treatment. J Trauma. 1977;17(7):526-31

[35] Hawkins RJ, Bell RH, Anisette G. Acute patellar dislocations. The natural history. Am J Sports Med. 1986;14(2):117-20

[36] Nikku R, Nietosvaara Y, Kallio PE, Aalto K, Michelsson JE. Operative versusclosed treatment of primary dislocation of the patella. Similar 2-year results in125 randomized patients. Acta Orthop Scand. 1997;68(5):419-23

[37] Nikku R, Nietosvaara Y, Aalto K, Kallio PE. Operative treatment of primary patellar dislocation does not improve medium-term outcome: A 7-year follow-up report and risk analysis of 127 randomized patients.Acta Orthop. 2005;76(5):699-704.

[38] Christiansen SE, Jakobsen BW, Lund B, Lind M. Isolated repair of the medialpatello-femoral ligament in primary dislocation of the patella: a prospectiverandomized study. Arthroscopy. 2008;24(8):881-7.

[39] Palmu S, Kallio PE, Donell ST, Helenius I, Nietosvaara Y. Acute patellardislocation in children and adolescents: a randomized clinical trial. J BoneJoint Surg Am. 2008;90(3):463-70.

[40] Sillanpää PJ, Mäenpää HM, Mattila VM, Visuri T, Pihlajamäki H. Arthroscopicsurgery for primary traumatic patellar dislocation: a prospective, nonrandomized study comparing patients treated with and without acute arthroscopicstabilization with a median 7-year follow-up. Am J Sports Med. 2008;36(12):2301-9.

[41] Lattermann C, Toth J, Bach BR Jr. The role of lateral retinacular release inthe treatment of patellar instability. Sports Med Arthrosc. 2007;15(2):57-60.

[42] Ricchetti ET, Mehta S, Sennett BJ, Huffman GR. Comparison of lateral releaseversus lateral release with medial soft-tissue realignment for the treatment ofrecurrent patellar instability: a systematic review. Arthroscopy. 2007;23(5):463-8.

[43] Mountney J, Senavongse W, Amis AA, Thomas NP. Tensile strength of the medialpatellofemoral ligament before and after repair or reconstruction. J Bone JointSurg Br. 2005;87(1):36-40.

[44] Sallay PI, Poggi J, Speer KP, Garrett WE. Acute dislocation of the patella. A correlative pathoanatomic study. Am J Sports Med. 1996;24(1):52-60.

[45] Nomura E. Classification of lesions of the medial patello-femoral ligament in patellar dislocation. Int Orthop. 1999;23(5):260-3.

[46] Burks RT, Desio SM, Bachus KN, Tyson L, Springer K. Biomechanical evaluationof lateral patellar dislocations. Am J Knee Surg. 1998;11(1):24-31

[47] Sillanpää PJ, Peltola E, Mattila VM, Kiuru M, Visuri T, Pihlajamäki H. Femoralavulsion of the medial patellofemoral ligament after primary traumatic patellardislocation predicts subsequent instability in men: a mean 7-year nonoperativefollow-up study. Am J Sports Med. 2009;37(8):1513-21

[48] Dodson CC, Shindle MK, Dines JS, Altchek DW. Arthroscopic suture anchor repairfor lateral patellar instability. Knee Surg Sports Traumatol Arthrosc. 2010;18(2):143-6.

[49] Mariani PP, Liguori L, Cerullo G, Iannella G, Floris L. Arthroscopic patellar reinsertion of the MPFL in acute patellar dislocations. Knee Surg SportsTraumatol Arthrosc. 2011;19(4):628-33.

[50] Ostermeier S, Holst M, Bohnsack M, Hurschler C, Stukenborg-Colsman C, WirthCJ. In vitro measurement of patellar kinematics following reconstruction of themedial patellofemoral ligament. Knee Surg Sports Traumatol Arthrosc. 2007;15(3):276-85

[51] Yamamoto RK. Arthroscopic repair of the medial retinaculum and capsule inacute patellar dislocations. Arthroscopy. 1986;2(2):125-31.

[52] Henry JE, Pflum FA Jr. Arthroscopic proximal patella realignment andstabilization. Arthroscopy. 1995;11(4):424-5.

[53] Halbrecht JL. Arthroscopic patella realignment: An all-inside technique.arthroscopy. 2001;17(9):940-5.

[54] Nomura E, Inoue M, Osada N. Augmented repair of avulsion-tear type medial patellofemoral ligament injury in acute patellar dislocation.knee Surg Sports Traumatol Arthrosc. 2005;13(5):346-51.

[55] Ahmad CS, Stein BE, Matuz D, Henry JH. Immediate surgical repair of the medial patellar stabilizers for acute patellar dislocation. A review of eight cases.am J Sports Med. 2000;28(6):804-10.

[56] Boring TH, O'Donoghue DH. Acute patellar dislocation: results of immediate surgical repair.Clin Orthop Relat Res. 1978;(136):182-5.

[57] Mäenpää H, Lehto MU. Surgery in acute patellar dislocation--evaluation of the effect of injury mechanism and family occurrence on the outcome of treatment.br J Sports Med. 1995;29(4):239-41.

[58] Camanho GL, Viegas Ade C, Bitar AC, Demange MK, Hernandez AJ.Conservative versus surgical treatment for repair of the medial patellofemoral ligament in acute dislocations of the patella.Arthroscopy. 2009;25(6):620-5.

[59] Schöttle PB, Scheffler SU, Schwarck A, Weiler A. Arthroscopic medial retinacular repair after patellar dislocation with and without underlying trochlear dysplasia: a preliminary report.Arthroscopy. 2006;22(11):1192-8.

[60] Arendt EA, Moeller A, Agel J. Clinical outcomes of medial patellofemoral ligament repair in recurrent (chronic) lateral patella dislocations. Knee Surg Sports Traumatol Arthrosc. 2011;19(11):1909-14.

[61] Camp CL, Krych AJ, Dahm DL, Levy BA, Stuart MJ. Medial patellofemoral ligament repair for recurrent patellar dislocation. Am J Sports Med. 2010;38(11):2248-54.

[62] Sillanpää PJ, Mattila VM, Visuri T, Mäenpää H, Pihlajamäki H. Patellofemoralosteoarthritis in patients with operative treatment for patellar dislocation: amagnetic resonance-based analysis. Knee Surg Sports Traumatol Arthrosc. 2011;19(2):230-5.

[63] Buckens CF, Saris DB. Reconstruction of the medial patellofemoral ligament for treatment of patellofemoral instability: a systematic review. Am J Sports Med. 2010;38(1): 181-8.

[64] Nomura E, Inoue M, Kobayashi S. Long-term follow-up and knee osteoarthritis change after medial patellofemoral ligament reconstruction for recurrent patellar dislocation.Am J Sports Med. 2007;35(11):1851-8.

[65] Ellera Gomes JL. Medial patellofemoral ligament reconstruction for recurrentdislocation of the patella: a preliminary report. Arthroscopy. 1992;8(3):335-40.

[66] Noyes FR, Butler DL, Grood ES, Zernicke RF, Hefzy MS.Biomechanical analysis of human ligament grafts used in knee-ligament repairs and reconstructions.J Bone Joint Surg Am. 1984;66(3):344-52.

[67] Drez D Jr, Edwards TB, Williams CS. Results of medial patellofemoral ligament reconstruction in the treatment of patellar dislocation. Arthroscopy. 2001;17(3):298-306.

[68] Schöttle PB, Fucentese SF, Romero J. Clinical and radiological outcome ofmedial patellofemoral ligament reconstruction with a semitendinosus autograft forpatella instability. Knee Surg Sports Traumatol Arthrosc. 2005;13(7):516-21.

[69] Nomura E, Horiuchi Y, Kihara M. A mid-term follow-up of medial patellofemoral ligament reconstruction using an artificial ligament for recurrent patellardislocation. Knee. 2000;7(4):211-215.

[70] Ellera Gomes JL, Stigler Marczyk LR, César de César P, Jungblut CF. Medialpatellofemoral ligament reconstruction with semitendinosus autograft for chronic patellar instability: a follow-up study. Arthroscopy. 2004;20(2):147-51.

[71] Steiner TM, Torga-Spak R, Teitge RA. Medial patellofemoral ligamentreconstruction in patients with lateral patellar instability and trochleardysplasia. Am J Sports Med. 2006;34(8):1254-61.

[72] Smith TO, Walker J, Russell N. Outcomes of medial patellofemoral ligamentreconstruction for patellar instability: a systematic review. Knee Surg SportsTraumatol Arthrosc. 2007;15(11):1301-14.

[73] Ahmad CS, Brown GD, Stein BS. The docking technique for medial patellofemoral ligament reconstruction: surgical technique and clinical outcome. Am J Sports Med. 2009;37(10):2021-7.

[74] Schöttle PB, Schmeling A, Rosenstiel N, Weiler A. Radiographic landmarks for femoral tunnel placement in medial patellofemoral ligament reconstruction.Am J Sports Med. 2007;35(5):801-4.

[75] Beck P, Brown NA, Greis PE, Burks RT. Patellofemoral contact pressures andlateral patellar translation after medial patellofemoral ligament reconstruction.Am J Sports Med. 2007;35(9):1557-63

[76] Elias JJ, Cosgarea AJ. Technical errors during medial patellofemoral ligament reconstruction could overload medial patellofemoral cartilage: a computationalanalysis. Am J Sports Med. 2006;34(9):1478-85.

[77] Carney JR, Mologne TS, Muldoon M, Cox JS. Long-term evaluation of the Roux-Elm-slie-Trillat procedure for patellar instability: a 26-year follow-up.Am J Sports Med. 2005;33(8):1220-3.

[78] Barber FA, McGarry JE. Elmslie-Trillat procedure for the treatment of recurrent pa-tellar instability. Arthroscopy. 2008;24(1):77-81.

[79] Endres S, Wilke A. A 10 year follow-up study after Roux-Elmslie-Trillat treatment for cases of patellar instability. BMC Musculoskelet Disord. 2011 Feb 18;12:48.

[80] Pidoriano AJ, Weinstein RN, Buuck DA, Fulkerson JP. Correlation of patellararticular lesions with results from anteromedial tibial tubercle transfer. Am J Sports Med. 1997;25(4):533-7.

[81] Palmer SH, Servant CT, Maguire J, Machan S, Parish EN, Cross MJ. Surgicalrecon-struction of severe patellofemoral maltracking. Clin Orthop Relat Res. 2004;(419): 144-8.

[82] Pritsch T, Haim A, Arbel R, Snir N, Shasha N, Dekel S. Tailored tibialtubercle trans-fer for patellofemoral malalignment: analysis of clinical outcomes. Knee Surg Sports Traumatol Arthrosc. 2007;15(8):994-1002.

[83] von Knoch F, Böhm T, Bürgi ML, von Knoch M, Bereiter H. Trochleaplasty for recur-rent patellar dislocation in association with trochlear dysplasia. A 4- to 14-year fol-low-up study. J Bone Joint Surg Br. 2006;88(10):1331-5.

Exercise Medicine

Chapter 4

Iron Supplementation and Physical Performance

Chariklia K. Deli, Ioannis G. Fatouros,
Yiannis Koutedakis and Athanasios Z. Jamurtas

Additional information is available at the end of the chapter

1. Introduction

Iron is one of the most abundant elements, essential for the completion of numerous important biological functions, including electron transfer reactions, gene regulation, binding and transport of oxygen, regulation of cell growth and differentiation. In the human body it is mainly found in the oxygen transport and storage proteins haemoglobin (Hb) (60 - 70%) and myoglobin (10%), in various iron-containing enzymes (2%), as well as in the liver, bone marrow and muscle in the form of the storage proteins ferritin (Ferr) and hemosiderin (20 - 30%) [1]. Only a minor quantity (0.1 - 0.2%) of total iron, mostly bound to the iron-transport protein transferrin, circulates in the plasma and other extracellular fluids [1, 2]. Besides its essential character, excessive free iron could adversely affect the human body, by augmenting oxidative stress, mainly via the Fenton and Haber-Weiss reactions. Ferritin, hemosiderin and transferrin, assist the system to maintain iron balance under tight control by keeping free iron levels low and hence restrain the conversion of hydrogen peroxide to the highly reactive hydroxyl radical [3] that disturbs cellular homeostasis when it is increased at toxic levels.

Iron absorption is the main mechanism through which iron balance is maintained. Nevertheless, iron losses may occur at multiple organs, such as the gastrointestinal tract [4-6], the skin [7, 8], the urinary tract [4], and additionally due to several physiological conditions such as the menstrual cycle in women [9, 10]. To compensate for these losses, as well as for satisfying the body's demands during growth and pregnancy, iron is absorbed from the diet. The percentage of food-iron that is absorbed from the intestine is approximately 10%, with heme-iron being absorbed in greater amounts compared with non-heme-iron [11-13]. Thus, from a typical daily diet of 2000 kcal that contains adequate quantities of meat, 1.8 mg of iron per day are absorbed [13]. In general, daily iron turnover (absorption and excretion) is approximately 1-2 mg per day [1, 2, 7].

There is a strong body of evidence suggesting that exercise affects iron status [14-17], although other studies do not support this association [18-20]. Iron plays a critical role in oxygen transport as it is necessary for the formation of Hb, the oxygen transport protein that is critical for aerobic capacity. Iron is also needed for the optimal function of many oxidative enzymes affecting the intracellular metabolism (i.e., the electron transport chain and oxidative phosphorylation pathway in mitochondria) [21]. Not only prolonged aerobic exercise but, to some extent, short duration activities (i.e. sprints), may influence the above mechanisms [22]. Consequently, a compromised iron status would negatively affect physical performance. On the other hand, iron deficiency is frequently attributed to exercise [14-16]. Therefore, iron supplementation is commonly used to avoid exercise-induced perturbations of iron homeostasis and maintain the required iron stores that are necessary to address exercise needs or enhance physical performance.

Numerous studies have attempted to clarify the effectiveness of enhanced iron intake, either through diet or through supplement consumption, to restore iron status or to enhance physical performance. Yet, no valid conclusions have been drawn. The results of these studies are contradictory as some of them produced positive effects [23, 24]) whereas others dispute such effects [25]. An important factor in iron absorption seems to be the previous iron status of the individual. This means that, several iron parameters are seen to be ameliorated following iron supplementation in situations of iron deficiency, whereas this is not always the case for individuals with normal iron status.

In this chapter, an attempt will be made, to clarify the effect of exercise on iron status in athletes. Furthermore, an effort will be made to address the role of dietary or supplemented iron on several indices of physical performance. Finally, the mechanisms through which exercise may alter iron homeostasis will also be discussed.

2. The importance of iron in physical activity

Exercise and/or physical activity is characterized by a substantial increase in oxygen needs. Iron is an indispensable factor for the formation of Hb, the protein responsible for oxygen transport from the respiratory organs to the peripheral tissues. Lack of adequate amounts of iron for the formation of Hb due to iron deficiency, can strongly affect physical work capacity, by reducing oxygen conveyance to the exercising muscles [21]. Iron is also a vital component for the formation of myoglobin, the iron-storage protein within the muscle that regulates the diffusion of oxygen from the erythrocytes to the cytoplasm and on to the mitochondria where it is used as the final acceptor of electrons processed by the respiratory chains producing water and forming energy in the process [26, 27]. The concentration of myoglobin in skeletal muscle is drastically reduced (40 - 60%) following iron deficiency, thus limiting the rate of oxygen diffusion from erythrocytes to mitochondria [28] which ultimately compromises the muscle's oxidative capacity.

Apart from oxygen transport and storage, iron is also needed for the optimal function of many oxidative enzymes and proteins regulating the intracellular metabolism [21, 27, 29]. The mitochondrial content of oxidative enzymes and proteins is an important factor regarding the muscle's capacity for work, as there is a strong association between the ability to maintain prolonged submaximal exercise and the activity of iron-dependent oxidative enzymes [29]. Iron deficiency negatively affects mitochondrial respiration mainly through the decline in heme iron-containing respiratory chain proteins cytochrome c and cytochrome c oxidase, as well as non-heme iron-containing enzymes succinate dehydrogenase and NADH dehydro-genase, but also the non-heme iron-sulfur protein content [27]. Therefore, iron deficiency may have detrimental effects, especially on endurance performance which is susceptible to, and negatively affected by disturbances in skeletal muscle's iron concentrations [27].

Besides athletes' training at sea level, iron deficiency could also affect athletes training at altitude. Staying at high altitude causes an increase in erythropoiesis in the bone marrow, stimulated by hypoxia. This increase in erythropoiesis is followed by an elevation in red blood cells volume and Hb concentration [30, 31]. Iron deficiency could negatively affect the above mechanism by limiting the rate of erythropoiesis and consequently aerobic performance. It has been demonstrated that athletes with low ferritin levels do not increase total red blood cell volume after 4 weeks at altitude, despite an acute increase in erythropoietin [32]. In contrast, a significant increase in erythropoietin but also in reticulocytes occurred in non-iron-deficient athletes during training at moderate altitude [30]. Such data suggests that iron sufficiency is critical for the favorable response of the athletes training to altitude, in an attempt to enhance their performance.

3. Iron needs in athletes

The need for iron supplementation in cases of iron deficiency anemia in athletes is indisputable. Nevertheless, the need for iron supplementation in situations of iron deficiency without anemia for enhanced performance is still under debate, despite the systematic use of iron supplements. The majority of studies do not report significant changes in physical capacity following iron supplementation [25, 33, 34]. Nevertheless, there are studies indicating an improvement of physical performance in iron depleted non anemic athletes following iron supplementation [23, 24].

Athletes at risk of iron deficiency include female and male middle and long distance runners, as well as all female athletes in other disciplines in which running is an important part of training or competition [17]. Iron demands during consecutive periods of intense training or competition are high, and may compromise iron status. In [15] is reported that a brief recovery following the in-season period may be insufficient to restore the reduced iron stores prior to the start of the subsequent high-intensity pre-season training. Additionally, even when the recommended dietary intake of iron is established through a controlled diet, iron status perturbations may be inevitable. In reference [35] the mean dietary intake of 16.3 mg per day was inadequate to prevent iron deficiency in female collegiate swimmers. Such disturbances however, if not treated, could be a threat, not only for athletic performance deterioration, but also for the athletes' health. In a recent study [36], female collegiate rowers, categorized as iron-depleted non-anemic (Hb $\geq$ 12 gIdL, Ferr < 20 µg/L), rowed about 4% slower than normal controls with a serum Ferr $\geq$ 20 µg/L in a self-reported best 2-km simulated race on an row ergometer. These findings point out that non-anemic iron depletion may impair performance.

On the other hand, unjustified and uncontrolled iron supplementation could lead to iron overload that could be toxic and hazardous for the athletes' health. Athletes with the homozygous form of hemochromatosis gene may be at risk of excessive iron storage due to excessive iron absorption [17]. According to the Department of Health and Human Services, Centers for Disease Control and Prevention (CDC) [37], hemochromatosis symptoms are non-specific, but the most commonly associated early hemochromatosis symptoms may include fatigue, weakness, weight loss, abdominal pain, and arthralgia. The simplest tests that indirectly indicate iron overloading are transferrin saturation (TS) and serum Ferr [37, 38]. TS levels >45% and Ferr >200 µg/L for premenopausal female or >300 µg/L for postmenopausal female and >300 µg/L for male, are indicative of iron overload. Nevertheless, the confirmation of hemochromatosis can be achieved indirectly by quantitative phlebotomy and hereditary hemochromatosis genotyping, or indirectly by liver biopsy [37, 38].

Taking the above under consideration, iron supplementation should be decided only after a thorough examination of athletes' hematological and iron status at the beginning, in the middle, as well as at the end of training or the competitive season. Controlled iron supplementation for all athletes with serum Ferr below 35µg/L is recommended for the replenishment of iron stores.

4. Evaluation of iron status in athletes

Due to the significant role of iron in optimal physical performance and health, the evaluation of iron status in athletes is of great importance in order to prevent iron deficiency. According to the World Health Organisation [39], iron deficiency progresses in three stages: in the first stage iron stores in bone marrow, liver, and spleen are depleted (serum Ferr concentrations <12µg/L); in the second stage, erythropoiesis decreases as iron supply to erythroid marrow is reduced (TS <16%); in the final stage Hb production falls drastically (Hb concentration <12g/L) resulting in anemia.

Iron status evaluation is not a single-parameter estimation. Day-to-day or acute phase response variations occur in several indices of iron status. Therefore, in order to make a valuable and more accurate assessment, the estimation of iron status indices and several hematological parameters is needed. These will be described in the following sections. Additionally, the reference range for the main indicators of iron status, as well as reported values in elite athletes is presented in Table 1.

4.1. Estimation of red blood cell parameters

The most commonly used hematological index is haemoglobin which reflects the effects of mechanisms that control the red cell mass (RCM) and plasma volume (PV). It is used as an indicator of anemia, that is when an individual's Hb concentration falls below the normal threshold of the person's corresponding age and sex category, (then the third stage of iron deficiency anemia has been developed [40]). Normal values lie between 11.7 - 155 g/dL and 12.8 - 17.3 g/dL for women and men, respectively [41, 42]. According to WHO the recommended Hb values (in g/100 ml of venous blood) below which anemia develops, are <13 g/dL for adult men, <12 g/dL and <11 g/dL for non-pregnant and pregnant adult females, respectively, while in children aged 6 months - 14 years the corresponding values are between 11 g/dL and 12 g/dL [40]. Haemoglobin concentrations are normally stable demonstrating a relatively low day-to-day variation of 2 - 4% [39]. Alongside Hb, hematocrit (Hct), the mean corpuscular haemoglobin concentration (MCHC), as well as the size and volume of red blood cells (RBC) are also useful markers for anemia [16,29].The classic Hb and Hct changes as a result of acute or chronic exercise should be kept in mind before a diagnosis is to be made. Namely, acute strenuous and prolonged exercise typically leads to an increase of Hb and Hematocrit due to hemoconcentration [43]. On the other hand, a decrease in the concentration of these indices may be seen within the first days of a regular cardiovascular training program due to hemodilution. This decrease is temporary and most athletes demonstrate normal Hb levels at the completion of training or the end of a competitive phase [43, 44]. Hence, when determining hematological changes in athletes the above changes should be also taken into account in order to avoid a misleading interpretation of "sports anemia" or "pseudoanemia".

4.2. Estimation of body iron stores

Serum Ferr concentration is one of the most frequently used indices in iron status examination. Serum concentration of Ferr and, in conditions of iron overload hemosiderin [2], serve as an indicator for body iron stores, available for protein and heme synthesis. Serum Ferr concentrations normally range within 10 - 300 µg/L [40, 42], whereas values lower than 12 µg/L reflect the absence of measurable iron stores in bone marrow, liver and spleen. Such values indicate the onset of a first stage iron deficiency [40]. Ferritin seems to be age- and sex-dependent, since lower values are reported for children and pre-menopause women as compared to adults and men, respectively.

Nevertheless, the expression and appearance of Ferr in serum are influenced by other factors as well. Ferritin is an acute-phase reactant and its serum concentration may be increased by liver disease, infections and other inflammatory conditions, malignant diseases, renal failure, cardiovascular diseases, high alcohol consumption, and aging [44-46]. Some types of physical activity are accompanied by inflammation-like reactions that can induce an acute phase response and increased Ferr levels for several days. In case of exercise-induced inflammation, normal Ferr levels could be deceptive, reflecting rather an acute phase response than the true efficiency of the athletes' iron stores. Day-to-day variability in Ferr has been estimated in the range of 13% - 75% in endurance athletes [19] and therefore, its serum concentrations cannot independently be equated to iron stores [47]. In summary, although serum Ferr concentration is commonly reported to be affected by training [4, 16, 35], there should be some caution before iron adequacy or inadequacy is diagnosed in athletes when ferritin is the only available evaluating index.

4.3. Estimation of plasma or serum iron status

Iron concentration, together with Total Iron Binding Capacity (TIBC) and TS provide information about iron status in plasma or serum.

Iron concentration expresses the total iron content per unit of serum volume, and its normal values typically range within 50 - 175 μg/dL [42, 48]. Iron concentration demonstrates a day-to-day variation of 15% - 26%, and a 10 - 20% variation during the day [49], and as a consequence, the measurement of serum iron concentration alone, cannot be rendered a valuable index of iron status.

Total Iron Binding Capacity (TIBC) reflects the total number of binding sites for iron atoms on transferrin per unit volume of plasma or serum [48]. The reference range for TIBC lies between 250-425 μg/dL (Tietz, 1995) and is a more stable indicator of iron status than iron concentration, with its day-to-day variation ranging within 8% - 12% while its diurnal variation is less than 5%. TIBC does not change before iron stores are depleted [48]. In depleted iron stores a rise in TIBC levels occurs as more free binding sites on transferrin are available for iron.

Transferrin is the iron binding protein that delivers iron to cells [48]. Transferrin levels are not affected by inflammatory reactions or other diseases and can therefore be used for diagnosing iron deficiency even under such conditions [44]. Transferrin saturation is the percentage of serum iron to TIBC, and values < 15% are indicative of a second stage iron deficiency. This stage is characterized by iron deficient erythropoiesis, with a restricted iron supply in the absence of anemia [40]. Its normal values range within 20% - 50% and 15% - 50% for men and women respectively [42]. Since TIBC is rather stable, any alteration in plasma TS will be the result of changes in iron concentration. Consequently, anything that alters iron concentration will alter TS as well [48]. Transferrin saturation in conjunction with serum Ferr concentration and Hb are the three critical parameters for the determination of the severity of iron deficiency.

4.4. Estimation of erythropoiesis into the bone marrow

Erythrocyte Protoporphyrin (EP) or Zinc Protoporphyrin (ZPP), and the soluble Transferrin Receptor (sTfR) reflect the adequacy or inadequacy of iron for erythropoiesis into the bone marrow and tissues.

Protoporphyrin is a carrier molecule and together with ferrous iron forms the heme group of Hb, myoglobin and other heme-containing enzymes. In cases of iron absence, instead of iron, zinc is incorporated to protoporphyrin and ZPP is formed. A rise in ZPP concentration is one of the first indicators of insufficient iron levels in bone marrow [50, 51]. Additionally, the ratio of EP to Hb is an excellent indicator of iron failure to meet the normal demands of bone marrow [50]. In healthy individuals, EP concentration is < 40 - 50 µg EP/dl of red blood cells. When TS falls below 15%, EP concentration increases rapidly to more than 70 - 100 µg/dl, whereas concentrations as high as 200 µg/dl may be reached in cases of prolonged or severe iron deficiency. Day-to-day variation of EP concentration is reported to fall around 6.5% [52].

The concentration of sTfR has also been used as an indicator of iron deficiency erythropoiesis [19, 41]. Plasma sTfR is a truncated form of the cellular receptor (TfR), which is responsible for binding and transferring iron into the cell. Transferrin receptor is upregulated when the cell needs more iron, and sTfR is proportional to the cellular TfR content. Normal concentration of sTfR ranges within 1.15 - 2.75 mg/L [41]. When iron stores become depleted and the functional pool of iron diminishes, the levels of sTfR increase [41, 53]. In contrast to Ferr, sTfR is not an acute phase protein, and its concentration is not affected by infections or other inflammatory conditions [16, 54]. Additionally, the much lower day-to-day recorded variability of 4% - 16% for the sTfR compared with the corresponding value of Ferr (13% - 75%) [19] may render sTfR a more accurate index for the estimation of athletes' iron status and the exercise-induced changes in iron metabolism [55]. The sTfR/log Ferr index with normal values ranging within 0.63 - 1.8 [41], is believed to be a more reliable index, as it is less variable and takes into account both the iron stores and the iron pool. Hence, it may reflect more accurately athletes' iron status.

4.5. Estimation of hemolysis

Haptoglobin (Hp) is used as an index of hemolysis. The destruction of the red blood cells membrane due to hemolysis allows Hb and its associated iron held within the cell to be released into the surrounding plasma. Haptoglobin binds free Hb released from erythrocytes, inhibiting its pro-oxidative activity [44]. The binding of Hb to Hp causes a decline in Hp levels, and the formed haemoglobin-haptoglobin complex is taken up exclusively by hepatocytes, thus preventing the excretion of free Hb in the urine [20]. Hence, the decline in Hp levels below normal values, which range between 15 - 200 mg/dL[42], reveals the occurrence of hemolysis. As a result, the regular return of catabolized red blood cells to the reticuloendothelial system (RES) is diminished. Therefore, the observed lower Hb concentration often seen in long distance runners may not always reflect iron deficiency. The shift of iron turnover from hepatocytes rather than the RES may represent an alternative explanation of the observed compromised iron status [20]. The estimation of Hp levels could be of great importance in the verification of true iron deficiency even when other parameters such as Hb, serum Ferr, or bone marrow hemosiderin appear to be lower than normal values.

Taking the above into consideration, an integral evaluation of an athlete's iron status should not be based on the estimation of one parameter alone. Additionally, day-to-day variations of the estimated indices, as well as exercise-induced changes in blood volume, acute phase reactions, infections, or other inflammatory conditions, should also be considered. This way, the assessment would be more integrated, and false conclusions about the effect of exercise on the athlete's iron status would be avoided.

		Hb g/dL	Hct %	RBC x 10^6 c/µL	MCV fL	MCH Pg/cell	MCHC g Hb/dL	RTC count % RBC
Reference values for non-athletes adults*	Males	13.2-17.3	39-49	4.3-5.7	80-99	27-34	32-37	0.5-1.5
	Females	11.7-15.5	35-45	3.8-5.1	81-100	27-34	32-36	0.1-1.5
Reported iron status indicators in elite Athletes (M±SD)								
Koehler et al. (2012)√ (several sports)	Males	14.7±1.1	42.3±2.6					
	Females	13.2±0.9	38.6±2.4					
Della Valle & Haas (2012)√	Females (N)	13.1±0.7	40.1±2.1				88.8±3.6	
	(D)	13.0±0.7	40.2±2.1				87.9±4.6	
Reinke et al. (2012) †	Males (CS)	12.2-17.1						
	(R)	11.6-17.2						
	(P)	12.4-16.5						
Schumacher et al. (2002)√	Males (EA)	15.7±1.0	46.6±3.3	5.24±0.52				
	(PA)	16.4±1.0	47.4±3.1	5.47±0.36				
Malczewska et al. (2001)√	Males (N)	16.38±1.1	0.49±0.0¥	5.26±0.36	90.9±3.9	31.2±2.4	34.3±4.5	
	(D)	15.92±1.1	0.47±0.0¥	5.12±0.32	91.7±3.3	31.2±1.7	33.7±1.5	
	Females (N)	14.5±0.9	0.42±0.0¥	4.5±0.37	91.8±4.9	32.3±3.0	35.0±2.9	
	(D)	13.8±0.8	0.42±0.0¥	4.6±0.33	88.9±3.3	29.9±1.8	33.2±1.6	
Rowland et al. (1987)	Males	14.7±1.0						
	Females	13.3±0.4						
Magnuson et al. (1984)	Males	14.6±0.9			87.9±7.2	31.3±2.1	35.8±1.8	

		Ferr µg/L	Iron µg/dL	TIBC µg/dL	TS %	sTFR mg/L	Hp mg/dL	EP µg EP/dL
Reference values for non-athletes adults*	Males	20-300	65-175	250-425	20-50	1.15-2.75	15-200	< 40-50
	Females	10-120	50-170	250-425	15-50	1.15-2.75	15-200	< 40-50
Reported iron status indicators in elite Athletes (M±SD)								
Koehler et al. (2012)√ (several sports)	Males	55.4±36.7						
	Females	35.4±22.0						
Della Valle & Haas (2012)√	Females (N)	43.0±20.3				6.4±2.5		
	(D)	13.9±5.1				6.4±2.1		

Reinke et al. (2012)†	Males (CS)	6-127			10.7-85.4			
	(R)	20-133			9.0-54.2			
	(P)	15-148			13.9-43.2			
Schumacher et al.	Males (EA)	125.6±91.5	125.0±50.2				73.0±38.9	
(2002)√	(PA)	82.3±61	105.5±38.6				55.2±30.7	
Malczewska et al.	Males (N)	65.9±1.83	104.3±28.2	310±36.7		1.78±1.3	1.29±0.58	
(2001)√	(D)	19.5±2.14	72.8±20.5	348±41.2		3.15±1.2	1.16±0.54	
	Females (N)	40.6±1.76	105.3±32.9	315±42.6		1.72±1.2	1.29±0.89	
	(D)	20.1±1.54	81.7±20.4	344±49.2		4.36±2.5	1.43±0.60	
Rowland et al.	Males	29.4±17.8						
(1987)	Females	26.6±11.4						
Magnuson et al. (1984)	Males	64.3±47.8	19.1±7.3 *		31.8±11.6		52.0±32	27±18

Hb: Haemoglobin, Hct: Hematocrit, RBC: Red blood cells, MCV: Mean corpuscular volume, MCH: Mean corpuscular Hemoglobin concentration; RTC: Reticulocytes count, Ferr: Ferritin, TIBC: Total iron binding capacity, TS: Transferrin saturation, sTfR: soluble transferrin receptor, Hp: Haptoglobin, EP: Erythrocyte protoporphyrin

√Values reported in Mean±SD, † the observed ranges, *Values reported in L/L, * Values reported in μmol/L

N: normal iron status, D: iron deficiency, CS: Competitive season, R: Recovery, P: Preparation, EA: Endurance trained athletes, PA: Power trained athletes

* WHO, Assessing the Iron Status of populations (2004); Suominen et al., 1998; Tietz, 1995; Lynch, 2004; Beard, 2004; Labbe et al., 1999;

Table 1. The main iron status indicators: reference values for non-athletes and reported values in elite athletes

5. Exercise-induced alterations of iron status in athletes

5.1. Chronic exercise

There is a great body of evidence indicating that several hematological and iron status parameters often appear altered as a result of chronic exercise (Table 2) giving the impression that athletes may be iron-deficient [14-17, 22, 43].

Several hematological variables in strength-trained athletes have been reported to be similarly low or even lower than that of endurance athletes [14, 56]. Nevertheless, it is mostly the endurance type of training that has been linked to lower values of several hematological indices [35, 43]. Actually, although within normal values, lower levels of RBC have been reported in endurance and/or power athletes as compared to sedentary individuals, while Hb and Hct were significantly lower in endurance athletes only when compared with power athletes [43]. These lower levels in endurance athletes have been attributed to reticulocytosis and expansion of plasma volume associated with chronic aerobic training [35, 43, 56]. However, abnormal Hb concentration (< 13 g/dL) was not only reported in endurance athletes, but in male athletes of combat sports as well [14]. What is more, even Hb levels below 12 g/dL, defining iron deficiency anemia, has been reported for female rowers, indicating that abnormal decrements in Hb concentration can be found in athletes other than runners [36].

While in the general population a serum Ferr concentration below 12µg/L is used for the identification of first stage iron deficiency, wider serum Ferr cut-offs values (ranging from 12 to 40 µg/L) have been adopted for the identification of diminished iron stores and iron deficiency in athletes [14, 15, 24, 33, 34 36]. Additionally, iron deficiency has also been distinguished to absolute, when serum Ferr is below 30µg/L, or functional, when serum Ferr is within 30 - 90µg/L or serum Ferr is within 100 - 299µg/L and TS is below 20% [15].

Although within normal range, athletes demonstrated lower values of serum Ferr but similar transferrin and Hp values compared with sedentary controls [43]. Similarly, in [56] significantly lower Ferr concentration in endurance athletes is reported compared with strength-trained athletes and controls, and Ferr levels below 50µg/L in 18% of endurance athletes as compared to 12% in controls.

Decreased serum Ferr values (< 35 µg/L) were recorded to one third of elite athletes [14]. These results are in agreement with those in reference [4] where decreased serum Ferr values (< 35 µg/L) and low, instead of normal, hepatic iron stores were also reported in male distance runners, indicating a true prelatent iron deficiency. The lower cut-off point of < 20 µg/L for Ferr adopted by the authors in reference [36], identified 30% of the rowers as being non-anemic iron-depleted at the beginning of a pre-training period, while another 10% were identified as anemic according to Hb values of less than 12.0 g/dl.

A very intense training or competitive period may lead to absolute (Ferr < 30µg/L) and functional (Ferr within 30 - 90µg/L or Ferr within 100 - 299 µg/L + TS <20%) iron deficiency in professional male soccer players [15, 57], elite rowers [15] and female swimmers [35]. In some cases, the allowed recovery period before the next training phase may not be sufficient for the replenishment of the depleted iron stores [15], and this point definitely needs closer attention.

Based on data of several investigations, iron status disturbances are more frequent in female than in male athletes. In reference [14], female athletes were about twice as likely to exhibit reduced Ferr levels. In that study, 58.8% of females had Ferr below 35 µg/L, whereas the corresponding percentage of their male counterparts was 31.2%. In another study [58], 45% of the female cross country runners became iron-deficient at the end of the competitive season, while in males only 17% of them were characterized as iron-deficient. Similarly, the prevalence of iron deficiency was greater in female athletes of several events, as compared to male athletes. Determination of the transferrin receptor-ferritin index (sTfR/logFerr) revealed values of 2.62±0.94 and 3.33±1.71 for iron-deficient male and female athletes, respectively [16]. Additionally, critically low Ferr levels below 15µg/L or even below 12µg/L have also been reported for female runners [58- 60].

The cause of reduced levels in Ferr or serum iron in athletes is not fully understood. Exercise-induced hemolysis, as documented by the reduced Hp values, may offer a plausible explanation. In reference [20], although no differences were observed in Hb concentration, the levels of iron concentration, Hct, Ferr, TS, and bone marrow hemosiderin were lower in athletes compared to controls. However, no true iron deficiency was established based on the normal mean cell volume (MCV) and EP values, as well as on the normal sideroblast count in bone marrow smears of all athletes, confirming an adequate supply of iron to normoblasts. The lower Hct and Ferr values in athletes could be explained by the simultaneous marked decline of Hp levels, indicating a shift of iron to the hepatocytes as a result of increased intravascular hemolysis. Thus, diagnosing iron deficiency solely based on reduced Ferr or hemosiderin levels, could lead to an underestimation of iron reserves and a possible false-positive diagnosis of "sports anemia".

5.2. Acute exercise

Not only chronic exercise, but also acute strenuous physical activity may alter several indices of iron status. A significant reduction in serum iron levels of 12.2 μmol/L was reported after a triathlon completion [61]. The authors proposed that heavy sweating or a prelatent iron deficiency may explain the observed severe reduction of serum iron. However, sweat iron concentration does not correlate with the increased whole body sweat rates [8].

A slight increase in sTfr, although within the normal range, has also been recorded after incremental running to exhaustion, but not after 45 min of submaximal exercise or after 3 consecutive days of aerobic training in highly trained endurance cyclists [55]. After the incremental running, an increase in Ferr, as well as in Hb and Packed Cell Volume (PCV) was also observed. This increase was mainly attributed to the concurrent hemoconcentration, as evidenced by the pronounced fall in plasma volume.

Regardless the acute or chronic character of exercise where most studies report variable responses in iron status, there are also studies that do not support significant differences in iron status between trained and untrained individuals. Indeed, similar incidence of iron deficiency between male endurance young athletes and non-athletes involved in several sport disciplines has been reported [18]. High physical activity of athletes did not affect iron stores, as it was found to be higher than in control subjects. It has to be mentioned though, that athletes had higher iron intake from the diet than controls, and that 18% of those that were iron-sufficient reported consumption of iron supplements. In a more recent study of the same institute [19] that involved female endurance athletes, lower incidence of iron deficiency was reported in athletes as compared to controls. These studies may lead to the assumption that the increased iron dietary intake and dietary factors involved in iron metabolism compensated for the augmented, exercise-induced losses of iron in young athletes. Regarding iron deficiency in athletes whose iron intake was sufficient, the authors attributed its prevalence in its diminished absorption for the male, and its leak to the blood due to menstrual cycle for the female athletes.

Taken together, these studies that attempted to evaluate the effects of exercise on iron status of athletes suggest that high volume training during a competitive season may compromise iron homeostasis. One determining factor that could help explain the reported discrepancies in iron status due to acute or chronic exercise is diet. Unfortunately, not many studies report athletes' daily dietary intake of iron, and since iron intake or absorption are determining factors for iron balance future studies need to address this issue.

Study	Study protocol	Subjects	Estimated indices	Results
Compromised iron status				
Chronic exercise				
Kohler et al (2012)	Retrospective estimation of iron status in athletes from 25 different events	96 males 16.1±2.3yo and 97 females 16.3±3yo elite athletes	Nutrition, Ferr, Fe, hematological parameters, CK, VO$_{2peak}$	**Dietary iron:** 81% of male and 39% of female athletes reached the RDA; iron density was lower in males; 57% of the females and 31% of the males had Ferr<35µg/L; similar VO$_{2peak}$ in athletes with low and normal iron status
Della Valle & Haas (2012)	Determination of the impact of iron depletion on performance at the beginning of a training season	165 female rowers (19.7±1.2yo)	Hb, Ferr, sTfR, 2-km TT	30%of the athletes were iron deficient (**Ferr** < 20µg/L) 10% of the athletes had iron deficiency anemia (**Hb** < 12 g/dL)
Reinke et al (2012)	Assessment of iron status after 3 seasons: championship, recovery, preseason training	10 professional male soccer players 20-36yo, 20 elite rowers 21-35yo	Hematological indices, Ferr, TS	27% of the athletes had iron deficiency after championship season which persisted in all time points in 14% of the athletes; **Ferr:** no significant increase during recovery; **sTransf:** ↑ in the recovery period, and ↓in the pre-season training; **Hb:** 10% of the athletes had apparent or border line anemia in all time points
Schumacher et al (2002)	Epidimiological study, estimation of hematological and iron status in endurance, mixed or power athletes	747 male athletes (24.2±8yo), 104 controls (29.9±6.9yo)	RBC,Hb, Hct, Fe, Ferr, Tf, Hp, VO$_{2peak}$	**Hb, Hct, RBC**: ↓in athletes than controls; ↓in endurance athletes **Ferr:** ↓in athletes than controls; **Fe, Tf, Hp:** no differences; **VO$_{2peak}$:** ↑in endurance athletes
Malczewska et al (2001)	Assessment of frequency of iron deficiency in athletes	131 males, 121 females of several events 16-36 years old	sTfR, Fe, TIBC, Ferr, Hp , TfR/log Ferr index	Latent iron deficiency in 29% of female and 11% of male athletes; higher sTfR and TIBC, lower Ferr levels in iron

Study	Study protocol	Subjects	Estimated indices	Results
				deficient compared with normal only in females
Nachtigall et al (1996)	Estimation of iron status and iron metabolism throughout a training period	45 male distance runners	Ferr, ^{59}Fe absorption	Ferr values <35μg in 51% of the athletes; up-regulated ^{59}Fe absorption, decreased liver iron concentration
Spodaryk et al (1993)	Estimation of hematological and iron status in endurance (E), strength-trained (S) athletes and controls (C)	39 male athletes from the 1988 Polish Olympic team (20.4 ± 2.2yo)	Hb, PCV, RBC, Ret, Fe, Ferr, Tf, Hp, TS	**Hb, PCV, RBC, TS:** ↓in E compared with C; **Ferr:** ↓in E compared with S and C; **Ret, GOT:** ↓in E compared with S
Brigham et al (1993)	Estimation of iron status during a competitive season	25 female varsity collegiate swimmers	Hb, Ferr	At baseline 17 athletes were iron depleted and 5 athletes were anemic. After 5 wk Hb decreased (≥6 g/L) in 44%, and Ferr (≥5 μg/L) in 24% of the athletes
Nickerson et al (1989)	Estimation of stage II iron deficiency (Ferr<12ng/ml and TS<16%) during the running session; iron supplementation or iron-rich diet or controls	41 female and 25 male cross-country runners and controls (15-18yo)	Ferr, TS, blood losses	**Iron deficiency:** 34% of females and 8% of males became iron deficient by the 45th or 75th day of running **Blood losses:** 14 stools in females and 1 stool in males with "/>4mg Hb/g of stool
Rowland et al (1987)	Estimation of iron status during a competitive season; supplementation of iron in the iron	30 male and 20 female cross country runners (14.3-18.6yo)	Ferr, Hb, RBC parameters	45%of females and 17% of males identified as iron deficient during the season;
Magnusson et al (1984)	Hematological and iron status comparison between distance runners	43 runners (19-46yo) and 119 controls (19-37yo)	Hb,Hct, MCV, MCHC, EP, Fe, TS, Ferr, BMHem, Sideroblasts, Hp	**Hb:** no differences between groups; **Hct, Fe, Ferr, TS, BMHem:** ↓in athletes; **Hp:** 0.52±0.32 g/L in athletes (11athletes had Hp<0.2g/L); **MCV, EP, MCHC:** no iron deficiency

Study	Study protocol	Subjects	Estimated indices	Results
Acute exercise				
Rogers et al (1986)	Evaluation pre, post, and 30 min, 24h, and 48h after a 160-km triathlon (canoeing, cycling, and running)	18 triathlon athletes	Fe, TIBC, lactoferrin, Ferr, Hp, cortisol, WCC, CRP, various enzymes	Post: ↑ in cortisol, WCC, lactoferrin and ↓ in Fe and TS; 24h: ↑by 300% in CRP, ↓ in Hp
Schumacher et al (2002)	Estimation of exercise on sTfR and other variables after an incremental running test till exhaustion (IRTTE), 45min submaximal running, 3d aerobic cycling	39 athletes (33 men, 6 women) (19.6 – 32.5yo)	Hb, Hct, BV, PV, RCV, sTfR, Ferr, Fe	**Hb, Hct:** ↑ after exercise; **PV, BV:** ↑after incremental and submaximal running; ↓after 3d aerobic cycling; **sTfR:** ↑after the incremental running; **Ferr:** ↑after incremental and submaximal running;
No alterations in iron status				
Malczewska et al (1997)	Estimation of iron status in endurance athletes	178 male athletes, 52 male controls 18-20 years old	Hb, PCV, RBC, WBC, MCHC, MCV, MCH, Fe, TS, TIBC, Ferr, Hp	Similar iron depletion in athletes (19%) and controls (20%); ↓ Ferr, Fe and ↑TIBC in the iron depleted subgroups
Malczewska et al (2000)	Estimation of iron status in endurance athletes	126 female athletes, 52 female controls 16-20 years old	Hb, Hct, RBC, WBC, MCHC, MCV, MCH, Fe, TIBC, TS, Ferr, Hp	Lower iron deficiency (26%) in athletes than controls (50%); ↓ Ferr, Fe and ↑TIBC in the iron deficient subgroups

VO_{2max}: Maximum Oxygen Consumption, TT: Time Trial, CK: Creatine Kinase, Ferr: Ferritin, Fe: Iron, Tf: Transferrin, TS: Transferrin Saturation, sTfR: Soluble Transferrin Receptor, TIBC: Total Iron Binding Capacity, Hb: Haemoglobin, Hct: Hematocrit, PCV: Packed Cell Volume, Ret: Reticulocytes, WCC: White Cells Count, RBC: Red Blood Cells, RCV: Red Cells Volume, WBC: White Blood Cells, MCH: Mean corpuscular Haemoglobin, MCHC: Mean Corpuscular Haemoglobin Concentration, MCV: Mean Corpuscular Volume, BMHem: Bone Marrow Hemosiderin, EP: Erythrocyte Protoporphyrin, Hp: Haptoglobin, PV: Plasma Volume, BV: Blood Volume, GOT: Glutamic Oxaloacetic Transaminase, CRP: C Reactive Protein

Table 2. Iron status in competitive athletes

6. Potential mechanisms for iron balance disturbances due to exercise

Iron absorption mainly, and to a lesser extent iron nutrition, are the two critical mechanisms by which iron balance is maintained since there is no other physiological process for iron excretion. The repletion of iron due to increased losses as well as the body's need during growth and pregnancy are covered by dietary iron intake. Consequently, a low dietary iron intake, could lead to compromised iron status [9]. According to values reported by the Institute of Medicine, Food & Nutrition Board [62], the recommended dietary intake (RDI) for total iron is 8 mg/day for adult men and 18 mg/day for menstruating women. Usually, male, but not female athletes achieve the RDI for iron [14, 17, 63]. The mechanism of iron absorption by the intestine is regulated by iron bioavailability in diet and by individual's iron status. Iron bioavailability has been found to be affected by the type of the diet and by the type of dietary iron [11]. Hence, mixed diet and heme iron provide greater bioavailability and absorption as compared to a vegetarian diet and nonheme iron, [11-13]. Furthermore, iron deficiency augments iron absorption.

Besides iron absorption and intake, several other mechanisms have been proposed to account for iron loss and iron balance disturbances, and ultimately the prevalence of iron deficiency in athletes. These mechanisms include increased gastrointestinal blood loss, hematuria, hemolysis [5, 6, 17, 64-67], increased iron loss in sweat [7, 8], as well as menstruation in women [9, 10, 68].

In athletes, gastrointestinal bleeding usually accompanied by occult blood, is a well-established phenomenon, mostly seen in distance runners [6, 60]. Gastrointestinal blood loss has shown to be the main contributor to the negative iron balance, as the excretion of ^{59}Fe in sweat and urine appears to be negligible compared to fecal excretion of 3 - 5 mg/day [4]. Running a marathon was associated with a gastrointestinal blood loss [67], and positive occult heme stools were found in runners after intensive training or competitive running [4, 5, 60, 67]. The origin of running-related intestinal bleeding has still to be clarified, but endoscopic examination has revealed bleeding lesions in the stomach and colon [65, 66]. Gastrointestinal bleeding is partly attributed to ischemic injury, and running has been shown to reduce visceral blood flow by up to 43% of pre-exercise levels [69] due to the diversion of blood flow from the splanchnic viscera to the working muscles. Exercise intensity, seems to play a significant role in the development of gastric ischemia [70], which increases mucosa permeability and enhances occult blood loss [6].

Increased iron loss through sweat has also been proposed as a mechanism related to the compromise of iron status as a result of increased sweat rates during exercise in athletes, or increased temperature in individuals living and exercising in hot climates. The daily loss of iron from the skin has been reported to be 0.24 mg/d [71] or 0.33 mg/d [72]. The reported 0.183 mg of iron loss during prolonged exercise at 50% of VO_{2max}, represented the 55% - 76% of the estimated daily iron loss from the skin, and the 23% for men and 10% for women of the estimated total daily iron loss [8]. It has to be mentioned that although the sweat rate increases during the 1st hour of exercise and remains constant thereafter, and males have higher sweat rates than females, the iron loss in males and females remains comparable. Additionally, the sweat iron loss declines in both genders during the 2nd hour of exercise [8], or after the first 30 min in a hot environment [7]. This reduction could be attributed to the initial sweat containing iron present in cellular debris [7], to the increased sweat rates while the total iron loss remains constant, or to a conservation mechanism that may prevent excessive iron loss during exercise [8]. Still, iron loss in sweat remains insignificant compared to that of the gastrointestinal tract.

Another explanation for compromised iron status in athletes is the shift of iron return to hepatocytes, rather than the RES, as a consequence of the increased intravascular hemolysis occurring mostly in weight-bearing activities, such as running. In these activities, hemolysis is due to the impact forces generated by the foot strike [73, 74]. Increased intravascular hemolysis has been reported in runners [20] and female artistic gymnasts [73]. However, foot strike cannot totally explain the exercise-induced hemolysis since hypohaptoglobinemia, a situation that reveals the presence of hemolysis, has also been observed in swimmers [75]. In non-weight-bearing activities hemolysis may result from the compression of the blood vessels caused by the vigorous contraction of the involved muscles [75].

Female athletes seem to be more prone to the development of iron deficiency [14, 16] and blood loss during menstruation may further explain this greater prevalence. Although menstrual blood loss in a single woman is very constant during menarche and throughout the fertile life, there is a large variation in blood loss among women [68]. Thus, in a mean cycle length of 28 days, menstrual blood loss may vary by as much as 26 - 44 ml, with a corresponding daily iron loss of about 0.5 - 0.7 mg [9, 76]. This great variation in blood and iron loss reported by these two studies could be associated with an extensive use of oral contraceptives which are known to reduce the amount of blood loss during menstruation [77]. Finally, menstrual iron loss in women has been shown to negatively correlate with serum Ferr, and iron status to significantly correlate with the duration and intensity of the menses in endurance athletes [19]. Taking into consideration the iron loss during menstruation along with the relative failure to achieve the daily RDI for iron the greater frequency of iron deficiency in female athletes can be justified.

7. Iron supplementation and exercise-induced alterations of iron status

7.1. Iron supplementation in iron-deficient individuals

Whether the increased uptake of iron through diet or supplements improves iron status in athletes is still under debate. This is mainly due to the great divergence of iron doses, intervention period, population, and exercise regimens used between studies. In situations of iron deficiency a proposed minimum therapeutic requirement corresponds to 100 mg/day of elemental iron, for a period of 12 weeks [17]. However, in several studies, much lower quantities of 20 - 50 mg/day of elemental iron for 12 weeks [10, 35] or smaller duration (of even two weeks) of iron supplementation have also been used and reported to be adequate to restore iron status to normal [78]. Table 3 summarizes the effects of iron supplementation on several indices of iron status.

A treatment with 100 mg/day of ferrous iron for 3 months, significantly increased the values of serum Ferr (from 34±11 to 54±18 µg/L) and liver iron (from 105±42 to 227±67 µg/g liver) [4]. In this study, 23 out of 45 athletes showed decreased baseline serum values (<35µg/L), and the typical iron deficiency in runners was confirmed in a subgroup of eight athletes in which iron metabolism was studied in detail using radio-iron labelling and liver iron quantification. These eight athletes showed up-regulated ^{59}Fe absorption and a decreased liver iron concentration as compared to a control group. The results of the eight athletes confirm that in cases of true iron deficiency, iron absorption is greater.

A moderate dose of 39 mg/day of elemental iron for 5 weeks effectively prevented the negative changes of iron status over the course of a competitive season in female collegiate swimmers

[35]. Absence of iron supplementation resulted in decreased Hb levels despite mean dietary iron intakes of 16.3 mg/day.

The ingestion of 105 mg/day of elemental iron combined with 500 mg of Vitamin C for 60 days resulted in the amelioration of iron status of previously iron-depleted, non-anemic elite female athletes [79]. The improved iron stores were reflected by the increase of Ferr in conjunction with the decrease of transferrin, sTfR and sTfR/log ferritin index.

Taken together the aforementioned results suggest that the initial stage of either iron sufficiency or iron deficiency, combined with the amount of iron ingested, plays a critical role in the absorption of iron from diet or supplementation.

7.2. Iron supplementation in individuals with normal iron status

Supplementation of iron is commonly used, not only in iron-deficient athletes, but also in athletes with normal iron status. The rationale behind this practice dictates that supplementation will preserve or enhance their performance. This concept is probably based on the catalytic role of iron on the oxygen transport and optimal function of oxidative enzymes and proteins during exercise. The hypothesis could be that with increased consumption of iron, the above mechanisms would be reinforced and exercise performance would be improved. Nevertheless, unlike the numerous studies addressing iron-deficient individuals, only few [25, 57, 63] have focused in iron-sufficient athletes.

The response of iron stores during a sports season was assessed in professional football players with normal iron stores at the beginning of the season [57]. The players consumed 50 mg/day of elemental iron over two periods during the training season. Supplementation took part for 15 days prior to the beginning of the season and 15 days during the middle season. Blood was collected three times during the season, one following the first supplementation period, another following the second supplementation period and a third time at the end of the season, where no iron supplementation had occurred. Ferritin, as well as calculated iron stores, showed a significant reduction at the end of the season which coincided with the absence of iron supplementation. In contrast, Ferr and iron store levels remained stable following supplementation regardless of the intensive training.

In another study, non-anemic, non-iron-deficient adolescent male and female swimmers aged 12-17 years old were either supplemented with 47 mg of elemental iron daily or consumed a diet rich in iron [25]. Both approaches failed to affect the athletes' iron status. In that study, despite the significant fluctuations during the six months of training, iron levels, TS and Ferr levels were similar at the end of the study as compared to baseline values. The authors attributed the failure of high iron intake to affect iron status to homeostatic mechanisms such as iron absorption. It could also be suggested that the quantity of elemental iron was not enough to improve iron status and that higher doses of iron are needed to achieve a favorable change in iron status. The younger age and the possible higher demands in reference [25] compared with that of reference [57], may have influenced the absorption of iron that resulted in different responses in these two studies.

Studies	Study protocol	Subjects	Estimated Indices	Results
Improvement in iron status				
Nachtigal et al. (1996)	100mg/d of elemental iron for 3 months, radio-iron labeling (^{59}Fe) in 8 iron deficient athletes	45 runners (23 out of 45 were iron deficient, Ferr<35 µg /L), and controls	Ferr, liver iron, iron absorption	Ferr: ↑ from 34±11 to 54±18 µg/L; liver Fe: ↑from 105 ±42 to 227±67 µg/g liver
Brigham et al. (1993)	39mg/d of elemental iron (IG) or placebo (PG) for 5 wks	25 female, iron depleted, varsity collegiate swimmers	Hb, Ferr	Hb:↑ in 24% of the subjects in the IG and in 12% in PG. Ferr: ↑ in 68% of the subjects in the IG and in 4% in PG
Pitsis et al. (2004)	105mg/d elemental iron + 500mg/d Vit C for 60 days	36 elite iron-depleted, non-anemic female athletes of several disciplines (13-26yo)	Red cell and reticulocyte parameters, Fe, Ferr, Tf, TS, sTfR	Ferr: ↑; Tf: ↓; sTfR: ↓; sTfR/ log Ferr: ↓ Red cell and reticulocyte parameters: no changes
Rowland et al. (1987)	Estimation of iron status during a competitive season; supplementation of iron in the iron deficient athletes (IG) in the midpoint of the season (the dose is not reported)	30 male and 20 female cross country runners (14.3-18.6yo)	Ferr, Hb, RBC, MCV, RBCDW,	Ferr: ↑in IG and ↓in untreated athletes at the end of the season; Hb, RBC, MCV, RBCDW: no changes
Escanero et al. (1997)	Variation of iron metabolism through a season; 50mg of iron/day for the last 15 days at the beginning (A) and the middle of (B), but not at the end (C) the season	9 soccer players at the 1st division (24±2.1yo)	RBC, MCV, MCH, MCHC, Fe, Tf, Ferr, TIBC, TS	Ferr, Iron stores: ↓at the end of the season (no iron supplement); remained stable at the beginning and the middle of the season (iron supplementation)
Improvement of performance				
Friedmann et al. (2001)	2 x 100mg/d elemental iron (IG) or placebo (PG) for 12 wks; the usual training	40 iron depleted endurance athletes (13.6-21.1yo, Ferr < 20 ng/mL) IG: 20 males and females (PG: 20	Hematological indices, Fe, Ferr, Trf, TS, BV, PV, VO$_2$, VCO$_2$, VE, MAOD, LA	IG: VO$_{2max}$, VO$_2$, TTE: ↑; Ferr: ↑ 20.1µg/ L, Tf: ↓ PG: no changes

Studies	Study protocol	Subjects	Estimated Indices	Results
		females and 8 males 14.5 -17.5yo)		
Rowland et al. (1988)	975mg/day ferrous sulfate (IG) or placebo (PG) for 4 wks (time C), after a 4wk control period (time B)	14 iron-deficient (Ferr < 20ng/mL) female cross-country runners (high-school age)	TTE, HR, VO_{2max}, VE, Hb, MCV, RBCDW, Ferr	TTE: ↑in both groups at time B, ↑ in IG and ↓in PG at time C; Ferr: ↓at time B in both groups, ↑at time C in IG; Hb, MCV, RBCDW: No changes in both groups
No changes in iron status or performance				
Peeling et al. (2007)	Intramuscular iron injections (5 x 2mL Ferrum H/day) (IG) or placebo for 20 days	16 iron depleted, female distance runners and controls	VO_{2max}, HR, LA, run-TTE, 10min submaximal economy test, Ferr	Ferr: ↑in IG; HR, LA, TTE: no differences between IG and PG
Tsalis et al. (2004)	47mg/d (IG) or dietary plan rich in iron (DIG) or regular diet for 6 months (endurance training: 3m; power training: 2m; tapering: 1m)	21 males and 21 females, 12-17yo, non-anemic, non-iron-deficient	Hematological indices; Fe, TIBC, TS, Ferr; swimming tests: 2000m, 800m, 200m and 25m sprint	Fe, TIBC, TS, Ferr: fluctuations within the phases; At m6: no differences from baseline; RBC, Hb and PVC: ↑at m6; performance tests: similar ↑in all groups
Klingshirn et al. (1992)	8wks of iron supplementation (IG), or placebo (PG)	18 iron depleted, female distance runners and controls 22-39yo	VO_{2max}, endurance run-TTE, LA, iron status	Ferr, TIBC: ↑ in IG compared with PG at wk 8 Endurance performance, LA: similar ↑ both groups
Powell & Tucker (1991)	130mg of elemental iron /day (IG) or placebo (PG), for 2wks; single blind design	10 female cross-country runners (20.2±1.3yo) with normal iron status	VO_{2max}, CO2, RER, VE, Fe, TIBC, Ferr, Hp, Hb, Hct, MCHC, MCV, WCC, LA	Hematological & iron status parameters: no significant changes; Metabolic parameters: no changes

VO_{2max}: Maximal Oxygen Consumption, VCO_2: Exhaled Carbon Dioxide, VE: Ventilation, MAOD: Maximal Accumulated Oxygen Deficit, TTE: Time to Exhaustion, HR: Heart Rate, CK: Creatine Kinase, LA: Lactate, Ferr: Ferritin, Fe: Iron, Tf: Transferrin, TS: Transferrin Saturation, sTfR: Soluble Transferrin Receptor, TIBC: Total Iron Binding Capacity, Hb: Haemoglobin, Hct: Hematocrit, PCV: Packed Cell Volume, MCHC: Mean Corpuscular Haemoglobin Concentration, BV: Blood volume, PV: Plasma Volume, MCV: Mean Corpuscular Volumes, RBC: Red Blood Cells Count, RBCDW: Red Blood Cell Distribution Width, WCC: White Cells Count, MAOD: Maximal Accumulated Oxygen Deficit

Table 3. The effect of dietary or supplemented iron on exercise-induced changes of iron status and physical performance

8. Iron supplementation and physical performance

8.1. Iron supplementation in iron-deficient individuals

There is no doubt that iron-deficiency anemia, which amongst other indicators (e.g. Ferr<12μg/L, TS<16%), is characterized by a decline in blood Hb concentration, clearly impairs physical performance by limiting oxygen transport to exercising muscles [22]. However, the need for iron supplementation in cases of depleted iron stores without observed anemia for optimal physical performance is still under debate (Table 3). Some studies have shown that iron supplementation improved physical performance [23, 24], whereas others report no alterations following iron supplementation [25, 34, 63].

The improvement of iron status due to iron supplementation has been accompanied by an improvement in endurance capacity [23, 24]. In young elite athletes with normal Hb concentrations, the return of low Ferr to normal values following supplementation of 200 mg/day of elemental iron for 12 weeks, even in the absence of increased erythropoiesis, has been shown to improve maximal aerobic capacity [23].

Iron supplementation also prevented the decline in performance that was associated with the progressive reduction of serum Ferr levels [24]. Iron deficient cross-country female runners were treated with 975 mg/d of ferrous sulfate or placebo for 4 weeks. Iron supplementation resulted in an increase in ferritin levels which was accompanied by an improvement of physical performance. Subjects not receiving iron therapy exhibited a decline in their performance [24].

Besides the aforementioned positive results in exercise performance there are studies reporting no beneficial effects due to iron supplementation [25, 34, 63]. In reference [63], no significant improvement of iron status or metabolic parameters related to running performance was found after 2 weeks of 130 mg elemental iron supplementation in non-anemic, iron-deficient female cross-country runners. Likewise, in [34], 8 weeks of iron supplementation in iron-depleted, non-anemic female distance runners, resulted in similar improvement of the endurance capacity in the supplemented and the placebo group, despite the improved iron status in the iron-supplemented group. In another study, the injection of 2 mL of Ferrum H (100mg of elemental iron) five times daily for 10 days did not result in any beneficial outcomes on submaximal economy, VO_{2max} and time to fatigue in non-anemic, iron-deficient female runners [33]. This study, failed to demonstrate any beneficial effect of iron supplementation on aerobic capacity, despite a significant rise in serum Ferr levels (from 19 to 65μg/L).

8.2. Iron supplementation in individuals with normal iron status

In one of the very few studies that used healthy, non-iron-depleted and non-anemic adolescent swimmers, the enhanced iron intake either through supplement or diet ranging from one to five times the RDA, did not change iron status or result in favorable changes of physical performance [25]. The authors attributed the observed fluctuations over the training period of six months to the different demands of each training phase irrespective of iron treatment. These observations strengthen the notion that the initial levels of iron status are of critical importance in the improvement of physical performance as a result of iron supplementation.

In [35], the mean dietary intake of 16.3 mg/day was not adequate to prevent the disturbance of iron status in female collegiate swimmers. Haemoglobin levels decreased at about 6 g/L in 44% of the athletes given placebo treatment, whereas the corresponding decrement in plasma Ferr was 5µg/L in 24% of the swimmers given the iron supplement. Consequently, the reductions in Hb and Ferr levels were lower in the athletes that were under iron supplementation.

9. Future research

Although the favorable effects of iron supplementation on physical capacity in iron-deficient anemic athletes has been well established, relatively little research has been conducted addressing iron-deficient non-anemic athletes. Therefore, further research is needed to clarify the necessity of iron supplementation in athletes with depleted iron stores, yet, normal Hb concentrations for improvement of their performance.

Despite the great importance of iron balance in athletes, no normative data for athletes exist and hence it is essential such norms are established. Such data would be more critical if appropriate discriminations were made, e.g. regarding the type of training (endurance or power-training athletes), sex, age, or seasonal demands and so on.

The commonly used parameters for the estimation of iron status in the general population (Hb, Hct, Ferr, iron concentration, TIBC, TS), may not always be adequately representative for athletes. Therefore, it would be useful if future studies incorporated additional parameters such as erythrocyte protoporphyrin, soluble transferrin receptor or haptoglobin, in order to get more accurate and complete estimation of iron status.

10. Conclusions

Iron is one of the most important elements for health and exercise performance. It is unclear whether iron intake by an athlete through diet is adequate in order to prevent iron balance disturbances and further research is needed to clarify dietary methods to prevent iron deficiency. It seems that exercise, acute or chronic, results in significant disturbances in iron balance due to different reasons. Changes in iron absorption and iron intake due to exercise, iron losses through the gastrointestinal tract, intravascular hemolysis, and to a lesser extent iron losses through sweat, are probable mechanisms for iron balance disturbances during exercise.

Alterations in iron status balance are reported as a result of exercise, especially in endurance trained, and women athletes. Iron-deficiency without anemia is a very commonly reported phenomenon among athletes, and occasionally iron deficiency anemia is also reported.

Iron balance is of great importance for optimal work capacity, and a compromise of iron status would have detrimental effects on physical performance in iron-depleted anemic athletes. In these situations, iron supplementation is required for restoration of iron levels and optimization of the athlete's performance and health. However, similar effects have not been well documented for athletes that are iron-deficient without the presence of anemia. Nevertheless, iron supplementation among athletes is a very common practice, despite the discrepancy regarding its beneficial effects in non-anemic, iron-depleted, or even normal iron status athletes. This discrepancy is attributed to the divergence in iron doses, athletic population, and the great variance in the intervention period, and exercise regimens that are used between studies.

Because of the different demands in iron through the several phases of training or competitive periods, evaluation of iron status of the athletes should be performed at the beginning, at the midpoint, and finally at the end of the season. Controlled iron supplementation for all athletes with serum Ferr below 35μg/L is recommended for the replenishment of iron stores.

Author details

Chariklia K. Deli[1,2], Ioannis G. Fatouros[2,3], Yiannis Koutedakis[1,2,4] and Athanasios Z. Jamurtas[1,2*]

*Address all correspondence to: ajamurt@pe.uth.gr

1 Department of Physical Education and Sport Science, University of Thessaly, Trikala, Greece

2 Institute of Human Performance and Rehabilitation, Center for Research and Technology - Thessaly, Trikala, Greece

3 Department of Physical Education and Sport Science, University of Thrace, Komotini, Greece

4 School of Sports, Performing Arts and Leisure, University of Wolverhampton, United Kingdom

References

[1] Fontecave M, Pierre JL. Iron - Metabolism, Toxicity and Therapy. Biochimie 1993;75(9): 767-773.

[2] Crichton RR, Ward RJ. An overview of iron metabolism: molecular and cellular criteria for the selection of iron chelators. Curr Med Chem 2003; 10(12): 997-1004.

[3] Bacic G, Spasojevic I, Secerov B, Mojovic M. Spin-trapping of oxygen free radicals in chemical and biological systems: new traps, radicals and possibilities. Spectrochim Acta A Mol Biomol Spectrosc 2008; 69(5): 1354-1366.

[4] Nachtigall D, Nielsen P, Fischer R, Engelhardt R, Gabbe EE. Iron deficiency in distance runners. A reinvestigation using Fe-labelling and non-invasive liver iron quantification. Int J Sports Med 1996; 17(7): 473-479.

[5] Stewart JG, Ahlquist DA, Mcgill DB, Ilstrup DM, Schwartz S, Owen, RA. Gastrointestinal Blood-Loss and Anemia in Runners. Annals of Internal Medicine 1984; 100(6): 843-845.

[6] de Oliveira EP, Burini RC. The impact of physical exercise on the gastrointestinal tract. Current Opinion in Clinical Nutrition and Metabolic Care 2009; 12: 533-553.

[7] Brune M, Magnusson B, Persson H, Hallberg L. Iron losses in sweat. Am J Clin Nutr 1986; 43: 438-443.

[8] DeRuisseau KC, Cheuvront SN, Haymes EM, Sharp RG. Sweat Iron and Zinc Losses During Prolonged Exercise. International Journal of Sport Nutrition and Exercise Metabolism 2002; 12: 428-437.

[9] Harvey LJ, Armah CN, Dainty JR, Foxall RJ, Lewis DJ, Langford NJ, Fairweather-Tait SJ. Impact of menstrual blood loss and diet on iron deficiency among women in the UK. British Journal of Nutrition 2005; 94(4): 557-564. doi: Doi 10.1079/Bjn20051493

[10] Lyle RM, Weaver CM, Sedlock DA, Rajaram S, Martin B, Melby CL. Iron status in exercising women: the effect of oral iron therapy vs increased consumption of muscle foods. Am J Clin Nutr 1992; 56(6): 1049-1055.

[11] Hurrell R, Egli I. Iron bioavailability and dietary reference values. Am J Clin Nutr 2010; 91(5): 1461S-1467S.

[12] Anschuetz S, Rodgers CD, Taylor AW. Meal Composition and Iron Status of Experienced Male and Female Distance Runners. J Exerc Sci Fit 2010; 8(1): 25-33.

[13] Herbert V. Recommended dietary intakes (RDI) of iron in humans. Am J Clin Nut 1987; 45(4): 679-686.

[14] Koehler K, Braun H, Achtzehn S, Hildebrand S, Predel HG, Mester J, Schnzer W. Iron status in elite young athletes: gender-dependent inXuences of diet and exercise. Eur J Appl Physiol 2012; 112(2): 513-523.

[15] Reinke S, Taylor WR, Duda GN, von Haehling S, Reinke P, Volk HD, Anker SD, Doehner W. Absolute and functional iron deficiency in professional athletes during training and recovery. Int J Cardiol 2012; 156(2): 186-191.

[16] Malczewska J. The Assessment of Frequency of Iron Deficiency in Athletes from the Transferrin Receptor-Ferritin Index. International Journal of Sports Nutrition and Exercise Metabolism 2001; 11: 42-52.

[17] Nielsen P, Nachtigall D. Iron supplementation in athletes. Current recommendations. Sports Med 1998; 26(4): 207-216.

[18] Malczewska J, Raczynski G. Iron status in male endurance athletes and in non-athletes. Biology of Sport 1997; 14(4): 259-273.

[19] Malczewska J, Raczynski G, Stupnicki R. Iron status in female endurance athletes and in non-athletes. International Journal of Sport Nutrition 2000; 10(3): 260-276.

[20] Magnusson B, Hallberg L, Rossander L, Swolin B. Iron-Metabolism and Sports Anemia .2. A Hematological Comparison of Elite Runners and Control Subjects. Acta Medica Scandinavica 1984; 216(2): 157-164.

[21] Beard JL. Iron biology in immune function, muscle metabolism and neuronal functioning. J Nutr 2001; 131: 2S-2.

[22] Rowland T. Iron Deficiency in Athletes: An Update. American Journal of Lifestyle Medicine 2012; OnlineFirst Version of Record. DOI: 10.1177/1559827611431541

[23] Friedmann B, Weller E, Mairbaurl H, Bartsch P. Effects of iron repletion on blood volume and performance capacity in young athletes. Medicine and Science in Sports and Exercise 2001; 33(5): 741-746.

[24] Rowland TW, Deisroth MB, Green GM, Kelleher JF. The Effect of Iron Therapy on the Exercise Capacity of Nonanemic Iron-Deficient Adolescent Runners. American Journal of Diseases of Children 1988; 142(2): 165-169.

[25] Tsalis G, Nikolaidis MD, Mougios V. Effects of Iron Intake Through Food or Supplement on Iron Status and Performance of Healthy Adolescent Suimmers During a Training Season. International Journal of Sports Medicine 2004; 25: 306-313.

[26] Dallman PR. Effects of Iron Deficiency Exclusive of Anemia. British joumal of Haematology 1978; 40: 179-184

[27] Hood DA, Kelton R, Nishio ML. Mitochondrial Adaptations to Chronic Muscle Use - Effect of Iron-Deficiency. Comparative Biochemistry and Physiology a-Physiology 1992; 101(3): 597-605.

[28] Beaton GH, Corey PN, Steele C. Conceptual and Methodological Issues Regarding the Epidemiology of Iron-Deficiency and Their Implications for Studies of the Functional Consequences of Iron-Deficiency. American Journal of Clinical Nutrition 1989; 50(3): 575-588.

[29] Beard J, Tobin B. Iron status and exercise. Am J Clin Nutr 2000; 72: 594-597.

[30] Friedmann B, Jost J, Rating T, Weller E, Werle E, Eckardt K-U, Bärtsch P, Mairbäurl H. Effects of Iron Supplementation on Total Body Hemoglobin During Endurance Training at Moderate Altitude. Int J Sports Med 1999; 20(2): 78-85.

[31] Chapman RF, Stray-Gundersen J, Levine BD. (). Individual variation in response to altitude training. J. Appl. Physiol 1998; 85(4): 1448-1456.

[32] Stray-Gundersen J, Alexander C, Hochstein A, deLemos D, Levine BD. Failure of red cell volume to increase with altitude exposure in iron deficient runners. Med. Sci. Sports Exerc 1992; 24: 90.

[33] Peeling P, Blee T, Goodman C, Dawson B, Claydon G, Beilby J, Prins A. Effect of iron injections on aerobic exercise performance of iron depleted female athletes. Int J Sport Nutr Ex Metab 2007; 17: 221-231.

[34] Klingshirn LA, Pate RR, Bourque SP, Davis JM, Sargent RG. Effect of Iron Supplementation on Endurance Capacity in Iron-Depleted Female Runners. Medicine and Science in Sports and Exercise 1992; 24(7): 819-824.

[35] Brigham DE, Beard J, Krimmel R, Kenney W. Changes in iron status during competitive season in female collegiate swimmers. Nutrition 1993; 9(5): 418-422.

[36] DellaValle DM, Haas JD. Impact of Iron Depletion Without Anemia on Performance in Trained Endurance Athletes at the Beginning of a Training Season: A Study of Female Collegiate Rowers. Int J Sport Nutr Exerc Metab 2011; 21(6): 501-506.

[37] CDC.Hemochromatosis: What every clinician and health care professional needs to know. CDC 2012; www.cdc.gov.

[38] Rossi E, Jeffrey GP. Clinical penetrance of C282Y homozygous HFE haemochromatosis. Clin Biochem Rev 2004; 25(3): 183-190.

[39] Worwood M. Indicators of the iron status of populations: ferritin. In WHO (Ed.) Assessing the Iron Status of populations. Second edition. Geneva, Switzerland: WHO; 2004.

[40] Lynch S. Indicators of the iron status of populations: red blood cell parameters. In WHO (Ed.) Assessing the Iron Status of populations. Second edition. Geneva, Switzerland: WHO; 2004

[41] Suominen P, Punnonen K, Rajamaki A, Irjala K. Serum transferrin receptor and transferrin receptor ferritin index identify healthy subjects with subclinical iron deficits. Blood 1998; 92(8): 2934-2939.

[42] Tietz NW. Clinical Guide to Laboratory Tests: Elsevier; 1995.

[43] Schumacher YO, Scmid A, Grathwohl D, Bultermann D, Berg A. Hematological indices and iron status in athletes of various sports and performances. Med. Sci. Sports Exerc. 2002; 34(5): 869-875.

[44] Zoller H, Vogel W. Iron supplementation in athletes - First do no harm. Nutrition 2004; 20(7-8): 615-619. doi: DOI 10.1016/j.nut.2004.04.006

[45] Hulthen L, Lindstedt G, Lundberg PA, Hallberg L. Effect of a mild infection on se-rum ferritin concentration - clinical and epidemiological implications. Eur J Clin Nutr 1998; 52(5): 376-379.

[46] Elin RJ, Wolff SM, Finch CA. Effect of Induced Fever on Serum Iron and Ferritin Concentrations in Man. Blood 1977; 49(1): 147-153.

[47] Hallberg L, Hulthen L. High serum ferritin is not identical to high iron stores. Ameri-can Journal of Clinical Nutrition 2003; 78(6): 1225-1226.

[48] Beard J. Indicators of the iron status of populations: free erythrocyte protoporphyrin and zinc protoporphyrin; serum and plasma iron, total iron binding capacity and transferrin saturation; and serum transferrin receptor. In WHO (Ed.) Assessing the Iron Status of populations.Second edition. Geneva, Switzerland: WHO; 2004

[49] Borel MJ, Smith SM, Derr J, Beard JL. Day-to-Day Variation in Iron-Status Indexes in Healthy-Men and Women. American Journal of Clinical Nutrition 1991; 54(4): 729-735.

[50] Labbe RF, Vreman HJ, Stevenson DK. Zinc protoporphyrin: A metabolite with a mis-sion. Clinical Chemistry 1999; 45(12): 2060-2072.

[51] Labbe RF, Dewanji A. Iron assessment tests: transferrin receptor vis-a-vis zinc proto-porphyrin. Clinical Biochemistry 2004; 37(3): 165-174.

[52] Romslo I, Talstad I. Day-to-Day Variations in Serum Iron, Serum Iron-Binding Ca-pacity, Serum Ferritin and Erythrocyte Protoporphyrin Concentrations in Anemic Subjects. European Journal of Haematology 1988; 40(1): 79-82.

[53] Skikne BS, Flowers CH, Cook JD. Serum Transferrin Receptor - a Quantitative Meas-ure of Tissue Iron-Deficiency. Blood 1990; 75(9): 1870-1876.

[54] Baynes RD. Assessment of iron status. Clinical Biochemistry 1996; 29(3): 209-215.

[55] Schumacher YO, Schmid A, Konig D, Berg A. Effects of exercise on soluble transfer-rin receptor and other variables of the iron status. British Journal of Sports Medicine 2002; 36(3): 195-199.

[56] Spodaryk K. Hematological and Iron-Related Parameters of Male Endurance and Strength Trained Athletes. European Journal of Applied Physiology and Occupation-al Physiology 1993; 67(1): 66-70.

[57] [57]. Escanero JF, Villanueva J, Rojo A, Herrera A, DelDiego ., Guerra M. Iron stores in professional athletes throughout the sports season. Physiology & Behavior 1997; 62(4): 811-814.

[58] Rowland TW, Black SA, Kelleher JF. Iron-Deficiency in Adolescent Endurance Ath-letes. Journal of Adolescent Health 1987; 8(4): 322-326.

[59] Gropper SS, Blessing D, Dcinham K, Barksdale JM. Iron status of female collegiate athletes involved in different sports. Biological Trace Element Research 2006; 109(1): 1-13.

[60] Nickerson HJ, Holubets MC, Weiler BR, Haas RG, Schwartz S, Ellefson ME. Causes of Iron-Deficiency in Adolescent Athletes. Journal of Pediatrics 1989; 114(4): 657-663.

[61] Rogers G, Goodman C, Mitchell D, Hattingh J. The Response of Runners to Arduous Triathlon Competition. European Journal of Applied Physiology and Occupational Physiology 1986; 55(4): 405-409.

[62] Institute of Medicine. Dietary Reference Intakes for Vitamin A, Vitamin K, Arsenic, Boron, Chromium, Copper, Iodine, Iron, Molybdenum, Nickel, Silicon, Vanadium, and Zinc. Food,and Nutrition Board. National Academy: Press; 2001

[63] Powell PD, Tucker A. Iron supplementation and running performance in female cross-country runners. Int J Sports Med 1991; 12(5): 462-467.

[64] Siegel AJ. Exercise-Related Hematuria - Reply. Jama-Journal of the American Medical Association 1979; 242(15): 1610-1610.

[65] Choi SC, Choi SJ, Kim JA, Kim TH, Nah Y, Etsuro Y, Evans DF. The role of gastrointestinal endoscopy in long-distance runners with gastrointestinal symptoms. European Journal of Gastrenterology & Hepatology 2001; 13: 1089-1094.

[66] Gaudin C, Zerath E, Guezennec CY. Gastric-Lesions Secondary to Long-Distance Running. Digestive Diseases and Sciences 1990; 35(10): 1239-1243.

[67] Mccabe ME, Peura DA, Kadakia SC, Bocek Z, Johnson LF. Gastrointestinal Blood-Loss Associated with Running a Marathon. Digestive Diseases and Sciences 1986; 31(11): 1229-1232.

[68] Hallberg L, Rossanderhulten L. Iron Requirements in Menstruating Women. American Journal of Clinical Nutrition 1991; 54(6): 1047-1058.

[69] Qamar MI, Read AE. Effects of Exercise on Mesenteric Blood-Flow in Man. Gut 1987; 28(5): 583-587.

[70] Otte JA, Oostveen E, Geelkerken RH, Groeneveld ABJ, Kolkman JJ. Exercise induces gastric ischemia in healthy volunteers: a tonometry study. Journal of Applied Physiology 2001; 91(2): 866-871.

[71] Green R, Charlton R, Seftel H, Bothwell T. Body Iron Excretion in Man. A Collaborative Study. American Journal of Medicine 1968; (45): 336-353.

[72] Jacob RA, Sandstead HH, Munoz JM, Klevay LM, Milne DB. Whole-Body Surface Loss of Trace-Metals in Normal Males. American Journal of Clinical Nutrition 1981; 34(7): 1379-1383.

[73] Sureira TM, Amancio OS, Braga JAP. Influence of Artistic Gymnastics on Iron Nutritional Status and Exercise-Induced Hemolysis in Female Athletes. International Journal of Sport Nutrition and Exercise Metabolism 2012; 22: 243 -250.

[74] Telford RD, Sly GJ, Hahn AG, Cunningham RB, Bryant C, Smith JA. Footstrike is the major cause of hemolysis during running. Journal of Applied Physiology 2003; 94(1): 38-42.

[75] Selby GB, Eichner ER. Endurance Swimming, Intravascular Hemolysis, Anemia, and Iron Depletion - New Perspective on Athletes Anemia. American Journal of Medicine 1986; 81(5): 791-794.

[76] Hallberg L, Hogdahl, A, Nilsson L, Rybo G. Menstrual blood loss - A Population study Acta obst. et gynec. scandinav 1966; 45: 320-351.

[77] Larsson G, Milsom I, Lindstedt G, Rybo G. The Influence of a Low-Dose Combined Oral-Contraceptive on Menstrual Blood-Loss and Iron Status. Contraception 1992; 46(4): 327-334.

[78] Schoene RB, Escourrou P, Robertson HT, Nilson KL, Parsons JR, Smith NJ. Iron Repletion Decreases Maximal Exercise Lactate Concentrations in Female Athletes with Minimal Iron-Deficiency Anemia. Journal of Laboratory and Clinical Medicine 1983; 102(2): 306-312.

[79] Pitsis GC, Fallon KE, Fallon SK, Fazakerley R. Response of soluble transferrin receptor and iron-related parameters to iron supplementation in elite, iron-depleted, nonanemic female athletes. Clinical Journal of Sport Medicine 2004; 14(5): 300-304.

Chapter 5

Exercise and Immunity

Hilde Grindvik Nielsen

Additional information is available at the end of the chapter

1. Introduction

Epidemiological evidence suggests a link between the intensity of the exercise and the occurrence of infections and diseases. The innate immune system appears to respond to chronic stress of intensive exercise by increased natural killer cell activity and suppressed neutrophil function. The measured effects of exercise on the innate immune system are complex and depend on several factors: the type of exercise, intensity and duration of exercise, the timing of measurement in relation to the exercise session, the dose and type of immune modulator used to stimulate the cell *in vitro* or *in vivo*, and the site of cellular origin. When comparing immune function in trained and non-active persons, the adaptive immune system is largely unaffected by exercise.

Physical activity in combination with infections is usually associated with certain medical risks, partly for the person who is infected and partly for the other athletes who may be infected. The risk of infection is greatest in team sports, but also in other sports where athletes have close physical contact before, during and after training and competitions.

This chapter starts with a short introduction of the immune system followed by a description of free radicals' and antioxidants' role in the immune system and how they are affected by physical activity. The chapter will also focus on need of antioxidant supplementation in combination with physical activity. The different theories regarding the effect of physical activity on the immune system will be discussed, along with advantages and disadvantages of being active, and finally effects of physical activity on the immune system are described.

2. The immune system

The immune system is large and complex and has a wide variety of functions. The main role of the immune system is to defend people against germs and microorganisms. Researchers are constantly making new discoveries by studying the immune system. There are several factors which influence or affect the daily functioning of the immune system: age, gender, eating habits, medical status, training and fitness level.

Bacteria and viruses can do harm to our body and make us sick. The immune system does a great job in keeping people healthy and preventing infections, but problems with the immune system can still lead to illness and infections. The immune system is separated in two functional divisions: the innate immunity, referred to as the first line of defense, and the acquired immunity, which, when activated, produces a specific reaction and immunological memory to each infectious agent.

2.1. The innate immune system

The innate immune system consists of anatomic and physiological barriers (skin, mucous membranes, body temperature, low pH and special chemical mediators such as complement and interferon) and specialized cells (natural killer cells and phagocytes, including neutrophils, monocytes and macrophages [1] (Table 1). When the innate immune system fails to effectively combat an invading pathogen, the body produces a learned immune response.

INNATE IMMUNITY		ADAPTIVE IMMUNITY	
Physical barriers	Epithelial cell barriers	Humoral	Antibody
	Mucus		Memory
Chemical barriers	Complement	Cell-mediated	Lymphocytes
	Lysozyme		T cells
	pH of body fluids		B cells
	Acute phase proteins		
White blood cells	Monocytes/macrophages		
	Granulocytes		
	Natural killer cells		

Table 1. Innate and adaptive immunity (Source: Modified after Mackinnon, 1999).

Leukocytes (also known as white blood cells) form a component of the blood. They are mainly produced in the bone marrow and help to defend the body against infectious disease and foreign materials as part of the immune system. There are normally between $4x10^9$ and $11x10^9$ white blood cells in a liter of healthy adult blood [2] (Table 2). The leukocytes circulate through the body and seek out their targets. In this way, the immune system works in a coordinated manner to monitor the body for substances that might cause problems. There are two basic types of leukocytes; the phagocytes, which are cells that chew up invading organisms, and the lymphocytes, which allow the body to remember and recognize previous invaders [1].

The granulocytes (a type of phagocyte that has small granules visible in the cytoplasm) consist of polymorphonuclear cells (PMN) which are subdivided into three classes; neutrophils, basophils, and eosinophils (Table 2). The neutrophils are the most abundant white blood cells, they account for 65 to 70% of all leukocytes [2]. When activated, the neutrophils marginate and undergo selectin-dependent capture followed by integrin-dependent adhesion, before migrating into tissues. Leukocytes migrate toward the sites of infection or inflammation, and undergo a process called chemotaxis. Chemotaxis is the cells' movement towards certain chemicals in their environment.

Granulocytes along with monocytes protect us against bacteria and other invading organisms, a process that is called phagocytosis (ingestion). Only cells participating in the phagocytosis are called phagocytes. The granulocytes are short lived. After they are released from the bone marrow they can circulate in the blood for 4 to 8 hours. Then they leave the blood and enter into the tissues and can live there for 3 to 4 days. If the body is exposed for serious infections, they live even shorter. The numbers of granulocytes in the blood depends on the release of mature granulocytes from the bone marrow and the body's need for an increased number of granulocytes (i.e. during infection). The neutrophil granulocytes are very important in the fight against infections. If a bacterial infection occurs, the neutrophils travel to the infected area and neutralize the invading bacteria. In those cases, the total number of neutrophil granulocytes is high. The eosinophil granulocytes do not phagocytize and are more important in allergic reactions. The same is the case with the basophil granulocytes; they contain histamine and heparin and are also involved in allergic reactions.

Monocytes (another type of white blood cell) are produced by the bone marrow from hematopoietic stem cell precursors called monoblasts. Monocytes make up between 3 and 8% of the leukocytes in the blood [2], and circulate in the blood for about 1 to 3 days before moving into tissues throughout the body. Monocytes are, like the neutrophil granulocytes, effective phagocytes, and are responsible for phagocytosis of foreign substances in the body. When the monocytes leave the blood barrier, they differentiate in the tissues and their size and characteristics change. These cells are named macrophages. Macrophages are responsible for protecting tissues from foreign substances but are also known to be the predominant cells involved in triggering atherosclerosis. Macrophages are cells that possess a large smooth nucleus, a large area of cytoplasm and many internal vesicles for processing foreign material.

Cells	Amount (cell/µL)
Leukocytes	4 500 – 11 000
-Neutrophils	4 000 – 7 000
-Lymphocytes	2 500 – 5 000
-Monocytes	100 – 1 000
-Eosinophils	0 – 500
-Basophils	0 - 100

Table 2. Normal values of circulating blood cell levels. Rhoades, 2003.

2.2. The acquired immune system

The second kind of protection is called adaptive (or active) immunity [2]. This type of immunity develops throughout our lives. Adaptive immunity involves the lymphocytes and develops from early childhood. Adults are exposed to diseases or are immunized against diseases through vaccination. The main cells involved in acquired immunity are the lymphocytes, and there are two kinds of them: B lymphocytes and T lymphocytes; both are capable of secreting a large variety of specialized molecules (antibodies and cytokines) to regulate the immune response. T lymphocytes can also be engaged in direct cell-on-cell warfare (Table 1). Lymphocytes start out in the bone marrow where they reside and mature into B cells. Lymphocytes can also leave and travel to the thymus gland and mature into T cells. B lymphocytes and T lymphocytes have separate functions: B lymphocytes are like the body's military intelligence system, seeking out their targets and organizing defenses, while T cells are like the soldiers, destroying the invaders that the intelligence system has identified [1].

3. C-Reactive Protein (CRP)

C-reactive protein (CRP) is an acute phase protein presented in the blood and rises in response to inflammation. Its physiological role is to bind to phosphocholine expressed on the surface of dead or dying cells to activate the complement system. The complement system is the name of a group of plasma proteins, which are produced by the liver, and is an important part of the innate immune system. The complement system has an important role in the fight against bacteria and virus infections.

A blood test is commonly used in the diagnosis of infections. The level of CRP rises when an inflammatory reaction starts in the body. Blood for analysis may be taken by a finger prick and can be analyzed quickly. The level of CRP increases in many types of inflammatory reactions, both infections, autoimmune diseases and after cellular damage. After an infection, it takes almost half a day before the CRP increase becomes measurable. During the healing process the level of CRP decreases in a relatively short time (½h ~ 12-24 hours in the blood).

The levels of CRP increase more during bacterial infections than viral and can thus be used to distinguish between these two types of infections. Bacterial infection can increase CRP to over 100 mg/L, while during viral infections the values are usually below 50 mg/L. This distinction between bacteria and viruses are often useful because antibiotics (such as penicillin) have no effect on viral infections, but can often be very useful in bacterial infections.

Recent investigations suggest that physical activity reduce CRP levels. Higher levels of physical activity and cardiorespiratory fitness are consistently associated with 6 to 35% lower CRP levels [3]. Longitudinal training studies have demonstrated reductions in CRP concentration from 16 to 41%, an effect that may be independent of baseline levels of CRP, body composition, and weight loss [3].

The mechanisms behind the role physical activity plays in reducing inflammation and suppressing CRP levels are not well defined [4]. Chronic physical activity is associated with reduced resting CRP levels due to multiple mechanisms including: decreased cytokine production by adipose tissue, skeletal muscles, endothelial and blood mononuclear cells, improved endothelial function and insulin sensitivity, and possibly an antioxidant effect [4]. A short-term increase in serum CRP has been observed after strenuous exercise [4]. This is due to an exercise-induced acute phase response, facilitated by the cytokine system, mainly through interleukin- 6 (IL-6). Exercise training may influence this response, whereas there is also a homeostatic, anti-inflammatory counter-acute phase response after strenuous exercise.

The most common infections in sports medicine are caused by bacteria or viruses. Infections are very common, particularly infections in the upper respiratory tract [5]. Asthma/airway hyper-responsiveness (AHR) is the most common chronic medical condition in endurance trained athletes (prevalence of about 8% in both summer and winter athletes) [6]. Inspiring polluted or cold air is considered a significant aetiological factor in some but not all sports people [6]. The symptoms of infections are healthy, which means that the body is reacting normally. The common cold is generally caused by virus infections and is self-healing and most of the times free of problems, but sometimes bacteria will follow and cause complications (e.g. ear infections). Mononucleosis ("kissing disease") and throat infections are usually caused by various viruses. Infections in the heart muscle (myocarditis) can be due to both virus and bacteria and represent a problematic area within the field of sports medicine [7].

4. Cytokines

Cytokines are substances secreted by certain immune system cells that carry signals locally between cells, and thus have an effect on other cells. Cytokines are the signaling molecules used extensively in cellular communication. The term cytokine encompasses a large and diverse family of polypeptide regulators that are produced widely throughout the body by cells of diverse embryological origin.

A pro-inflammatory cytokine is a cytokine which promotes systemic inflammation, while an anti-inflammatory cytokine refers to the property of a substance or treatment that reduces inflammation. TNF-α, IL-1β and IL-8 are some examples of pro-inflammatory cytokines. IL-6 and IL-10 belong to the anti-inflammatory category. IL-6 can be both pro-inflammatory and anti-inflammatory.

Heavy physical activity produces a rapid transient increase in cytokine production and entails increases in both pro-inflammatory (IL-2, IL-5, IL-6, IL-8, TNFα) and anti-inflammatory (IL-1ra, IL-10) cytokines. Interleukin-6 (IL-6) is the most studied cytokine associated with physical exercise [8]. Many studies have investigated the effects of different forms and intensities of exercise on its plasma concentration and tissue expression [9-11]. The effects of physical exercise seem to be mediated by intensity [10] as well as the duration of effort, the muscle mass involved and the individual's physical fitness level [12].

Increases in IL-6 over 100 times above resting values have been found after exhaustive exercise such as marathon races, moderate exercise (60–65% VO_{2max}) and after resistance exercise, and may last for up to 72 h after the end of the exercise [13]. One explanation for the increase in IL-6 after exhaustive exercise is that IL-6 is produced by the contracting muscle and is released in large quantities into the circulation. Studies have shown that prolonged exercise may increase circulating neutrophils' ability to produce reactive oxygen metabolites, but the release of IL-6 after exercise has been associated with neutrophil mobilization and priming of the oxidative activity [14]. Free radical damaging effects on cellular functions are for IL-6 seen as a key mediator of the exercise-induced immune changes [13].

5. Free radicals

Free radicals are any atom with an unpaired electron. Reactive oxygen species (ROS) are all free radicals that involve oxygen. ROS formation is a natural ongoing process that takes place in the body, while the antioxidant defense is on duty for collecting and neutralizing the excess production of oxygen radicals. Many sources of heat, stress, irradiation, inflammation, and any increase in metabolism including exercise, injury, and repair processes lead to increased production of ROS [15]. ROS have an important function in the signal network of cellular processes, including growth and apoptosis, and as killing tools of phagocytising cells [15]. The granulocytes and the monocytes produce ROS like superoxide anion (O_2^-), hydrogen peroxide (H_2O_2), peroxynitrite ($ONOO^-$), and hydroxyl radical (OH).

Superoxide anion (O_2^-), an unstable free radical that kills bacteria directly, is produced through the nicotinamide adenine dinucleotide phosphate (NADPH) oxidase-mediated oxidative burst reaction [16]. The superoxide anion also participates in the generation of secondary free radical reactions to generate other potent antimicrobial agents, *e.g.*, hydrogen peroxide [16]. Superoxide anion is generated in both intra- and extracellular compartments and when nitric oxide (NO) and O_2^- react with each other, peroxynitrite ($ONOO^-$) can form very rapidly [17]. Peroxynitrite is a strong oxidation which damages DNA, proteins and other cellular elements. The stability of $ONOO^-$ allows it to diffuse through cells and hit a distant target. Intracellular $ONOO^-$ formation will usually minimize by increased intracellular superoxide dismutase (SOD) activity [17] (Figure 1).

Regular physical activity and exercise at moderate levels are important factors for disease prevention [18]. Strenuous exercise leads to the activation of several cell lines within the immune system, such as neutrophils, monocytes, and macrophages, which all are capable of producing ROS [19]. During resting conditions, the human body produces ROS to a level which is within the body's capacity to produce antioxidants. During endurance exercise, there is a 15- to 20-fold increase in whole body oxygen consumption, and the oxygen uptake in the active muscles increases 100- to 200-fold [20]. This elevation in oxygen consumption is thought to result in the production of ROS at rates that exceed the body's capacity to detoxify them. Oxidative stress is a result of an imbalance between the production of ROS and the body's ability to detoxify the reactions (producing antioxidants). In the literature, there is disagreement whether or not oxidative stress and subsequent damage associated with exercise is harmful or not. This ambiguity may partly be explained by the methods chosen for the different investigations [18]. Experimental and clinical evidence have linked enhanced production of ROS to certain diseases of the cardiovascular system including hypertension, diabetes and atherosclerosis [21]. Oxidized LDL inhibits endothelial ability to produce nitric oxide (NO). This is unfortunate since NO increases blood flow, allows monocytes to adhere to the endothelium, decreases blood clots and prevents oxidation of LDL. High amount of free radicals promotes the atherosclerosis process by oxidation of LDL. Free radicals react with substances in the cell membrane and damage the cells that line the blood vessels. This means that the fat in the blood can more easily cling to a damaged vessel wall. If there are sufficient antioxidants present, it is believed that the harmful processes in the blood vessels can be slowed down. On the other hand, free radicals are not always harmful, but can serve a useful purpose in the human body. The oxygen radicals are necessary compounds in the maturation process of the cellular structure. Complete elimination of the radicals would not only be impossible, but also harmful [22].

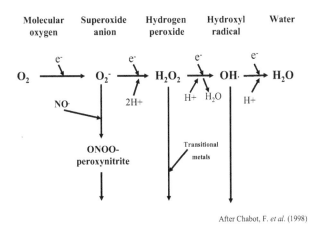

After Chabot, F. *et al.* (1998)

Figure 1. A simplified overview of the generation of ROS.

6. Antioxidants

An antioxidant is a chemical compound or a substance such as vitamin E, vitamin C, or beta carotene, thought to defend body cells from the destructive effects of oxidation. Antioxidants are important in the context of organic chemistry and biology: all living cells contains a complex systems of antioxidant compounds and enzymes, which prevent the cells by chemical damages due to oxidation. There are many examples of antioxidants: e.g. the intracellular enzymes like superoxide dismutase (SOD), glutathione peroxidase, glutathione reductase, catalase, the endogenous molecules like glutathione (GSH), sulfhydryl groups, alpha lipoic acid, Q 10, thioredoxin, the essential nutrients: vitamin C, vitamin E, selenium, N-acetyl cysteine, and the dietary compounds: bioflavonoids, pro-anthocyanin.

The task of antioxidants is to protect the cell against the harmful effects of high production of free radicals. We can influence our own antioxidant defenses by eating food that contains satisfactory amounts of antioxidants (Table 3). A diet containing polyphenol antioxidants from plants is necessary for the health of most mammals [23]. Antioxidants are widely used as ingredients in dietary supplements that are used for health purposes, such as preventing cancer and heart diseases [23]. However, while many laboratory experiments have suggested benefits of antioxidant supplements, several large clinical trials have failed to clearly express an advantage of dietary supplements. Moreover, excess antioxidant supplementation may be harmful [22].

Different types of antioxidants	Food with a high content of antioxidants
Vitamin C	Fruit and vegetables
Vitamin E	Oils
Polyphenols/flavonoids	Tea, coffee, soya, fruit, chocolates, red wine and nuts
Carotenoids	Fruit and vegetables

Table 3. Examples of food with a high content of antioxidants.

Neutrophils are protected against ROS by SOD, catalase, glutathione peroxidase, and gluta-thione reductase. The exogenous antioxidants include among others vitamin E (∞-tocopherol), vitamin C and coenzyme Q. The lipid-soluble α-tocopherol is considered the most efficient among the dietary antioxidants, because it contributes to membrane stability and fluidity by preventing lipid peroxidation. Coenzyme Q or ubiquinon is also lipid-soluble, and has the same membrane stabilization effect as vitamin E. Ascorbic acid or vitamin C (water-soluble) is, however, the predominant dietary antioxidant in plasma. The apprehension of increased rates of ROS production during exercise is part of the rationale why many athletes could theoretically profit by increasing their intake of antioxidant supplements beyond recommend-ed doses. Table 4 shows an overview of the localization and function to the enzymatic antioxidants which protects the cell against oxidative stress.

Non-enzymatic antioxidant reserve is the first line of defense against free radicals (Table 5). Three non-enzymatic antioxidants are of particular importance. 1) Vitamin E, the major lip-id-soluble antioxidant which plays a vital role in protecting membranes from oxidative damage, 2) Vitamin C or ascorbic acid which is a water-soluble antioxidant and can reduce radicals from a variety of sources. It also appears to participate in recycling vitamin E radi-cals. Interestingly, vitamin C can also function as a pro-oxidant under certain circumstances.

3) Glutathione, which is seen as one of the most important intracellular defense against damage by reactive oxygen species.

Enzymatic antioxidants	Localisation	Function
Superoxid oxidase	Mitochondria, cytosol	Superoxid anion
Glutathion peroxidase	Mitochondria, cytosol, cell membrane	Reduces H_2O_2
Catalase	Perisosomes	Reduces H_2O_2
Glutaredoksine	Cytolsol	Protects and repair proteins and no-proteins thioles

Table 4. An overview of enzymatic antioxidants and associated free radicals.

In addition to these "big three", there are numerous small molecules that function as antioxidants. Examples include bilrubin, uric acid, flavonoids, and carotenoids.

Non-enzymatic antioxidants	Localisation	Function
Vitamin C	Aqueous	Scavenger free radicals
Vitamin E	Cell membrane	Reduces free radicals to less active substances
Carotenes	Cell membrane	Scavenger free radicals
Glutathione	Non- proteins thiols	Scavenger free radicals
Flavenoids/polyphenoles	Cell membrane	Scavenger free radicals
Ubuquinon	Cell membrane	Scavenger free radicals

Table 5. An overview of non-enzymatic antioxidants and associated free radicals.

The optimal aim is an equal production of free radicals together with equal production of antioxidants (Figure 2). There is broad evidence suggesting that physical exercise affects the generation of ROS in leukocytes [3,15] which may induce muscle damage [12,23] and may explain phenomena like decreased physical performance, muscular fatigue, and overtraining [16]. Detrimental influences of free radicals are due to their oxidizing effects on lipids, proteins, nucleic acids, and the extracellular matrix. However, the available data to support the role of ROS in relation to physical exercise are highly inconsistent and partly controversial. These controversies are probably due to the different methodologies used to assess ROS, generally including time-demanding and laborious cell isolation procedures and subsequent cell culturing that most certainly affects the ROS status of these cells in an uncontrolled and unpredictable manner. The type of physical activity studied also varied considerably and probably influenced the results presented.

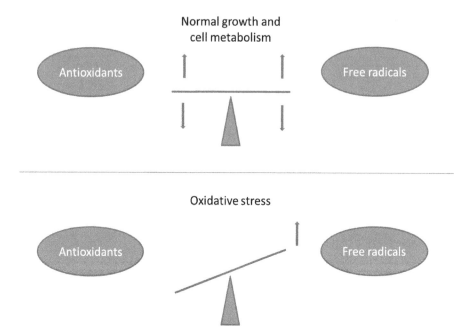

Figure 2. The balance between antioxidants and the amount of free radicals.

7. Physical activity and antioxidant supplementation

A very important question in this context is whether exercise-induced oxidative stress is associated with an increased risk of diseases. The great disparities as to whether ROS production increases or decreases after physical exercise should be considered when comparing different studies of antioxidant supplementation and exercise-induced oxidative stress; likewise the differences in antioxidant dosages used, the biological potency of different forms of the same antioxidant and the different manufacturers' products. The main explanations for the inconsistencies of the effect of antioxidant supplementation on oxidative stress seems to be due to the different assay techniques used to measure in vitro neutrophil ROS production, the exercise mode [22], and the fitness levels of participants.

The human body has an elaborate antioxidant system that depends on the endogenous production of antioxidant compounds like enzymes, as well as the dietary intake of antioxidant vitamins and minerals. Still, there is not enough knowledge at present as to whether the body's natural antioxidant defense system is sufficient to counteract the induced increase of free
r

Until now, the majority of investigations address the effects of exercise on markers of oxidative stress, and not the occurrence of disease. However, most research points to a beneficial effect of regular moderate-to-vigorous physical activity on disease prevention [22] [27].

8. Different methods for detection of free radicals and antioxidants

The work of getting reliable and validated measures of both free radicals and anti-oxidants is still ongoing. The most common methods for detecting free radicals are: 1) Electron spin resonance (ESR) and "spin trapping", which quantify and generate free radicals. This technique makes it possible to identify the cells in their own milieu. 2) Flow cytometry, which is a technique for counting, examining and sorting microscopic particles suspended in a stream of fluid, and 3) Chemiluminiscence Luminol, which is a method used to detect free radicals with chemical reactions (Table 6).

Method	Free radicals
Electron spin resonance	Free radicals; $O_2^{\cdot-}$, $OH^{\cdot-}$ - intra cellular
Flow cytometry	Free radicals; $O_2^{\cdot-}$, H_2O_2, $ONOO^-$ - intra cellular
Cheluminiscence	Free radicals - extra cellular

Table 6. An overview of some of the methods used for detection of free radicals.

Part of the problem with measuring free radicals is that cells are very reactive and short-lived. Most methods used today are not sensitive enough and it is not unusual to find false signals and interference from other substances. It is therefore difficult to compare various studies involving the use of different methods, because it is difficult to know if the different laboratories have measured the same substances (Figure 3).

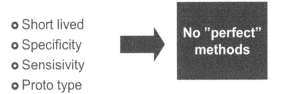

- Short lived
- Specificity
- Sensisivity
- Proto type

No "perfect" methods

Figure 3. No "perfect" methods.

Several methods have been introduced to measure the plasma total antioxidant capacity (TAC) [24], and there are several techniques for quantifying TAC. The most widely used methods for TAC measurements are 1) the colorimetric method (a method for determining concentrations of colored compounds in a solution), 2) the fluorescence method (a method for detecting particular components with exquisite sensitivity and selectivity) and 3) the chemiluminescence method (a method for observation of a light (luminescence) as a result of a chemical reaction) [24-26].

9. Effect of exercise on immunity

9.1. The J- curve

Although the consensus is lacking in some areas, there is sufficient agreement to make some conclusions about the effects of exercise on the immune system. Numerous publications before 1994 resulted in assumption that a J-shaped relationship [27] best described the relationship between infection sensitivity and exercise intensity. The hypothesis is based on cross-section analysis of a mixed cohort of marathon runners, sedentary men and women as well as longitudinal studies on athletes and non-athletes [28-30] that showed increased immunity with increased exercise training. However, one study [31] observed a lower risk for upper respiratory tract infections (URTI) in over-trained compared with well-trained athletes. Previous infections, pathogen exposure, and other stressors apart from exercise may also influence immune response and therefore interpretations of the results of such studies need to be made with care. According to the J-shaped curve, moderate amounts of exercise may enhance immune function above sedentary levels, while excessive amounts of prolonged high intensity exercise may impair immune function [13] (Figure 4).

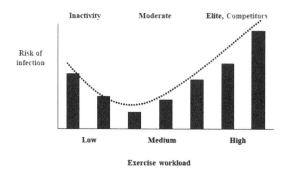

Figure 4. The risk of infection in relation to physical activity. Nieman *et al.*,1994.

9.2. The S-curve

With regard to induced infections in animals, the influence of any exercise intervention appears to be pathogen specific, and dependent on the species, age, and sex of the animals selected for study, and the type of exercise paradigm. Individuals exercising moderately may lower their risk of upper respiratory tract infections (URTI) while those undergoing heavy exercise regimens may have higher than normal risk. When including elite athletes in the J-curve model, the curve is suggested to be S-shaped [30] (Figure 5). This hypothesis states that low and very high exercise loads increases the infection odds ratio, while moderate and high exercise loads decreases the infection odds ratio, but this needs to be verified by compiling data from a larger number of subjects [30].

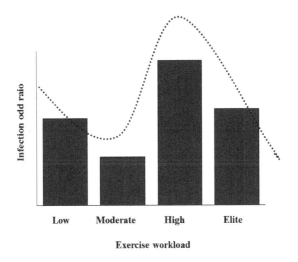

Figure 5. S-shaped relationship between training load and infection rate. Malm et al., 2006.

10. The open window theory

The J-curve relationship has been established among scientists, coaches, and athletes. However, the immunological mechanism behind the proposed increased vulnerability to upper respiratory tract infections (URTI) after strenuous physical exercise is not yet described [32]. The phenomenon is commonly referred to as the "open window" for pathogen entrance [33] (Figure 6). The "open window" theory means that there is an 'open window' of altered immunity (which may last between 3 and 72 hours), in which the risk of clinical infection after exercise is excessive [34, 35]. This means that running a marathon or simply engaging in a prolonged bout of running, increases your risk of contracting an upper-respiratory system infection. Fitch [6] reported that Summer Games athletes who undertake endurance training have a much higher prevalence of asthma compared to their counterparts that have little or no endurance training. Years of endurance training seems to incite airway injury and inflammation [6]. Such inflammation varies across sports and the mechanical changes and dehydration within the airways, in combination with levels of noxious agents like airborne pollutions, irritants or allergens may all have an effect [6].

It is well known that exhausting exercise can result in excessive inflammatory reactions and immune suppression, leading to clinical consequences that slow healing and recovery from injury and/or increase your risk of disease and/or infection [18]. Comparing the immune responses to surgical trauma and stressful bouts of physical activity, there are several parallels; activation of neutrophils and macrophages, which accumulate free radicals [18] [33], local release of proinflammatory cytokines [34], and activation of the complement, coagulation and fibrinolytic cascades [35]. Both physical and psychological stress have been regarded as potent suppressors of the immune system [36], which leaves us with many unanswered questions about whether or not physical exercise is beneficial or harmful for the immune system [37].

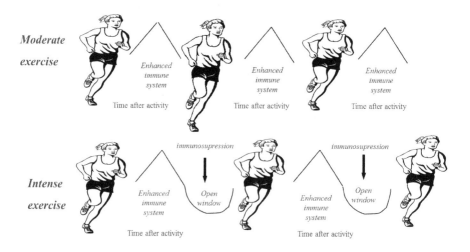

Figure 6. The open window theory. Pedersen & Ullum, 1994.

One of the most studied aspects of exercise and the immune system is the changes in leukocyte numbers in circulating blood [36-39]. The largest changes occur in the number of granulocytes (mainly neutrophils). The mechanisms that cause leukocytosis can be several: an increased release of leukocytes from bone marrow storage pools, a decreased margination of leukocytes onto vessel walls, a decreased extravasation of leukocytes from the vessels into tissues, or an increase in number of precursor cells in the marrow [2]. During exercise, the main source of circulatory neutrophils are primary (bone marrow) and secondary (spleen, lymph nodes, gut) lymphoid tissues, as well as marginated neutrophils from the endothelial wall of peripheral veins [40, 41]. Fry et al., [38] observed that neutrophil number increases proportionally with exercise intensity following interval running over a range of intensities.

Exercise intensity, duration and/or the fitness level of the individual may all play a role in regards to the degree of leukocytosis occurring [42-44]. One way to cure physical stress for the immune system is to increase the total number of leukocytes for fighting the infection and for normalizing the homeostasis. The argument that exercise induces an inflammation like response is also supported by the fact that the raised level of cytokines result in the increased secretion of adrenocorticotrophic hormone (ACTH), which induces the enhancement of systemic cortisol level. Monocytes and thrombocytes are responsible for the initiation of exercise induced acute phase reaction [41].

11. Physical activity – A stimulator and an inhibitor to the immune system

Primarily physical activity stimulates the immune system and strengthens the infection defense. There are indications that untrained people who start exercising regularly get a progressively stronger immune system and become less susceptible to infections [45]. Intensive endurance training or competition which last for at least one hour stimulates the immune system sharply in the beginning, but a few hours after exercise/competition, a weakened immune system results [46]. This means that the immune system in the hours after hard exercise/competition has a weakened ability to fight against bacteria and viruses and the susceptibility to infection is temporarily increased [47]. This effect is seen in both untrained and trained individuals. How long this period lasts for is partly dependent of the intensity and duration of the exercise, and is very individual. The "open period" can last from a few hours up to a day. If such a long-term activity session happens too frequently, it can cause prolonged susceptibility to infections and increased risk of complications if an infection is acquired. Planning of training/activity/competition and rest periods is therefore very important and should be done on an individual basis.

12. Summary

The body's immune system fights all that it perceives as a foreign body. The immune system is separated in two functional divisions: the innate immunity, referred to as the first line of defense, and acquired immunity, which produces a specific reaction and immunological memory to each infectious agent.

Free radicals are any atom with an unpaired electron. Reactive oxygen species (ROS) are all free radicals that involve oxygen. ROS formation is a natural ongoing process that takes place in the body, while the antioxidant defense is on duty for collecting and neutralizing the excess production of oxygen radicals. Many sources of heat, stress, irradiation, inflammation, and any increase in metabolism including exercise, injury, and the repair processes lead to increased production of ROS.

An antioxidant is a chemical compound or a substance such as vitamin E, vitamin C, or beta carotene, thought to defend body cells from the destructive effects of oxidation. Antioxidants are important in the context of organic chemistry and biology: all living cells contain a complex systems of antioxidant compounds and enzymes, which prevent the cells death by chemical damages due to oxidation.

A very important question in this context is whether exercise-induced oxidative stress is associated with an increased risk of disease. The great disparities as to whether ROS production increases or decreases after physical exercise should be considered when comparing different studies of antioxidant supplementation and exercise-induced oxidative stress; likewise the differences in antioxidant dosages used, the biological potency of different forms of the same antioxidant and the different manufacturers products. The main explanations for the inconsistencies as to the effect of antioxidant supplementation on oxidative stress seems to be due to the different assay techniques used to measure the ROS production, the exercise mode, and the fitness levels of participants.

The J-curve theory describes that moderate exercise loads enhance immune function above sedentary levels, while excessive amounts of prolonged high intensity exercise may impair immune function. However, the immunological mechanism behind the proposed increased vulnerability to upper respiratory tract infections (URTI) after strenuous physical exercise is not yet described. This phenomenon is referred to as the "open window". The "open window" theory means that there is an 'open window' of altered immunity (which may last between 3 and 72 hours) in which the risk of clinical infection after exercise is excessive. When including elite athletes in the J-curve model, the curve is suggested to be S-shaped. This hypothesis states that low and very high exercise load increases the infection odds ratio, while moderate and high exercise loads decreases the infection odds ratio, but this needs to be verified by compiling data from a larger number of subjects.

- Exercise has anti-inflammatory effects, which means that moderate amounts of exercise may enhance immune function above sedentary levels.

- Physical activity is associated with reduced resting C-reactive protein (CRP) levels.

- Heavy physical activity produces a rapid, transient increases in cytokine production and entails increases in both pro-inflammatory and anti-inflammatory cytokines.

- Physical exercise affects the generation of reactive oxygen species (ROS) in leukocytes, which may induce muscle damage, decreased physical performance, muscular fatigue, and overtraining.

- It is currently not known whether the body's natural antioxidant defense system is sufficient to counteract the induced increase of ROS during physical exercise or if additional supplements are needed.

- There are three main theories describing the effects of exercise on immunity: 1) the J-curve theory, 2) the "open window" theory and 3) the S-curve theory.

Author details

Hilde Grindvik Nielsen*

Address all correspondence to: hilde.nielsen@nhck.no

University College of Health Sciences – Campus Kristiania, Oslo, Norway

References

[1] Mackinnon LT. Advances in Exercise Immunology. Human Kinetics 1999.

[2] Roitt IB, J; Male, D. Immunology: Mosby; 2001.

[3] Plaisance EP, Grandjean PW. Physical activity and high-sensitivity C-reactive protein. Sports Medicine. 2006;36(5):443-58.

[4] Kasapis C, Thompson PD. The effects of physical activity on serum C-reactive protein and inflammatory markers: a systematic review. Journal of the American College of Cardiology. 2005;45(10):1563-9.

[5] Nieman DC. Risk of upper respiratory tract infection in athletes: an epidemiologic and immunologic perspective. Journal of Athletic Training. 1997;32(4):344-9.

[6] Fitch KD. An overview of asthma and airway hyper-responsiveness in Olympic athletes. British Journal of Sports Medicine. 2012;46(6):413-6.

[7] Friman G, Wesslen L, Karjalainen J, Rolf C. Infectious and lymphocytic myocarditis: epidemiology and factors relevant to sports medicine. Scandinavian Journal of Medicine & Science in Sports. 1995;5(5):269-78.

[8] Chaar V, Romana M, Tripette J, Broquere C, Huisse MG, Hue O, et al. Effect of strenuous physical exercise on circulating cell-derived microparticles. Clinical Hemorheology and Microcirculation. 2011;47(1):15-25.

[9] Santos RV, Tufik S, De Mello MT. Exercise, sleep and cytokines: is there a relation? Sleep Medicine Reviews. 2007;11(3):231-9.

[10] Moldoveanu AI, Shephard RJ, Shek PN. The cytokine response to physical activity and training. Sports Medicine. 2001;31(2):115-44.

[11] Ostrowski K, Rohde T, Asp S, Schjerling P, Pedersen BK. Pro- and anti-inflammatory cytokine balance in strenuous exercise in humans. Journal of Physiology. 1999;515 (Pt 1):287-91.

[12] Fischer CP. Interleukin-6 in acute exercise and training: what is the biological relevance? Exercise Immunology Review. 2006;12:6-33.

[13] Gleeson M. Immune function in sport and exercise. Journal of Applied Physiology (Bethesda, Md : 1985). 2007;103(2):693-9.

[14] Santos VC, Levada-Pires AC, Alves SR, Pithon-Curi TC, Curi R, Cury-Boaventura MF. Changes in lymphocyte and neutrophil function induced by a marathon race. Cell Biochemistry and Function. 2012. [Epub ahead of print].

[15] Fehrenbach E, Northoff H. Free radicals, exercise, apoptosis, and heat shock proteins. Exercise Immunology Review.2001;7:66-89.

[16] Konig D, Wagner K-H, Elmadfa I, Berg A. Exercise and Oxidative Stress: Significance of Antioxidants With Reference to Inflammatory, Muscular and Systemic stress. Exercise Immunology Review. 2001;7:108-33.

[17] Murphy MP, Packer MA, Scarlett JL, Martin SW. Peroxynitrite: a biologically significant oxidant. General Pharmacology. 1998;31(2):179-86.

[18] Williams SL, Strobel NA, Lexis LA, Coombes JS. Antioxidant requirements of endurance athletes: implications for health. Nutrition Reviews. 2006;64(3):93-108.

[19] Cannon JG, Blumberg JB. Acute phase immune response in exercise. In: Sen CK, Packer L, Hanninen O, editors. Handbook of oxidants and antioxidants in exercise. Amsterdam: Elsevier; 2000. p. 177-94.

[20] Åstrand P-O, Rodahl K. Textbook of Work Physiology. Third Edition ed. Singapore: McGraw-Hill Book Company; 1986.

[21] Clarkson PM, Thompson HS. Antioxidants: what role do they play in physical activity and health?. American Journal of Clinical Nutrition. 2000;72(2 Suppl):637S-46S.

[22] Ji LL. Antioxidants and Oxidative stress in Exercise. Proceedings of the Society for Experimental Biology and Medicine. 1999;222:283-92.

[23] R B. Dietary antioxidants and cardiovascular disease. Current Opinion in Lipidology. 2005;16:8.

[24] Janaszewska AB, G. Assay of total antioxidant capacity: comparison of four methods as applied to human blood plasma. Scandinavian Journal of Clinical Laboratory Investigation. 2002;62:231.

[25] Schlesier K, Harwat M, Bohm V, Bitsch R. Assessment of antioxidant activity by using different in vitro methods. Free Radical Research. 2002;36(2):177-87.

[26] Prior RL, Cao G. In vivo total antioxidant capacity: comparison of different analytical methods. Free Radical Biology & Medicine. 1999;27(11-12):1173-81.

[27] Nieman DC. Exercise, infection, and immunity. International Journal of Sports Medicine 1994;15Suppl3:S131-41.

[28] Peters EM, Bateman ED. Ultramarathon running and upper respiratory tract infections. An epidemiological survey. South African Medical Journal. 1983;64(15):582-4.

[29] Nieman DC, Johanssen LM, Lee JW. Infectious episodes in runners before and after a roadrace. Journal of Sports Medicine & Physical Fitness. 1989;29(3):289-96.

[30] Ekblom B, Ekblom O, Malm C. Infectious episodes before and after a marathon race. Scandinavian Journal of Medicine & Science in Sports. 2006;16(4):287-93.

[31] Mackinnon LT, Hooper SL. Plasma glutamine and upper respiratory tract infection during intensified training in swimmers. Medicine and Science in Sports Exercise. 1996;28(3):285-90.

[32] Nieman DC. Is infection risk linked to exercise workload? Medicine and Science in Sports Exercise. 2000;32(7 Suppl):S406-11.

[33] Pedersen BK, Ullum H. NK cell response to physical activity: possible mechanisms of action. Medicine and Science in Sports Exercise. 1994;26(2):140-6.

[34] Shephard RJ. Sepsis and mechanisms of inflammatory response: is exercise a good model?. British Journal of Sports Medicine 2001;35(4):223-30.

[35] Nieman DC, Nehlsen-Cannarella SL, Fagoaga OR, Henson DA, Utter A, Davis JM, et al. Effects of mode and carbohydrate on the granulocyte and monocyte response to intensive, prolonged exercise. Journal of Applied Physiology. 1998;84(4):1252-9.

[36] Ronsen O. Immune, endocrine and metabolic changes related to exhaustive and repeated exercise session. Oslo: University of Oslo; 2003.

[37] Pedersen BK, Hoffman-Goetz L. Exercise and the immune system: regulation, integration, and adaptation. Physiology Review. 2000;80(3):1055-81.

[38] Fry RW, Morton AR, Crawford GP, Keast D. Cell numbers and in vitro responses of leucocytes and lymphocyte subpopulations following maximal exercise and interval training sessions of different intensities. European Journal of Applied Physiology and Occupational Physiology. 1992;64(3):218-27.

[39] McCarthy DA, Dale MM. The leucocytosis of exercise. A review and model. Sports Medicine 1988;6(6):333-63.

[40] van Eeden SF, Granton J, Hards JM, Moore B, Hogg JC. Expression of the cell adhesion molecules on leukocytes that demarginate during acute maximal exercise. Journal of Applied Physiology. 1999;86(3):970-6.

[41] Muir AL, Cruz M, Martin BA, Thommasen H, Belzberg A, Hogg JC. Leukocyte kinetics in the human lung: role of exercise and catecholamines. Journal of Applied Physiology. 1984;57(3):711-9.

[42] Nieman DC, Nehlsen-Caranella S. Effects of Endurance Exercise on the Immune Response. In: Shepard RJ, Åstrand P-O, editors. Endurance in Sport. London: Blackwell Science Ltd; 1992. p. 487-504.

[43] Peake JM. Exercise-induced alterations in neutrophil degranulation and respiratory burst activity: possible mechanisms of action. Exercise Immunology Review. 2002;8:49-100.

[44] Alessio HM, Goldfarb AH, Cao G. Exercise-induced oxidative stress before and after vitamin C supplementation. International Journal of Sport Nutrition. 1997;7(1):1-9.

[45] Nash MS. Exercise and immunology. Medicine and Science in Sports and Exercise. 1994;26(2):125-7.

[46] Friman G, Wright JE, Ilback NG, Beisel WR, White JD, Sharp DS, et al. Does fever or myalgia indicate reduced physical performance capacity in viral infections? Acta Medica Scandinavica. 1985;217(4):353-61.

[47] Waninger KN, Harcke HT. Determination of safe return to play for athletes recovering from infectious mononucleosis: a review of the literature. Clinical Journal of Sport Medicine. 2005;15(6):410-6.

Chapter 6

The Positive and Negative Aspects of Reactive Oxygen Species in Sports Performance

Guolin Li

Additional information is available at the end of the chapter

1. Introduction

Physical exercise, especially moderate physical exercise, can benefit health in a wide range of ways [1-3]. Evidence from different age groups, genders and races has revealed that regular physical exercise is associated with high levels of physical fitness and a reduced risk of mortality, while sedentary habits are related to low levels of physical fitness and an increased threat of all-cause mortality [1-8]. However, the physiological mechanism of physical exercise-induced physical fitness remains only partly understood.

During physical exercise, the metabolic rate increases greatly, as quantified by oxygen consumption and heat production, which results in an enhanced generation of reactive oxygen species (ROS). ROS describe both oxygen-centred free radicals and reactive non-radical derivatives of oxygen resulting from a sequential reduction of oxygen through the addition of electrons. Table 1 shows the representative ROS. The role of ROS in physical exercise is frequently misunderstood. Most people tend to either overemphasize the deleterious role of ROS by maintaining that any ROS generation in vivo during exercise would damage cellular constituents, or underemphasize the beneficial effect of exercise-induced ROS by assuming that the body has enough ROS in vivo that it needs. Two breakthroughs, the identification of ROS in redox regulation and findings on the role of antioxidant supplementation in preventing health-promoting effects of physical exercise, have led scientists to re-examine the role of ROS, especially their positive influence. The goal of this chapter is to outline the current evidence on the sites of ROS generation during exercise, the role of exercise-induced ROS, the effects of antioxidant supplementation on physical-exercise-induced physical fitness, and the mechanism of ROS in exercise-induced adaptation.

Oxygen-centred free radicals	Reactive non-radical derivatives of oxygen
superoxide anion ($O_2^{\cdot-}$)	hydrogen peroxide (H_2O_2)
hydroxyl radical ($HO^{\cdot}$)	singlet oxygen ($1\Delta g$)
peroxyl radical ($RO_2^{\cdot}$)	ozone (O_3)
alkoxyl radical ($RO^{\cdot}$)	

Table 1. Name (Radical depiction) of reactive oxygen species (ROS)

2. Evidence of ros generation in exercise

Exercise has been shown to alter oxidative stress in a wide range of body fluids, cells and/or tissues in human beings, rodents and other animals. These include commonly used model tissues, such as blood [9-11] and skeletal muscle [9, 12-14], along with many other models less often used for laboratory research, such as neutrophils [15-17], lymphocytes [18-20], the diaphragm [21, 22], liver [23-25], heart [23, 26-28], lung [22, 29], brain [30-32], kidney [33, 34], spleen [35, 36], and thymus [35, 37, 38], as well as urine [39-41] and exhaled breath [42, 43].

Although oxidative stress is a common response of cells or tissues to exercise, this does not suggest that all models respond in a similar way to the same exercise. In fact, the levels of ROS generation are different across tissues and/or cells even at rest, let alone during exercise. There is some good evidence that the basal rate of superoxide anion production within the liver of the sperm whale is the highest, more than fourfold higher than that in the brain, about threefold higher than in the heart and muscle, and twofold higher than in the kidney [44]. Another indirect piece of evidence indicates that the heart contains about a tenfold higher level of lipid peroxide than the liver in rats [45]. Moreover, different forms of exercise result in different levels of oxidative stress depending on organ or tissue types. The responses to oxidative stress in the heart and muscle caused by eight-week treadmill running (chronic exercise) or treadmill running to exhaustion (acute exercise) are quite different from those in the brain and liver of rats [46]. This is possibly due to the differences in mitochondrial biogenesis and the occurrence of oxidant-induced degeneration.

The following sections therefore present the evidence on ROS generation during exercise in different tissues or organs.

2.1. Muscle

To explore the relationships between oxidative stress and sports medicine, the majority of researchers have focused on muscles for the reason that their contractions are primarily responsible for all force production and movement, as well as maintenance of and changes in posture.

ROS are hard to be detected because they are highly unstable and short-lived. In early studies, due to the limitations in the analytical techniques and approaches available to detect ROS directly, the levels of ROS are commonly evaluated through indirect and nonspecific methods, such as the analysis of thiobarbituric acid reactive substances (TBARS) or end products of lipid peroxidation [47, 48]. As indicated by these indirect methods, a significant number of studies suggest an increase of ROS during exercise, especially during bouts of intensive exercise [47-49]. Some studies have found that, in comparison to sedentary control, the muscular malondialdehyde (MDA) levels of muscle homogenates in rats exposed to periods of exhaustive exercise increased by more than 100% [47]. The administration of vitamin E can reduce the damage to skeletal muscle [50-52], and muscles from vitamin-E-deficient mice or rats are more likely to be damaged during contractile activity [47, 53]. Based on these early studies, some researchers have suggested that mitochondria are the predominant site for generating ROS during exercise [47], and that the generating rate is related to mitochondrial oxygen consumption [54, 55].

Confusingly, some studies have found little or no change in muscular TBARS or MDA levels after exercise. The results from Alessio et al. have demonstrated that the levels of TBARS do not increase significantly with exhaustive aerobic or nonaerobic isometric exercise [56]. Other studies also show that moderate-intensity resistance exercise had no effects on serum MDA concentration in both resistance-trained and untrained subjects [57], and graded exercise to fatigue did not promote an increase in MDA levels [58]. Though the exact reason is still unclear, the methodical variation between studies, the nonspecific nature of TBARS assay [59, 60], the reactivity of MDA and other aldehydes [61], or even the rapid clearance of TBARS from plasma [62], may account for this issue.

Still, it cannot be concluded that exercise does not alter the levels of ROS even if the TBARS or MDA levels do not change. In fact, there is much evidence for oxidative stress after exhaustive exercise, although the levels of TBARS do not increase [56]. Therefore, if the direct evidence that indicates increasing ROS levels during exercise is lacking, it is difficult to conclude that the damage incurred during contractile activity is mediated by ROS.

The emergence of new technologies, especially electron spin resonance/electron paramagnetic resonance (ESR or EPR) spectroscopy, has made the direct detection of free radicals *in vivo* possible. To our knowledge, though EPR/ESR is not sensitive to the concentrations of free radicals typically found in biological systems, it is the only direct method to assay free radicals. In 1982, Davies and collaborators provided the first direct proof that high-intensity exercise enhances free radical production as indicated by a heightened ESR signal (around g=2.004) in muscle and liver homogenates [47]. Other studies have provided further evidence to suggest that exercise promotes ROS generation. Intriguingly, the increase of ROS seems to play some roles in muscle damage caused by extensive muscular activity, as 30 minutes of excessive contractile activity of rat hind-limb muscles shows an average 70% increase in the amplitude of the major ESR signal, and also a leakage of intracellular creatine kinase enzyme into the blood plasma [63].

These observations have prompted researchers to look for more details on the kinds of ROS that are formed in muscles during or after exercise. Based on ESR/EPR signals, Davies and collaborators have found that the concentration of two ubisemiquinone free radicals (presumably Qi and Qo) is very high in exercised animals [64]. A result from extracellular fluid by microdialysis has also shown that a 15-min protocol of 180 isometric contractions can induce a rapid increase in superoxide anion concentrations and hydroxyl radical activity [65].

Based on the well-characterized *in vitro* models of single isolated muscles or cultured myotubes, researchers have identified a series of ROS and provided evidence that muscles are under considerable oxidative stress after contractile activities, especially lengthening contractile activities. Reid and colleagues have shown that muscular contraction increases intracellular levels of superoxide anion radicals and hydrogen peroxide (H_2O_2), and these ROS promote low-frequency fatigue [66]. Subsequent data from the same group also identify superoxide anion in the extracellular space of diaphragm muscle fibres, and the level is enhanced by fatiguing muscular contractions [67]. When the cultured myotubes are stimulated to contract with different frequencies of electrical stimulation, there is a release of superoxide anion and nitric oxide (NO) into the extracellular medium and an increase in extracellular hydroxyl radical activity [68]. Through loading fluorescein probes with single intact muscle fibres, other studies have developed a method to measure the intracellular ROS generation *in situ* by real-time fluorescence microscopy and illustrated a net increase of ROS by contractions of isolated fibres [69]. It is now possible to analyse different ROS by using different fluorescein probes. The intracellular NO production is visualized in real time using the fluorescent NO probe 4-amino-5-methylamino-2',7'-difluorofluorescein diacetate [70]. With the use of 2',7'-dichloro-dihydrofluorescein as an intracellular probe, researchers have confirmed the dynamic changes of ROS levels during contractile activity in skeletal muscle myotubes [71]. The rate of ROS generation does not change significantly over 30 min in resting myotubes, but it is increased approximately fourfold during 10 min of repetitive contractile activities [71], and the superoxide scavenger Tiron can effectively negate the rise in intracellular fluorescence [71]. Recently, several other probes have also been developed, which permit the monitoring of different ROS in specific cells or organelles [69-74], and will provide more detailed evidence for the exercise-induced increase of ROS. Of note is that, since there are limitations to the most widely used fluorescent probes for detecting and measuring ROS, researchers should be cautious with regard to the optimal use of selected fluorescent probes and interpretation of results [75].

Despite the challenges of detection and the inconsistent results from different methods or models, significant studies have provided evidence for exhaustive exercise promoting extensive ROS formation in muscles (for reviews, see [76-78]).

2.2. Liver

A great deal of research has detected an alteration of ROS in the liver during or after exercise. When Davies *et al.* provided the first direct evidence for ROS generation in muscles after exhaustive exercise, they also found a rise of free radicals in liver homogenates [47]. TBARS, an indicator of lipid peroxidation, has also been reported to increase in the liver and muscles subsequent to exercise, and dietary vitamin E supplementation can reduce (but not eliminate) the increase of TBARS in the liver [79]. Endurance training shows a decreased level of MDA and protein carbonylation, and a significant increase in the activity of superoxide dismutase in mice [80]. Consistent with the effects of exercise on oxidative stress in muscles, most of the other available studies have also suggested that acute exercise, especially intensive or exhaustive acute exercise, indiscriminately induces oxidative stress in the liver, while endurance or long-term training shows a beneficial role in ameliorating oxidative stress.

Important to note is that the liver is distinct from muscles that directly participate in contractile activity or produce forces to support movement. It is logical to consider that the impact of exercise on hepatic oxidative stress should not be the same as the impact on muscles. Results from acute sprint exercise in mice have confirmed this concept. Although the exercise causes an increase in TBARS levels in skeletal muscle, there is no change in the liver [81]. Furthermore, exercise training appears to have little effect on hepatic or myocardial enzyme systems, but can cause adaptive effects in skeletal muscle antioxidant enzymes [82]. A study to investigate the responses to oxidative stress induced by chronic or acute exercise in the brain, liver, heart, kidney, and muscles of rats has also shown that the responses from the brain and liver to oxidative stress are quite different from those in the heart and muscles, and the difference may be attributed to the organ or tissue types and endogenous antioxidant levels [46].

Although the potential mechanism for generating ROS induced by exercise in muscles has been explored in depth, the related mechanism in the liver has not been extensively studied. Based on the above evidence, the mechanism for ROS production in the liver should be greatly different from that in muscles. Further research is needed to reveal the detailed mechanisms, and the energy stress and hepatic ischemia reperfusion should be given particular attention.

2.3. Brain

Exercise has been reported to benefit the brain or nervous system in a wide range of ways, while oxidative stress is involved in the pathogenesis of several age-related nervous diseases. Therefore, the links between exercise-induced alteration of ROS generation in the brain and the potential beneficial effects of exercise on the brain have attracted great attention from researchers in recent years.

Intense physical training can significantly increase TBARS levels and decrease the levels of the brain-derived neurotrophic factors (BDNF) in the brain cortex of mice, which promotes brain mitochondrial dysfunction [83]. Acute and exhaustive swimming exercise has also been reported to elevate the lipid peroxidation and ROS formation in the brain tissue of rats [84, 85], while long-term dietary restriction or selenium supplementation protects against the oxidative stress [84, 85]. Vitamin E deficiency may promote mitochondrial H_2O_2 generation, lipid peroxidation and protein oxidation in the brain [86]. However, vitamin C supplementation has been shown to offer no protection against exercise-induced oxidative damage in brain tissue [87]. Swimming does not significantly influence the oxidative damage, nor is it reflected in the carbonyl content [88], and even over-training does not significantly change the levels of TBARS, 8-hydroxydeoxyguanosine or other biomarkers of oxidative stress in rat brains significantly [89]. Aerobic exercise does not affect lipid peroxidation of the brain, but a diabetic condition improves the activities of several antioxidant enzymes [90]. Though different brain regions of rats react differentially in response to acute exercise-induced oxidative stress, as reported by Somani et al. [91, 92], and this may explain some of the discrepancies, differences in the type of exercise, the analytic technique and the age, sex and strain of animals should be the key issues.

Under conditions of aging or stress, or pathological conditions, the oxidative stress in the brain increases rapidly. Exercise may improve these conditions through strengthening the function of antioxidant defence systems and/or decreasing oxidative stress. Habitual exercise has been reported to overcome the age-related deficit in antioxidant enzymes and prevent oxidative damage in aged brain [93, 94]. There is considerable evidence for physical exercise playing an important preventive and therapeutic role in oxidative stress-associated diseases, such as in reducing oxidative stress after traumatic brain injury [32], increasing thioredoxin-1 levels [95] and the activities of antioxidant enzymes [90] in diabetic brains, and restoring the antioxidant system in the brain of hyperphenylalaninemic rats [96]. Furthermore, exercise-induced modulation of the redox state is an important means to withstand oxidative stress under stress conditions. It has been suggested that exercise may promote mitochondrial function, expressions of mitofusin and antioxidant enzymes against chronic unpredictable mild stress in the brain [97], and reverse the decrease in BDNF and the increase in ROS induced by consuming a high-fat diet [98].

In summary, the effect of exercise on the brain is complex. Although the current data on exercise-induced redox alternation in the brain is still conflicted, there is overwhelming evidence that habitual and regular exercise is an important way to improve brain function by enhancing resistance against oxidative stress and facilitating recovery from oxidative stress. Further investigation is needed to identify the biological basis for the association of exercise, ROS and brain functions.

2.4. Others

Muscular contractile activity has been proven to promote the generation of ROS, and the redox status in the brain and liver may also be altered after physical exercise. However, the effect of exercise on the oxidative stress of other tissues or cells is not consistent. This discrepancy in the findings may be attributed to the differences in exercise type, duration and intensity across protocols, as well as the differences in cells and/or tissues.

Oxidative damage occurs in lymphoid tissues after exhaustive exercise [35], and vigorous exercise has also been reported to result in a transient increase of oxidative stress in lymphocytes [18]. For cigarette smokers, maximal exercise induces pulmonary oxidative stress and leads to oxidative damage in the lungs [42], while in normal lungs exercise neither leads to significant oxidative stress, nor alters mitochondrial respiration [22]. For trained men, even strenuous bouts of exercise do not cause a significant increase in blood oxidative stress, which may be related to the attenuation in ROS production as an adaptation to chronic exercise training [11].

Intriguingly, in rat kidneys exercise training has been noted to prevent oxidative stress and inflammation and to preserve antioxidant status, which mediates the effects of chronic exercise on preserving renal haemodynamics and structure [33, 34]. In rat hearts, prolonged exercise could upregulate the mRNA expression and activity of uncoupling protein 2 (UCP2), which may reduce cross-membrane potential and thus ROS production [27]. However, endurance training can blunt exercise-induced UCP2 activation, and increase removal of ROS [27]. In white blood cells, exercise results in substantial improvements in markers of DNA and RNA damage [39].

The impacts of gender on exercise-induced oxidative stress should not be ignored. Females seem to be more protected against oxidative stress induced by swimming. H_2O_2 is mainly produced in males, which subsequently leads to the increase of MnSOD gene expression and activity [20].

3. Sites of ROS generation in exercise

3.1. ROS generation by mitochondria

Mitochondria have often been cited as the major site of ROS generation in tissues. Based on the classic works by Chance and his collaborators, when mitochondria are in state 4, about 2% of total oxygen consumed by mitochondria is converted into H_2O_2 and other ROS [99, 100]. As oxygen consumption increases greatly during exercise, many researchers have assumed that mitochondria should be a key site of ROS formation, and the extent of ROS generation may be related to the oxygen consumption by mitochondria [54, 55]. When Davies and colleagues found the first direct evidence for exercise-induced ROS formation, they also suggested mitochondria as the predominant source [47]. This hypothesis seems to be confirmed by subsequent data. Davies and Hochstein did identify two free radicals, that is, two forms of semistabilized mitochondrial ubisemiquinone (presumably Qi and Qo) [64]. They found that the concentration of the two free radicals was obviously higher in exercised animals than in control animals, which has actually provided the first evidence for the mitochondrial genera-tion of free radicals induced by exercise *in vivo* [64]. Other EPR signal studies also supported the importance of mitochondria in ROS production [63, 101].

In vitro experiments have indicated that mitochondrial ROS generation is lower in state 3 than in state 4 respiration [100]. There is considerable evidence that muscular mitochondria are predominant in state 3 rather than in state 4 during aerobic contractile activity, which would limit the ROS formation during contractions [102, 103]. This has led other researchers to support the above hypothesis of mitochondria as a main site of ROS generation. To explore the specific site of exercise associated with ROS production, Puente-Maestu *et al.* isolated mitochondria from skeletal muscle of chronic obstructive pulmonary disease (COPD) patients at rest and after exercise, and analysed mitochondrial oxygen consumption and ROS produc-tion [49]. Then, they related the *in vitro* ROS production during the state 3 respiration with skeletal muscle oxidative stress after exercise [49]. They found that mitochondrial complex III was the main site of producing H_2O_2 in mitochondria of skeletal muscle, and the mitochondrial production of H_2O_2 in the state 3 respiration contributed to exercise-induced muscle oxidative damage [49].

Another argument regards the semiquinone radicals. McArdle and his colleagues assayed the effects of repeated lengthening contractions on semiquinone-derived free radical signal, oxidation of protein thiols and glutathione, and lipid peroxidation in the extensor digitorum longus muscles of rats. Although they found the oxidation of protein thiols and glutathione was enhanced after contractions, the magnitude of the semiquinone-derived free radical signal observed by ESR was the same in exercised and non-exercised skeletal muscles [104]. To further explore the site of ROS generation during exercise, another study [65] isolated the gastrocnemius muscles from MnSOD knockout heterozygous (Sod2$^{+/-}$) and wild-type (Sod2$^{+/+}$) mice, and measured the concentrations of superoxide anions and hydroxyl radical activity in the extracellular space by microdialysis. They found that isometric contractions induced a rapid, equivalent increase in superoxide anion concentrations in the extracellular space of both Sod2$^{+/-}$ and Sod2$^{+/+}$ mice, whereas hydroxyl radical activity increased only in the extracellular space of muscles of Sod2$^{+/+}$ mice [65]. In other words, a reduction in MnSOD activity did not change the concentration of superoxide anions in the extracellular space, but decreased the concentration of hydroxyl radicals in the extracellular space. Considering that MnSOD is located in the mitochondrial matrix, these results suggest that mitochondria are the key sites in converting superoxide anions to hydroxyl radicals. Furthermore, mice with skeletal-muscle-specific deficiency of MnSOD (muscle-Sod2$^{-/-}$) also demonstrated a severe disturbance in exercise activity, increased oxidative damage and reduced ATP content in their muscle tissue, while a single administration of the antioxidant EUK-8 significantly improved the exercise activity and ATP level [14]. These findings indicate that even if the mitochondrion is not the major site, it is at least an important site in generating superoxide anions in muscles during exercise.

In light of the above observations, the electron transport associated with the mitochondrial respiratory chain is considered the central process leading to ROS production during exercise.

3.2. ROS generation by xanthine oxidase

Another possible site for ROS generation during exercise, especially intensive or exhaustive exercise, is xanthine oxidase (XO). As an intensive or exhaustive exercise can result in ischemia or hypoxia in certain regions of the body, massive ATP depletion occurs and ATP will be converted to adenosine diphosphate, adenosine monophosphate, inosine, and finally hypoxanthine. Under normal physiological conditions, xanthine dehydrogenase is the dominant form of XO, which can catalyse the oxidation of hypoxanthine to xanthine or further the oxidation of xanthine to uric acid by using NAD$^+$ as an electron acceptor. However, under ischemia conditions, the xanthine dehydrogenase can be converted to XO by reversible sulfhydryl oxidation or by irreversible proteolytic modification [105, 106], and XO can no longer utilize NAD$^+$ as the electron acceptor, instead using molecular oxygen as the electron acceptor and yielding four units of superoxide anions per unit of transformed substrate. As a result, under reperfusion conditions, a burst of superoxide anions and H$_2$O$_2$ can result [107].

XO has been thought to be responsible for the production of ROS and tissue damage during or after intensive exercise, and the inhibition of XO by allopurinol or oxypurinol can reduce the production of ROS. Ryan and collaborators measured XO activity, H$_2$O$_2$ levels, lipid peroxidation, the activities of antioxidant enzymes, and skeletal muscle function in aged mice with or without administration of allopurinol. In addition to finding inhibition of XO by allopurinol treatment, they found the treatment could prevent the increase of catalase and

CuZnSOD activities, reduce oxidative stress and improve skeletal muscle function in response to electrically stimulated isometric contractions [108]. In most cases in other animals, evidence has also been provided for the beneficial effects of allopurinol or oxypurinol in inhibiting XO and thus attenuating the generation of ROS. Lipid hydroperoxides, GSSG and the formation of ROS during exercise are reduced significantly in an allopurinol-treated horse [109]. Exercise could cause an increase in blood XO activity in rats, and inhibiting XO with allopurinol could prevent exercise-induced oxidation of glutathione in both rats and human beings [110]. Furthermore, allopurinol has also been shown to decrease oxidative stress and ameliorate the morbidity and mortality of congestive heart failure patients (for reviews, see [111]). In the light of these observations, some researchers have suggested that XO may play a more important role in generating ROS than mitochondria do [112].

However, results from Capecchi *et al.* have shown that allopurinol has no effect on superoxide anion generation or enzyme release from neutrophils stimulated *in vitro* with formyl-me-thionyl-leucyl-phenylalanine [113]. Nor do more recent observations support the critical role of XO in generating ROS during intensive exercise. Olek and colleagues tested the effects of allopurinol ingestion on the slow component of VO_2 kinetics (the dynamic behaviour of O_2 uptake in the transition from rest to exercise) and the alternations of plasma oxidative stress markers during severe intensity exercise. They found short-term intensive exercise could induce oxidative stress, and although allopurinol intake might cause an increase in resting xanthine and hypoxanthine plasma concentrations (supporting XO inhibition by allopurinol), it neither modified the kinetics of oxygen consumption nor altered ROS overproduction [114].

Gomez-Cabrera *et al.* [115] examined the effects of allopurinol on the inhibition of ROS production and on the activation of nuclear factor kappaB (NFκB) in rats subjected to exhaustive exercise. They found that exercise did result in considerably more glutathione oxidation in the control rat than in the rat administered with allopurinol before exercise. However, the administration of allopurinol could also negate the exercise-induced activation of NFκB, which is an important signalling pathway involved in upregulating the expression of important enzymes for cell defence (superoxide dismutase) and adaptation to exercise. That is to say, at the same time as allopurinol decreases XO-mediated oxidative stress, it also prevents useful cellular adaptations to exercise in rats.

3.3. Other sites and current understanding

Except for mitochondria and XO, there should be other sites of ROS production during and after exercise. When tissue damage has occurred, several cells in the immune system (including macrophages/monocytes, eosinohpils and neutrophils) may also generate large quantities of ROS [116]. For example, circulating neutrophils has been reported to produce ROS due to the facilitation of myeloperoxidase degranulation after exhaustive exercise [17]. Although more investigation is needed to fully elucidate the mechanism and site of ROS formation in exercise, at the present time mitochondria and XO are still worth focusing on.

4. Role of ROS in exercise: Foe or friend?

Sedentary habits are associated with low levels of cardiorespiratory fitness and an increased threat of all-cause mortality, while physically active habits are associated with fitness improvement and reduced mortality risk [1, 7, 117]. However, the detailed mechanism of physical activity-induced physical fitness remains only partly understood.

Since 1982, when Davies *et al.* provided the first direct proof that high-intensity exercise enhances free radical production [47], further evidence has emerged for exercise promoting ROS formation. Besides mitochondria, XO and phagocytes in skeletal muscle have also been reported to be potentially responsible for generating ROS in response to exercise [77]. Here, it is necessary to substantiate the role of ROS in sports medicine and in exercise-induced effects.

4.1. Harmful effect of ROS in exercise

ROS form as a natural by-product of normal energy metabolism. They have been considered as toxic molecules due to their high reactivity to most of the biological macromolecules, which generally include DNA damage, oxidations of polyunsaturated fatty acids and amino acids, and oxidative inactivation of specific enzymes.

As aerobic exercise will undoubtedly increase the metabolic rate in the body, the harmful effects of exercise and exercise-induced ROS are well documented. Exercise localized to a peripheral muscle group in COPD patients has been shown to induce systemic oxidative stress [118]. Acute exercise-induced oxidative stress contributes to post-exercise proteinuria in untrained rats [119]. A maximal bicycle exercise results in DNA strand breaks and oxidative DNA damage [120]. High-competition swimming imposes high and sustained oxidative and proteolytic stress on adolescents, which may increase potential risk of cardiovascular disease in the future [121]. A run-to-exhaustion exercise leads to an increase in oxidative damage of lymphoid tissues in rats [122].

In summary, strenuous exercise under conditions of disease or overtraining would significantly elevate respiration rate, lead to a dramatic and sustained increase in ROS that is more than the antioxidant defence system can scavenge, and eventually result in oxidative stress and damage to physiological functions. Therefore, though regular exercise is important to improve cardiorespiratory fitness, extreme or exhaustive physical activities should be avoided, especially under certain disease conditions.

4.2. Beneficial role of ROS in exercise

4.2.1. Oxidative stress and beneficial effect of exercise

There is growing evidence for the healthy role of exercise. Some studies indicate its beneficial effect is associated with the attenuation of oxidative stress. It is reported that regular training can ameliorate ethanol-induced oxidative injury in the liver [123], endurance training may attenuate exercise-induced oxidative stress [25], and chronic exercise can improve antioxidant status and induce a reduction in arterial hypertension development in rats [124]. Athletes participating in regular and adequate training would enhance antioxidant capacity and bring about improvement in both peripheral resistance to insulin and all the functional metabolic interchanges in cellular membranes [125]. Intriguingly, leisure time, moderate occupational or household physical activities are also positively related to total antioxidant capacity, and can decrease the risk of cardiovascular disease [126].

In particular conditions, however, although exercise prevents some pathologic processes, it increases oxidative stress. As illustrated in elderly people, sustained exercise enhances cardiorespiratory function and reduces the risk of cardiovascular disease, but it also significantly enhances some biomarkers of oxidative stress [127]. This is also the case in atherogenic mice. Exercise lowered plasma cholesterol and atherosclerotic lesions, with a concomitant increase in oxidative stress and endothelial NO synthase [128]. In this condition, though vitamin E supplementation can decrease the exercise-induced oxidative stress, it also counteracts the beneficial effects of exercise on atherosclerosis and hinders the induction of arterial antioxidant response [128]. These findings have led to researchers beginning to consider the positive effects of ROS themselves.

4.2.2. Beneficial role of ROS in exercise

Early studies in this area have focused on the oxidative damage induced by augmented formation of ROS. Subsequent data, however, have shown that ROS also participate in redox regulation, and it has been widely accepted that the moderate concentrations of ROS *in vivo* function as regulatory mediators in signalling processes and as initiators in re-establishing "redox homeostasis" [129, 130]. There are now a significant number of studies suggesting that regular exercise can enhance the capacity of antioxidant defence systems to lower oxidative stress or the levels of ROS. In this context, some researchers have begun to speculate a positive role of a transient high level of ROS induced by exercise. This hypothesis has been confirmed in a rat diaphragm. In this study, fibre bundles from a rat diaphragm were incubated with exogenous catalase or SOD to decrease the tissue level of ROS, and then the peak twitch stress, time-to-peak tension and half-relaxation time were measured. The results showed that either selective removal of H_2O_2 with catalase or selective removal of superoxide anions with SOD depressed submaximal contractile activities in a dose-dependent way [131]. These findings indicate the ROS present in non-fatigued muscle can promote excitation-contraction coupling and are responsible for optimal contractile function [131]. Subsequently, many studies have documented a role of ROS as second messengers responsible for the prevention of diseases by stimulating antioxidant response [128], or other adaptations to exercise by activating useful cellular redox signalling pathways including peroxisome proliferator-activated receptor-gamma coactivator-1alpha [132], mitogen-activated protein kinase and NFκB [115, 133].

Moreover, it is now clear that ROS not only play an important role in regulating muscle contractile activity, but are also involved in promoting muscle regeneration in recovery from muscle damage [134], improving insulin sensitivity [135], and mediating the vasodilatory response during exercise [136]. As a result, ROS generated in response to exercise and other physiological or pathological stimuli might be important signalling molecules rather than solely by-products of energy metabolism.

4.3. Current understanding

Thanks to evidence gathered over the last three decades, we now understand the effects of exercise and the role of exercise-induced ROS more clearly. During exercise, although oxygen consumption in the body increases more than tenfold, the intracellular H_2O_2 concentrations in skeletal muscle induced by contractile activities only increase by approximately 100 nM [78]. This modest increase of H_2O_2 can only be enough to assume the functions of the signalling molecule and to stimulate some of the adaptations of muscle to exercise. ROS are not only toxic but also involved in cell signalling and in regulating several redox-sensitive transcription factors [115, 132, 133]. An inhibition of ROS generation would also modify cellular redox signalling pathways associated with adaptations to exercise [115, 132, 133]. It is now clear that physical activities cause oxidative stress only when exhaustive. ROS induced by moderate exercise may serve as signalling molecules to increase the expression of cytoprotective proteins and to maintain some other normal functions. Habitual and regular exercise is a useful strategy for improving physical fitness and reducing mortality risk.

5. Antioxidant supplementation in exercise: Beneficial or detrimental?

ROS are unavoidable by-products of energy metabolism, and cells continuously generate ROS in metabolic processes. High metabolic rates during exercise have led to the assumption that exercise leads to excessive production of ROS in skeletal muscle, which is associated with muscle damage and impaired muscle function. As a result, the supplementation of antioxidants may offer some protection against exercise-induced oxidative damage, and improve muscle function and physical performance. In this context, numerous antioxidants are marketed, and antioxidant supplementation has become very common with athletes or other physically active individuals. However, there is not enough scientific evidence to support their efficacy and long-term safety.

5.1. Antioxidant supplementation and oxidative stress

The majority of studies have illustrated that antioxidants attenuate the oxidative stress induced by exercise, although oxidative stress is estimated through measuring its indirect outcomes, such as by-products of lipid peroxidation, protein oxidation and DNA damage. A study by Alessio *et al.* tested the effects of vitamin C supplementation for one day and two weeks on oxidative stress in subjects with or without exercise. When the subjects were at rest, they found that vitamin C supplementations did not affect the levels of TBARS or oxygen radical absorbance capacity, but with the same subjects after 30 minutes of exercise, the supplementation did prevent the increase of oxidative stress [137]. Oral ingestion of vitamin C has been reported to effectively prevent exercise-induced lipid peroxidation in patients with type 1 diabetes mellitus [138]. The supplementation of vitamin E can diminish the increase of lipid hydroperoxides and TBARS in the plasma and muscle fibres of rats following aerobic exercise [139]. The combined administration of vitamin E and C improves indices of oxidative stress associated with repetitive loading exercise and aging, and ameliorates the positive work output of muscles in aged rodents [140]. Although the most widely studied antioxidants are vitamin E and ascorbic acid (vitamin C), the effects on suppressing exercise-induced oxidative stress have also demonstrated in other antioxidants, including β-carotene [141], N-acetylcysteine (NAC) [142], L-arginine [143], coenzyme Q [144], α-lipoic acid [145], resveratrol [146], several other compounds [147, 148], selenium [149], teas [150], and concentrates from fruit, berry and vegetable [151].

However, many studies show that the administration of antioxidants, alone or in combination, does not significantly affect exercise-induced oxidative stress [134, 152-157]. Several observations even indicate an increase of oxidative stress following antioxidant supplementation pre- or post-exercise, especially with high doses [158-162]. Moreover, some investigations that have confirmed the beneficial effects of antioxidants on oxidative stress did not demonstrate a significant improvement in performance [163] or the functions related to pain and muscle damage [151]. Therefore, the health-promoting effects of antioxidants should be explored in more detail.

5.2. Antioxidant supplementation and fatigue

The role of antioxidant supplementation in protecting against fatigue remains highly controversial. One reason for this controversy is the lack of strong evidence for oxidative stress involved in muscle fatigue. Some studies have displayed an association between oxidative stress and muscle fatigue [164, 165], and the anabolic androgenic steroid stanozolol, a drug used in sport to enhance muscle mass and strength and to increase muscle fatigue resistance, can protect against acute exercise-induced oxidative stress by reducing mitochondrial ROS production [13]. However, the association has been challenged by other observations that suggest that graded exercise to fatigue does not promote an increase in oxidative stress in the blood of exercise-trained heart transplant recipients [58], and an enhanced running time to exhaustion does not lead to attenuation of lipid peroxidation [166]. As a result, although NAC supplementation has been reported to improve muscle fatigue in rats [167], it does not affect the time to fatigue in a group of untrained men [168], or in those participating in submaximal cycling exercises [169].

5.3. Antioxidant supplementation and muscle damage

The processes of force production during repetitive eccentric exercise have been widely accepted to result in muscle damage, which is specifically the case when the exercise is unaccustomed. Given that high levels of ROS generated during contractile activities may contribute to the muscle damage (for reviews, see [170, 171]), and antioxidants may scavenge ROS, the potential preventive effects of antioxidant supplementation on muscle damage have been explored in depth, with variations in dosage, timing and duration of administration. Most of the research has focused on the effects of vitamin C and E. Some studies do find some protecting role of the two antioxidants against oxidative stress, while there is no strong evidence for their role in preventing muscle damage (for reviews, see[172]). However, some findings do not support a major role for antioxidant supplementation to reduce markers of oxidative stress [134, 152, 173, 174]. There appears to be no independent or combined effect of vitamin C, vitamin E and other antioxidants supplementation on facilitating recovery of muscle function after exercise-induced muscle damage [152], protecting against the delayed onset of muscle soreness and markers of muscle damage [173], or attenuating muscular damage induced by exhaustive exercise such as a marathon run [174]. On the contrary, a number of investigations suggest that the administration of antioxidants may promote cellular damage [161], transiently increase tissue damage [162], and hinder the recovery of muscle damage [134]. Therefore, recent studies have cast doubt on the benign effects of antioxidant supplementation.

5.4. Antioxidant supplementation and exercise performance

Similar to equivocal effects of antioxidant administration on muscle damage, present results regarding the role of antioxidant supplementation in exercise performance are inconsistent. There is some evidence to display that the supplementation of antioxidant can benefit exercise performance, while the majority of studies do not support it. Even the combined supplementation of vitamins E, C, NAC, coenzyme Q10, polyprenols and other antioxidants in different subject populations and exercise protocols fails to improve exercise performance. Moreover, there is increasing evidence suggesting a deleterious effect of antioxidant supplementation on exercise performance. For more details on this issue, readers are recommended to read an excellent recently published review by Peternelj and Coombes [136].

5.5. Current understanding

ROS formation during exercise may have dual effects. High levels of ROS produced during strenuous exercise may be related to oxidative damage and impaired muscle function. However, the moderate or transient high levels of ROS induced by exercise may act as signalling molecules to stimulate adaptive responses through redox-sensitive signalling pathways to maintain cellular redox homeostasis during exercise. This scenario explains why subjects involved in exercise training have shown an increase of resistance to oxidative stress under a wide range of physiological and pathological stresses.

Although the majority of studies on the supplementation of antioxidants have supported their beneficial effects on attenuating exercise-induced oxidative stress, there is limited evidence for antioxidant treatment offering any protection against exercise-induced muscular function damage or exercise performance. A plausible explanation is that the attenuation of ROS by antioxidant supplementation may block some useful cell signalling pathways and gene expression involved in adaptations to exercise, which may preclude the health-promoting effects of exercise in subjects.

6. The mechanism of ROS for exercise-induced physical fitness

Despite great progress made in sports medicine, the mechanism of exercise-induced physical fitness remains only partly understood. Combined with the hormetic characteristic of physical activity and the property of allostasis, we have assumed that hormesis-induced allostatic buffering capacity enhancement is a physiological mechanism to explain exercise-induced physical fitness [130]. This hypothesis seems to be a good framework to illustrate the role of ROS in exercise-induced physical fitness.

6.1. Exercise, ROS and hormesis

Hormesis is basically characterized by biphasic dose-response –low-dose stimulation and high-dose inhibition [175-177]. This is often used to refer to the beneficial effects of low doses of potentially harmful substances [175-177]. As described in section 2, exercise is associated with the increased generation of ROS. This may be the reason for early studies considering aerobic exercise as a mild oxidative stressor [139, 178]. Indeed, sustained high doses of ROS are unquestionably deleterious, whereas a large amount of evidence emerging in recent years has suggested that a mild increase of ROS may evoke a cellular adaptive response to exercise. Therefore, ROS-induced response has the typical bi-phasic features of hormesis.

6.2. ROS-induced enhancement of allostatic buffering capacity

6.2.1. ROS and allostatic buffering capacity

More than two decades ago, Sterling and Eyer coined the term allostasis from the Greek "allo" meaning "variable", and "stasis" meaning "stable". Thus, allostasis means "remaining stable by being variable" [179], that is, maintaining stability through a multi-point. Since in organisms, especially in higher animals, the stability of the internal milieu is associated with many rhythms, such as daily rhythm of body temperature, daily rhythmic secretion of serotonin, melatonin and other hormones, and many other rhythms, allostasis should be a more accurate concept than homeostasis (remaining stable by staying the same). Although there is no evidence at present to show that redox *in vivo* remains stable by being variable, numerous studies have suggested that the increased formation of ROS, whether induced by aging, exercise, or other stress conditions, is initiated to re-establish "redox homeostasis" (for review, see [129]). From a rigorous scientific point of view, the term "redox homeostasis" used here should be replaced by "redox allostasis".

Based on the multi-point property of allostasis, we have postulated the allostatic system as a special "buffering system": it has a basal level and certain buffering capacity that can maintain dynamic stability. Therefore, we have coined the term "allostatic buffering capacity (ABC)" with five components: basal level, peak level, buffering range, increase rate and recovery rate, to give a good picture of the capacity of an allostatic system to maintain dynamic stability. The action model of exercise on ABC has also been addressed. For more details, readers are recommended to read our review published in 2009 [130].

6.2.2. Present evidence of exercise-induced ROS to enhance redox ABC

Regular exercise can promote mitochondrial biogenesis and enhance muscle oxidative capacity [180, 181], and the molecular signals are mainly the increased ROS, such as H_2O_2 [180, 181]. In addition, exercise training has been reported to decrease ROS production through reducing the electronic leakage with better-regulated mitochondrial electron-transport chain [182] and a larger pool of functional mitochondria [183], which is critical to maintain health and delay the onset and progressive course of some diseases [184]. Moreover, the SOD activity has consistently been shown to increase with exercise in an intensity-dependent manner [185]. Long-term athletic training can increase the activity of proteasome complexes, which increase the degradation and turnover rate of oxidative modified proteins [186].

These findings indicate that regular exercise can enhance the redox ABC through: (a) lowering the basal ROS level by reducing ROS production, decreasing resting respiration rate and re-establishing redox allostasis, (b) increasing the peak level and oxidative buffering range by promoting mitochondrial biogenesis, and (c) decreasing the oxidative stress rate and increasing recovery rate by re-establishing redox allostasis and enhancing the antioxidant defensive system and damage repair system. In contrast, intense and prolonged exercise may damage redox ABC.

7. Summary and perspectives

Most currently available evidence clearly demonstrates that physical activity is associated with an increase of ROS generation in almost all studied cells, tissues and organs. There are many sites for producing ROS during or after exercise (Figure 1]. During moderate aerobic exercise, mitochondria are the predominant site for generating ROS. When energy depletion or ischemia-reperfusion occurs, especially during or after exhaustive exercise, XO may be an important site for ROS production. Macrophages, eosinophils, neutrophils and other cells in the immune system may also contribute to the ROS formation after exercise when tissue damage occurs. With the advance of analytical methods and techniques for assaying ROS *in situ*, more evidence would be produced to fully elucidate the mechanism and site of ROS formation during or after exercise.

ROS formation during exercise has dual effects. Based on the free radical theory of aging, ROS are toxic molecules due to their high reactivity to most biological macromolecules. Supplementation with antioxidants should offer some preventive effects against exercise-induced oxidative damage, and improve muscular function and physical performance. However, growing evidence shows that exercise-induced ROS may act as signalling molecules to mediate useful cellular adaption to exercise, mainly through regulating the expression of cytoprotective proteins and/or several redox-sensitive transcription factors. Although the supplementation of antioxidants may attenuate exercise-induced oxidative stress, there is insufficient evidence that it protects against exercise-induced muscular function damage or exercise performance.

Combined with the hormetic characteristic of exercise-induced ROS and the property of allostasis, hormesis-induced ABC enhancement should be a physiological mechanism to explain ROS-induced physical fitness (Figure 1). Different intensities or types of physical exercise would cause different levels of ROS generation. Too-small or too-large ROS will introduce too-weak eustress ("good stress") or too-strong distress ("bad stress") and result in allostasis load through weakening ABC or damaging ABC, respectively. However, moderate and transient high levels of ROS induced by physical exercise will introduce eustress *in vivo* and contribute to the hormesis-induced ABC enhancement, which benefits physical fitness. Further work is needed to substantiate the exact mechanisms of ROS in physical fitness.

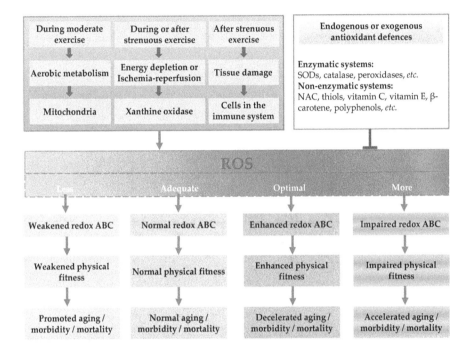

Figure 1. The sources and potential effects of reactive oxygen species (ROS). During or after exercise, ROS are generated as a result of aerobic metabolism in mitochondria, as well as from the activation of xanthine oxidase (XO). In addition, a variety of cells in the immune system can contribute to ROS production. A sophisticated enzymatic and non-enzymatic antioxidant defence system regulates overall ROS levels. Adequate ROS levels are necessary to maintain redox allostatic buffering capacity (ABC). Optimal higher levels of ROS can enhance redox ABC, which improves physical fitness and subsequently delays the aging process and reduces morbidity or mortality of all-cause diseases. Lowering ROS levels below the allostatic set point may interrupt the physiological role of ROS in maintaining redox ABC and cellular adaption to exercise. Similarly, an excessive rise in ROS levels may also constitute a stress signal that damages redox ABC, and ultimately accelerate the aging process and age-related diseases.

Acknowledgements

Very grateful to Dr. Dazhong Yin and Ms. Fang Lei for their constructive suggestions during preparation of the paper. This work has been supported by National Science Funds of China (30800207, 31271257) and Scientific Research Funds of Hunan Provincial Education Department.

List of abbreviations

ROS: reactive oxygen species

TBARS: thiobarbituric acid reactive substances

MDA: malondialdehyde

ESR: electron spin resonance

EPR: electron paramagnetic resonance

NO: nitric oxide

BDNF: brain-derived neurotrophic factor

UCP2: uncoupling protein 2

COPD: chronic obstructive pulmonary disease

ATP: adenosine triphosphate

XO: xanthine oxidase

NFκB: nuclear factor kappaB

NAC: N-acetylcysteine

ABC: allostatic buffering capacity

Author details

Guolin Li*

Address all correspondence to: hnsdlgl@hunnu.edu.cn

College of Life Sciences, Hunan Normal University, Changsha, Hunan, China

References

[1] Blair SN, Kohl HW, III, Barlow CE, Paffenbarger RS, Jr., Gibbons LW, Macera CA. Changes in physical fitness and all-cause mortality. A prospective study of healthy and unhealthy men. JAMA: The Journal of the American Medical Association. 1995;273(14):1093-8.

[2] Church TS, Earnest CP, Skinner JS, Blair SN. Effects of different doses of physical activity on cardiorespiratory fitness among sedentary, overweight or obese postmeno-

pausal women with elevated blood pressure: a randomized controlled trial. JAMA: The Journal of the American Medical Association. 2007;297(19):2081-91.

[3] Kokkinos P, Myers J, Kokkinos JP, Pittaras A, Narayan P, Manolis A, et al. Exercise capacity and mortality in black and white men. Circulation. 2008;117(5):614-22.

[4] Blair SN, Kampert JB, Kohl HW, III, Barlow CE, Macera CA, Paffenbarger RS, Jr., et al. Influences of cardiorespiratory fitness and other precursors on cardiovascular disease and all-cause mortality in men and women. JAMA: The Journal of the American Medical Association. 1996;276(3):205-10.

[5] Ekelund LG, Haskell WL, Johnson JL, Whaley FS, Criqui MH, Sheps DS. Physical fitness as a predictor of cardiovascular mortality in asymptomatic North American men. The Lipid Research Clinics Mortality Follow-up Study. NEnglJ Med. 1988;319(21):1379-84.

[6] Lee IM. Dose-response relation between physical activity and fitness: even a little is good; more is better. JAMA: The Journal of the American Medical Association. 2007;297(19):2137-9.

[7] Myers J, Prakash M, Froelicher V, Do D, Partington S, Atwood JE. Exercise capacity and mortality among men referred for exercise testing. NEnglJ Med. 2002;346(11): 793-801.

[8] Paffenbarger RS, Jr., Hyde RT, Wing AL, Hsieh CC. Physical activity, all-cause mortality, and longevity of college alumni. NEnglJ Med. 1986;314(10):605-13.

[9] Rodriguez DA, Kalko S, Puig-Vilanova E, Perez-Olabarria M, Falciani F, Gea J, et al. Muscle and blood redox status after exercise training in severe COPD patients. Free radical biology & medicine. 2012 Jan 1;52(1):88-94. PubMed PMID: 22064359. Epub 2011/11/09. eng.

[10] Nikolaidis MG, Kyparos A, Dipla K, Zafeiridis A, Sambanis M, Grivas GV, et al. Exercise as a model to study redox homeostasis in blood: the effect of protocol and sampling point. Biomarkers : biochemical indicators of exposure, response, and susceptibility to chemicals. 2012 Feb;17(1):28-35. PubMed PMID: 22288504. Epub 2012/02/01. eng.

[11] Farney TM, McCarthy CG, Canale RE, Schilling BK, Whitehead PN, Bloomer RJ. Absence of blood oxidative stress in trained men following strenuous exercise. Medicine and science in sports and exercise. 2012 Apr 19. PubMed PMID: 22525774. Epub 2012/04/25. Eng.

[12] Smuder AJ, Kavazis AN, Min K, Powers SK. Exercise protects against doxorubicin-induced oxidative stress and proteolysis in skeletal muscle. Journal of applied physiology (Bethesda, Md : 1985). 2011 Apr;110(4):935-42. PubMed PMID: 21310889. Pubmed Central PMCID: 3075128. Epub 2011/02/12. eng.

[13] Saborido A, Naudi A, Portero-Otin M, Pamplona R, Megias A. Stanozolol treatment decreases the mitochondrial ROS generation and oxidative stress induced by acute

exercise in rat skeletal muscle. Journal of applied physiology (Bethesda, Md : 1985). 2011 Mar;110(3):661-9. PubMed PMID: 21164155. Epub 2010/12/18. eng.

[14] Kuwahara H, Horie T, Ishikawa S, Tsuda C, Kawakami S, Noda Y, et al. Oxidative stress in skeletal muscle causes severe disturbance of exercise activity without muscle atrophy. Free radical biology & medicine. 2010 May 1;48(9):1252-62. PubMed PMID: 20156551. Epub 2010/02/17. eng.

[15] Syu GD, Chen HI, Jen CJ. Severe exercise and exercise training exert opposite effects on human neutrophil apoptosis via altering the redox status. PloS one. 2011;6(9):e24385. PubMed PMID: 21931703. Pubmed Central PMCID: 3170310. Epub 2011/09/21. eng.

[16] Tauler P, Aguilo A, Gimeno I, Noguera A, Agusti A, Tur JA, et al. Differential response of lymphocytes and neutrophils to high intensity physical activity and to vitamin C diet supplementation. Free radical research. 2003 Sep;37(9):931-8. PubMed PMID: 14670000. Epub 2003/12/13. eng.

[17] Suzuki K, Sato H, Kikuchi T, Abe T, Nakaji S, Sugawara K, et al. Capacity of circulating neutrophils to produce reactive oxygen species after exhaustive exercise. Journal of applied physiology (Bethesda, Md : 1985). 1996 Sep;81(3):1213-22. PubMed PMID: 8889756. Epub 1996/09/01. eng.

[18] Turner JE, Bosch JA, Drayson MT, Aldred S. Assessment of oxidative stress in lymphocytes with exercise. Journal of applied physiology (Bethesda, Md : 1985). 2011 Jul; 111(1):206-11. PubMed PMID: 21493722. Epub 2011/04/16. eng.

[19] Fisher G, Schwartz DD, Quindry J, Barberio MD, Foster EB, Jones KW, et al. Lymphocyte enzymatic antioxidant responses to oxidative stress following high-intensity interval exercise. Journal of applied physiology (Bethesda, Md : 1985). 2011 Mar; 110(3):730-7. PubMed PMID: 21127208. Epub 2010/12/04. eng.

[20] Sureda A, Ferrer MD, Tauler P, Tur JA, Pons A. Lymphocyte antioxidant response and H2O2 production after a swimming session: gender differences. Free radical research. 2008 Apr;42(4):312-9. PubMed PMID: 18404530. Epub 2008/04/12. eng.

[21] Smuder AJ, Min K, Hudson MB, Kavazis AN, Kwon OS, Nelson WB, et al. Endurance exercise attenuates ventilator-induced diaphragm dysfunction. Journal of applied physiology (Bethesda, Md : 1985). 2012 Feb;112(3):501-10. PubMed PMID: 22074717. Epub 2011/11/15. eng.

[22] Caillaud C, Py G, Eydoux N, Legros P, Prefaut C, Mercier J. Antioxidants and mitochondrial respiration in lung, diaphragm, and locomotor muscles: effect of exercise. Free radical biology & medicine. 1999 May;26(9-10):1292-9. PubMed PMID: 10381202. Epub 1999/06/25. eng.

[23] Salo DC, Donovan CM, Davies KJ. HSP70 and other possible heat shock or oxidative stress proteins are induced in skeletal muscle, heart, and liver during exercise. Free

radical biology & medicine. 1991;11(3):239-46. PubMed PMID: 1937141. Epub 1991/01/01. eng.

[24] Hoene M, Franken H, Fritsche L, Lehmann R, Pohl AK, Haring HU, et al. Activation of the mitogen-activated protein kinase (MAPK) signalling pathway in the liver of mice is related to plasma glucose levels after acute exercise. Diabetologia. 2010 Jun; 53(6):1131-41. PubMed PMID: 20195842. Epub 2010/03/03. eng.

[25] Taysi S, Oztasan N, Efe H, Polat MF, Gumustekin K, Siktar E, et al. Endurance training attenuates the oxidative stress due to acute exhaustive exercise in rat liver. Acta physiologica Hungarica. 2008 Dec;95(4):337-47. PubMed PMID: 19009910. Epub 2008/11/18. eng.

[26] Frasier CR, Sloan RC, Bostian PA, Gonzon MD, Kurowicki J, Lopresto SJ, et al. Short-term exercise preserves myocardial glutathione and decreases arrhythmias after thiol oxidation and ischemia in isolated rat hearts. Journal of applied physiology (Bethesda, Md : 1985). 2011 Dec;111(6):1751-9. PubMed PMID: 21940849. Epub 2011/09/24. eng.

[27] Bo H, Jiang N, Ma G, Qu J, Zhang G, Cao D, et al. Regulation of mitochondrial uncoupling respiration during exercise in rat heart: role of reactive oxygen species (ROS) and uncoupling protein 2. Free radical biology & medicine. 2008 Apr 1;44(7): 1373-81. PubMed PMID: 18226608. Epub 2008/01/30. eng.

[28] Nie J, Close G, George KP, Tong TK, Shi Q. Temporal association of elevations in serum cardiac troponin T and myocardial oxidative stress after prolonged exercise in rats. European journal of applied physiology. 2010 Dec;110(6):1299-303. PubMed PMID: 20711602. Epub 2010/08/17. eng.

[29] Prigol M, Luchese C, Nogueira CW. Antioxidant effect of diphenyl diselenide on oxidative stress caused by acute physical exercise in skeletal muscle and lungs of mice. Cell biochemistry and function. 2009 Jun;27(4):216-22. PubMed PMID: 19382129. Epub 2009/04/22. eng.

[30] Falone S, D'Alessandro A, Mirabilio A, Petruccelli G, Cacchio M, Di Ilio C, et al. Long term running biphasically improves methylglyoxal-related metabolism, redox homeostasis and neurotrophic support within adult mouse brain cortex. PloS one. 2012;7(2):e31401. PubMed PMID: 22347470. Pubmed Central PMCID: 3275619. Epub 2012/02/22. eng.

[31] Lima FD, Oliveira MS, Furian AF, Souza MA, Rambo LM, Ribeiro LR, et al. Adaptation to oxidative challenge induced by chronic physical exercise prevents Na+,K+-ATPase activity inhibition after traumatic brain injury. Brain research. 2009 Jul 7;1279:147-55. PubMed PMID: 19422810. Epub 2009/05/09. eng.

[32] Griesbach GS, Hovda DA, Gomez-Pinilla F, Sutton RL. Voluntary exercise or amphetamine treatment, but not the combination, increases hippocampal brain-derived neurotrophic factor and synapsin I following cortical contusion injury in rats. Neuro-

science. 2008 Jun 23;154(2):530-40. PubMed PMID: 18479829. Pubmed Central PMCID: 2441485. Epub 2008/05/16. eng.

[33] Agarwal D, Elks CM, Reed SD, Mariappan N, Majid DS, Francis J. Chronic exercise preserves renal structure and hemodynamics in spontaneously hypertensive rats. Antioxidants & redox signaling. 2012 Jan 15;16(2):139-52. PubMed PMID: 21895524. Pubmed Central PMCID: 3222098. Epub 2011/09/08. eng.

[34] George L, Lokhandwala MF, Asghar M. Exercise activates redox-sensitive transcription factors and restores renal D1 receptor function in old rats. American journal of physiology Renal physiology. 2009 Nov;297(5):F1174-80. PubMed PMID: 19759268. Pubmed Central PMCID: 2781333. Epub 2009/09/18. eng.

[35] Azenabor AA, Hoffman-Goetz L. Intrathymic and intrasplenic oxidative stress mediates thymocyte and splenocyte damage in acutely exercised mice. Journal of applied physiology (Bethesda, Md : 1985). 1999 Jun;86(6):1823-7. PubMed PMID: 10368344. Epub 1999/06/16. eng.

[36] Kruger K, Frost S, Most E, Volker K, Pallauf J, Mooren FC. Exercise affects tissue lymphocyte apoptosis via redox-sensitive and Fas-dependent signaling pathways. American journal of physiology Regulatory, integrative and comparative physiology. 2009 May;296(5):R1518-27. PubMed PMID: 19261913. Epub 2009/03/06. eng.

[37] Quadrilatero J, Hoffman-Goetz L. Mouse thymocyte apoptosis and cell loss in response to exercise and antioxidant administration. Brain, behavior, and immunity. 2005 Sep;19(5):436-44. PubMed PMID: 16061151. Epub 2005/08/03. eng.

[38] Moraska A, Deak T, Spencer RL, Roth D, Fleshner M. Treadmill running produces both positive and negative physiological adaptations in Sprague-Dawley rats. American journal of physiology Regulatory, integrative and comparative physiology. 2000 Oct;279(4):R1321-9. PubMed PMID: 11004000. Epub 2000/09/27. eng.

[39] Hofer T, Fontana L, Anton SD, Weiss EP, Villareal D, Malayappan B, et al. Long-term effects of caloric restriction or exercise on DNA and RNA oxidation levels in white blood cells and urine in humans. Rejuvenation research. 2008 Aug;11(4):793-9. PubMed PMID: 18729811. Pubmed Central PMCID: 2724865. Epub 2008/08/30. eng.

[40] Radak Z, Pucsuk J, Boros S, Josfai L, Taylor AW. Changes in urine 8-hydroxydeoxy-guanosine levels of super-marathon runners during a four-day race period. Life sciences. 2000 Mar 24;66(18):1763-7. PubMed PMID: 10809173. Epub 2000/05/16. eng.

[41] McAnulty SR, Nieman DC, Fox-Rabinovich M, Duran V, McAnulty LS, Henson DA, et al. Effect of n-3 fatty acids and antioxidants on oxidative stress after exercise. Medicine and science in sports and exercise. 2010 Sep;42(9):1704-11. PubMed PMID: 20164809. Epub 2010/02/19. eng.

[42] Taito S, Sekikawa K, Domen S, Konishi K, Kimura T, Takahashi M, et al. Pulmonary oxidative stress is induced by maximal exercise in young cigarette smokers. Nicotine

& tobacco research : official journal of the Society for Research on Nicotine and To-bacco. 2012 Feb;14(2):243-7. PubMed PMID: 22080589. Epub 2011/11/15. eng.

[43] Font-Ribera L, Kogevinas M, Zock JP, Gomez FP, Barreiro E, Nieuwenhuijsen MJ, et al. Short-term changes in respiratory biomarkers after swimming in a chlorinated pool. Environmental health perspectives. 2010 Nov;118(11):1538-44. PubMed PMID: 20833607. Pubmed Central PMCID: 2974690. Epub 2010/09/14. eng.

[44] Cantu-Medellin N, Byrd B, Hohn A, Vazquez-Medina JP, Zenteno-Savin T. Differential antioxidant protection in tissues from marine mammals with distinct diving capacities. Shallow/short vs. deep/long divers. Comparative biochemistry and physiology Part A, Molecular & integrative physiology. 2011 Apr;158(4):438-43. PubMed PMID: 21147244. Epub 2010/12/15. eng.

[45] Arguelles S, Garcia S, Maldonado M, Machado A, Ayala A. Do the serum oxidative stress biomarkers provide a reasonable index of the general oxidative stress status? Biochimica et biophysica acta. 2004 Nov 1;1674(3):251-9. PubMed PMID: 15541294. Epub 2004/11/16. eng.

[46] Liu J, Yeo HC, Overvik-Douki E, Hagen T, Doniger SJ, Chyu DW, et al. Chronically and acutely exercised rats: biomarkers of oxidative stress and endogenous antioxidants. Journal of applied physiology (Bethesda, Md : 1985). 2000 Jul;89(1):21-8. PubMed PMID: 10904031. Epub 2000/07/25. eng.

[47] Davies KJ, Quintanilha AT, Brooks GA, Packer L. Free radicals and tissue damage produced by exercise. Biochemical and biophysical research communications. 1982 Aug 31;107(4):1198-205. PubMed PMID: 6291524. Epub 1982/08/31. eng.

[48] Jackson MJ, Jones DA, Edwards RH. Vitamin E and skeletal muscle. Ciba Foundation symposium. 1983;101:224-39. PubMed PMID: 6557905. Epub 1983/01/01. eng.

[49] Puente-Maestu L, Tejedor A, Lazaro A, de Miguel J, Alvarez-Sala L, Gonzalez-Aragoneses F, et al. Site of Mitochondrial ROS Production in Skeletal Muscle of COPD and its Relationship with Exercise Oxidative Stress. American journal of respiratory cell and molecular biology. 2012 Apr 5. PubMed PMID: 22493009. Epub 2012/04/12. Eng.

[50] Phoenix J, Edwards RH, Jackson MJ. The effect of vitamin E analogues and long hydrocarbon chain compounds on calcium-induced muscle damage. A novel role for alpha-tocopherol? Biochimica et biophysica acta. 1991 Oct 21;1097(3):212-8. PubMed PMID: 1932145. Epub 1991/10/21. eng.

[51] Phoenix J, Edwards RH, Jackson MJ. Effects of calcium ionophore on vitamin E-deficient rat muscle. The British journal of nutrition. 1990 Jul;64(1):245-56. PubMed PMID: 2119221. Epub 1990/07/01. eng.

[52] Phoenix J, Edwards RH, Jackson MJ. Inhibition of Ca2+-induced cytosolic enzyme efflux from skeletal muscle by vitamin E and related compounds. The Biochemical

journal. 1989 Jan 1;257(1):207-13. PubMed PMID: 2493242. Pubmed Central PMCID: 1135557. Epub 1989/01/01. eng.

[53] Quintanilha AT, Packer L. Vitamin E, physical exercise and tissue oxidative damage. Ciba Foundation symposium. 1983;101:56-69. PubMed PMID: 6557908. Epub 1983/01/01. eng.

[54] Boveris A, Chance B. The mitochondrial generation of hydrogen peroxide. General properties and effect of hyperbaric oxygen. The Biochemical journal. 1973 Jul;134(3): 707-16. PubMed PMID: 4749271. Pubmed Central PMCID: 1177867. Epub 1973/07/01. eng.

[55] Loschen G, Azzi A, Richter C, Flohe L. Superoxide radicals as precursors of mito-chondrial hydrogen peroxide. FEBS letters. 1974 May 15;42(1):68-72. PubMed PMID: 4859511. Epub 1974/05/15. eng.

[56] Alessio HM, Hagerman AE, Fulkerson BK, Ambrose J, Rice RE, Wiley RL. Genera-tion of reactive oxygen species after exhaustive aerobic and isometric exercise. Medi-cine and science in sports and exercise. 2000 Sep;32(9):1576-81. PubMed PMID: 10994907. Epub 2000/09/20. eng.

[57] Dixon CB, Robertson RJ, Goss FL, Timmer JM, Nagle EF, Evans RW. The effect of acute resistance exercise on serum malondialdehyde in resistance-trained and un-trained collegiate men. Journal of strength and conditioning research / National Strength & Conditioning Association. 2006 Aug;20(3):693-8. PubMed PMID: 16937984. Epub 2006/08/30. eng.

[58] Jimenez L, Lefevre G, Richard R, Duvallet A, Rieu M. Exercise does not induce oxida-tive stress in trained heart transplant recipients. Medicine and science in sports and exercise. 2000 Dec;32(12):2018-23. PubMed PMID: 11128845. Epub 2000/12/29. eng.

[59] Halliwell B, Chirico S. Lipid peroxidation: its mechanism, measurement, and signifi-cance. Am J Clin Nutr. 1993 May;57(5 Suppl):715S-24S; discussion 24S-25S. PubMed PMID: 8475889. Epub 1993/05/01. eng.

[60] Gutteridge JM, Halliwell B. The measurement and mechanism of lipid peroxidation in biological systems. Trends in biochemical sciences. 1990 Apr;15(4):129-35. PubMed PMID: 2187293. Epub 1990/04/01. eng.

[61] Li G, Liu L, Hu H, Zhao Q, Xie F, Chen K, et al. Age-related carbonyl stress and er-ythrocyte membrane protein carbonylation. Clinical hemorheology and microcircula-tion. 2010 2010/12/28;46(4):305-11. PubMed PMID: 21187579. Epub 2010/12/29. eng.

[62] Jenkins RR. Exercise and oxidative stress methodology: a critique. Am J Clin Nutr. 2000 Aug;72(2 Suppl):670S-4S. PubMed PMID: 10919973. Epub 2000/08/02. eng.

[63] Jackson MJ, Edwards RH, Symons MC. Electron spin resonance studies of intact mammalian skeletal muscle. Biochimica et biophysica acta. 1985 Nov 20;847(2): 185-90. PubMed PMID: 2998478. Epub 1985/11/20. eng.

[64] Davies KJ, Hochstein P. Ubisemiquinone radicals in liver: implications for a mito-chondrial Q cycle in vivo. Biochemical and biophysical research communications. 1982 Aug 31;107(4):1292-9. PubMed PMID: 6291526. Epub 1982/08/31. eng.

[65] McArdle A, van der Meulen J, Close GL, Pattwell D, Van Remmen H, Huang TT, et al. Role of mitochondrial superoxide dismutase in contraction-induced generation of reactive oxygen species in skeletal muscle extracellular space. American journal of physiology Cell physiology. 2004 May;286(5):C1152-8. PubMed PMID: 15075214. Epub 2004/04/13. eng.

[66] Reid MB, Haack KE, Franchek KM, Valberg PA, Kobzik L, West MS. Reactive oxygen in skeletal muscle. I. Intracellular oxidant kinetics and fatigue in vitro. Journal of ap-plied physiology (Bethesda, Md : 1985). 1992 Nov;73(5):1797-804. PubMed PMID: 1474054. Epub 1992/11/01. eng.

[67] Reid MB, Shoji T, Moody MR, Entman ML. Reactive oxygen in skeletal muscle. II. Ex-tracellular release of free radicals. Journal of applied physiology (Bethesda, Md : 1985). 1992 Nov;73(5):1805-9. PubMed PMID: 1335453. Epub 1992/11/01. eng.

[68] Pattwell DM, McArdle A, Morgan JE, Patridge TA, Jackson MJ. Release of reactive oxygen and nitrogen species from contracting skeletal muscle cells. Free radical biol-ogy & medicine. 2004 Oct 1;37(7):1064-72. PubMed PMID: 15336322. Epub 2004/09/01. eng.

[69] Palomero J, Pye D, Kabayo T, Spiller DG, Jackson MJ. In situ detection and measure-ment of intracellular reactive oxygen species in single isolated mature skeletal mus-cle fibers by real time fluorescence microscopy. Antioxidants & redox signaling. 2008 Aug;10(8):1463-74. PubMed PMID: 18407749. Pubmed Central PMCID: 2536563. Epub 2008/04/15. eng.

[70] Pye D, Palomero J, Kabayo T, Jackson MJ. Real-time measurement of nitric oxide in single mature mouse skeletal muscle fibres during contractions. The Journal of physi-ology. 2007 May 15;581(Pt 1):309-18. PubMed PMID: 17331997. Pubmed Central PMCID: 2075220. Epub 2007/03/03. eng.

[71] McArdle F, Pattwell DM, Vasilaki A, McArdle A, Jackson MJ. Intracellular genera-tion of reactive oxygen species by contracting skeletal muscle cells. Free radical biolo-gy & medicine. 2005 Sep 1;39(5):651-7. PubMed PMID: 16085183. Epub 2005/08/09. eng.

[72] Belousov VV, Fradkov AF, Lukyanov KA, Staroverov DB, Shakhbazov KS, Terskikh AV, et al. Genetically encoded fluorescent indicator for intracellular hydrogen perox-ide. Nature methods. 2006 Apr;3(4):281-6. PubMed PMID: 16554833. Epub 2006/03/24. eng.

[73] Zuo L, Christofi FL, Wright VP, Liu CY, Merola AJ, Berliner LJ, et al. Intra- and ex-tracellular measurement of reactive oxygen species produced during heat stress in

diaphragm muscle. American journal of physiology Cell physiology. 2000 Oct; 279(4):C1058-66. PubMed PMID: 11003586. Epub 2000/09/26. eng.

[74] Robinson KM, Janes MS, Pehar M, Monette JS, Ross MF, Hagen TM, et al. Selective fluorescent imaging of superoxide in vivo using ethidium-based probes. Proceedings of the National Academy of Sciences. 2006 Oct 10;103(41):15038-43. PubMed PMID: 17015830. Pubmed Central PMCID: 1586181. Epub 2006/10/04. eng.

[75] Kalyanaraman B, Darley-Usmar V, Davies KJ, Dennery PA, Forman HJ, Grisham MB, et al. Measuring reactive oxygen and nitrogen species with fluorescent probes: challenges and limitations. Free radical biology & medicine. 2012 Jan 1;52(1):1-6. PubMed PMID: 22027063. Epub 2011/10/27. eng.

[76] Powers SK, Jackson MJ. Exercise-induced oxidative stress: cellular mechanisms and impact on muscle force production. Physiol Rev. 2008 Oct;88(4):1243-76. PubMed PMID: 18923182. Pubmed Central PMCID: 2909187. Epub 2008/10/17. eng.

[77] Jackson MJ. Free radicals generated by contracting muscle: by-products of metabolism or key regulators of muscle function? Free RadicBiolMed. 2008;44(2):132-41.

[78] Jackson MJ. Control of reactive oxygen species production in contracting skeletal muscle. Antioxidants & redox signaling. 2011 Nov 1;15(9):2477-86. PubMed PMID: 21699411. Pubmed Central PMCID: 3176346. Epub 2011/06/28. eng.

[79] Brady PS, Brady LJ, Ullrey DE. Selenium, vitamin E and the response to swimming stress in the rat. The Journal of nutrition. 1979 Jun;109(6):1103-9. PubMed PMID: 448449. Epub 1979/06/01. eng.

[80] da Silva LA, Pinho CA, Rocha LG, Tuon T, Silveira PC, Pinho RA. Effect of different models of physical exercise on oxidative stress markers in mouse liver. Applied physiology, nutrition, and metabolism = Physiologie appliquee, nutrition et metabolisme. 2009 Feb;34(1):60-5. PubMed PMID: 19234586. Epub 2009/02/24. eng.

[81] Kayatekin BM, Gonenc S, Acikgoz O, Uysal N, Dayi A. Effects of sprint exercise on oxidative stress in skeletal muscle and liver. European journal of applied physiology. 2002 Jun;87(2):141-4. PubMed PMID: 12070624. Epub 2002/06/19. eng.

[82] Ji LL. Antioxidant enzyme response to exercise and aging. Medicine and science in sports and exercise. 1993 Feb;25(2):225-31. PubMed PMID: 8450725. Epub 1993/02/01. eng.

[83] Aguiar AS, Jr., Tuon T, Pinho CA, Silva LA, Andreazza AC, Kapczinski F, et al. Intense exercise induces mitochondrial dysfunction in mice brain. Neurochemical research. 2008 Jan;33(1):51-8. PubMed PMID: 17619145. Epub 2007/07/10. eng.

[84] Akil M, Bicer M, Menevse E, Baltaci AK, Mogulkoc R. Selenium supplementation prevents lipid peroxidation caused by arduous exercise in rat brain tissue. Bratislavske lekarske listy. 2011;112(6):314-7. PubMed PMID: 21692404. Epub 2011/06/23. eng.

[85] Aydin C, Sonat F, Sahin SK, Cangul IT, Ozkaya G. Long term dietary restriction ameliorates swimming exercise-induced oxidative stress in brain and lung of middle-aged rat. Indian journal of experimental biology. 2009 Jan;47(1):24-31. PubMed PMID: 19317348. Epub 2009/03/26. eng.

[86] Jolitha AB, Subramanyam MV, Asha Devi S. Modification by vitamin E and exercise of oxidative stress in regions of aging rat brain: studies on superoxide dismutase iso-enzymes and protein oxidation status. Experimental gerontology. 2006 Aug;41(8): 753-63. PubMed PMID: 16843630. Epub 2006/07/18. eng.

[87] Coskun S, Gonul B, Guzel NA, Balabanli B. The effects of vitamin C supplementation on oxidative stress and antioxidant content in the brains of chronically exercised rats. Molecular and cellular biochemistry. 2005 Dec;280(1-2):135-8. PubMed PMID: 16311914. Epub 2005/11/29. eng.

[88] Toldy A, Stadler K, Sasvari M, Jakus J, Jung KJ, Chung HY, et al. The effect of exercise and nettle supplementation on oxidative stress markers in the rat brain. Brain Res Bull. 2005 May 30;65(6):487-93. PubMed PMID: 15862920. Epub 2005/05/03. eng.

[89] Ogonovszky H, Berkes I, Kumagai S, Kaneko T, Tahara S, Goto S, et al. The effects of moderate-, strenuous- and over-training on oxidative stress markers, DNA repair, and memory, in rat brain. Neurochemistry international. 2005 Jun;46(8):635-40. PubMed PMID: 15863241. Epub 2005/05/03. eng.

[90] Ozkaya YG, Agar A, Yargicoglu P, Hacioglu G, Bilmen-Sarikcioglu S, Ozen I, et al. The effect of exercise on brain antioxidant status of diabetic rats. Diabetes & metabolism. 2002 Nov;28(5):377-84. PubMed PMID: 12461474. Epub 2002/12/04. eng.

[91] Somani SM, Husain K, Diaz-Phillips L, Lanzotti DJ, Kareti KR, Trammell GL. Interaction of exercise and ethanol on antioxidant enzymes in brain regions of the rat. Alcohol (Fayetteville, NY). 1996 Nov-Dec;13(6):603-10. PubMed PMID: 8949956. Epub 1996/11/01. eng.

[92] Somani SM, Ravi R, Rybak LP. Effect of exercise training on antioxidant system in brain regions of rat. Pharmacology, biochemistry, and behavior. 1995 Apr;50(4):635-9. PubMed PMID: 7617712. Epub 1995/04/01. eng.

[93] Devi SA, Kiran TR. Regional responses in antioxidant system to exercise training and dietary vitamin E in aging rat brain. Neurobiology of aging. 2004 Apr;25(4):501-8. PubMed PMID: 15013571. Epub 2004/03/12. eng.

[94] Asha Devi S. Aging brain: prevention of oxidative stress by vitamin E and exercise. TheScientificWorldJournal. 2009;9:366-72. PubMed PMID: 19468659. Epub 2009/05/27. eng.

[95] Lappalainen Z, Lappalainen J, Oksala NK, Laaksonen DE, Khanna S, Sen CK, et al. Diabetes impairs exercise training-associated thioredoxin response and glutathione

status in rat brain. Journal of applied physiology (Bethesda, Md : 1985). 2009 Feb; 106(2):461-7. PubMed PMID: 19074570. Epub 2008/12/17. eng.

[96] Mazzola PN, Terra M, Rosa AP, Mescka CP, Moraes TB, Piccoli B, et al. Regular exercise prevents oxidative stress in the brain of hyperphenylalaninemic rats. Metabolic brain disease. 2011 Dec;26(4):291-7. PubMed PMID: 21947687. Epub 2011/09/29. eng.

[97] Liu W, Zhou C. Corticosterone reduces brain mitochondrial function and expression of mitofusin, BDNF in depression-like rodents regardless of exercise preconditioning. Psychoneuroendocrinology. 2012 Jan 12;37(7):1057-70. PubMed PMID: 22244747. Epub 2012/01/17. Eng.

[98] Molteni R, Wu A, Vaynman S, Ying Z, Barnard RJ, Gomez-Pinilla F. Exercise reverses the harmful effects of consumption of a high-fat diet on synaptic and behavioral plasticity associated to the action of brain-derived neurotrophic factor. Neuroscience. 2004;123(2):429-40. PubMed PMID: 14698750. Epub 2003/12/31. eng.

[99] Chance B, Sies H, Boveris A. Hydroperoxide metabolism in mammalian organs. Physiol Rev. 1979 Jul;59(3):527-605. PubMed PMID: 37532. Epub 1979/07/01. eng.

[100] Boveris A, Oshino N, Chance B. The cellular production of hydrogen peroxide. The Biochemical journal. 1972 Jul;128(3):617-30. PubMed PMID: 4404507. Pubmed Central PMCID: 1173814. Epub 1972/07/01. eng.

[101] Richardson RS, Donato AJ, Uberoi A, Wray DW, Lawrenson L, Nishiyama S, et al. Exercise-induced brachial artery vasodilation: role of free radicals. American journal of physiology Heart and circulatory physiology. 2007 Mar;292(3):H1516-22. PubMed PMID: 17114239. Epub 2006/11/23. eng.

[102] Herrero A, Barja G. ADP-regulation of mitochondrial free radical production is different with complex I- or complex II-linked substrates: implications for the exercise paradox and brain hypermetabolism. Journal of bioenergetics and biomembranes. 1997 Jun;29(3):241-9. PubMed PMID: 9298709. Epub 1997/06/01. eng.

[103] Di Meo S, Venditti P. Mitochondria in exercise-induced oxidative stress. Biological signals and receptors. 2001 Jan-Apr;10(1-2):125-40. PubMed PMID: 11223645. Epub 2001/02/27. eng.

[104] McArdle A, van der Meulen JH, Catapano M, Symons MC, Faulkner JA, Jackson MJ. Free radical activity following contraction-induced injury to the extensor digitorum longus muscles of rats. Free radical biology & medicine. 1999 May;26(9-10):1085-91. PubMed PMID: 10381177. Epub 1999/06/25. eng.

[105] Nishino T, Okamoto K, Kawaguchi Y, Hori H, Matsumura T, Eger BT, et al. Mechanism of the conversion of xanthine dehydrogenase to xanthine oxidase: identification of the two cysteine disulfide bonds and crystal structure of a non-convertible rat liver xanthine dehydrogenase mutant. The Journal of biological chemistry. 2005 Jul 1;280(26):24888-94. PubMed PMID: 15878860. Epub 2005/05/10. eng.

[106] Saksela M, Lapatto R, Raivio KO. Irreversible conversion of xanthine dehydrogenase into xanthine oxidase by a mitochondrial protease. FEBS letters. 1999 Jan 25;443(2): 117-20. PubMed PMID: 9989587. Epub 1999/02/16. eng.

[107] Engerson TD, McKelvey TG, Rhyne DB, Boggio EB, Snyder SJ, Jones HP. Conversion of xanthine dehydrogenase to oxidase in ischemic rat tissues. The Journal of clinical investigation. 1987 Jun;79(6):1564-70. PubMed PMID: 3294898. Pubmed Central PMCID: 424467. Epub 1987/06/01. eng.

[108] Ryan MJ, Jackson JR, Hao Y, Leonard SS, Alway SE. Inhibition of xanthine oxidase reduces oxidative stress and improves skeletal muscle function in response to electrically stimulated isometric contractions in aged mice. Free radical biology & medicine. 2011 Jul 1;51(1):38-52. PubMed PMID: 21530649. Epub 2011/05/03. eng.

[109] Mills PC, Smith NC, Harris RC, Harris P. Effect of allopurinol on the formation of reactive oxygen species during intense exercise in the horse. Research in veterinary science. 1997 Jan-Feb;62(1):11-6. PubMed PMID: 9160417. Epub 1997/01/01. eng.

[110] Vina J, Gimeno A, Sastre J, Desco C, Asensi M, Pallardo FV, et al. Mechanism of free radical production in exhaustive exercise in humans and rats; role of xanthine oxidase and protection by allopurinol. IUBMBLife. 2000;49(6):539-44.

[111] Kelkar A, Kuo A, Frishman WH. Allopurinol as a cardiovascular drug. Cardiology in review. 2011 Nov-Dec;19(6):265-71. PubMed PMID: 21983313. Epub 2011/10/11. eng.

[112] Vina J, Gomez-Cabrera MC, Lloret A, Marquez R, Minana JB, Pallardo FV, et al. Free radicals in exhaustive physical exercise: mechanism of production, and protection by antioxidants. IUBMB life. 2000 Oct-Nov;50(4-5):271-7. PubMed PMID: 11327321. Epub 2001/05/01. eng.

[113] Capecchi PL, Pasini FL, Pasqui AL, Orrico A, Ceccatelli L, Acciavatti A, et al. Allopurinol prevents ischaemia-dependent haemorheological changes. European journal of clinical pharmacology. 1988;35(5):475-81. PubMed PMID: 2853054. Epub 1988/01/01. eng.

[114] Olek RA, Safranow K, Jakubowska K, Olszewska M, Chlubek D, Laskowski R. Allopurinol intake does not modify the slow component of V(.)O(2) kinetics and oxidative stress induced by severe intensity exercise. Physiological research / Academia Scientiarum Bohemoslovaca. 2012 Mar 6;61(1):89-96. PubMed PMID: 22188105. Epub 2011/12/23. eng.

[115] Gomez-Cabrera MC, Borras C, Pallardo FV, Sastre J, Ji LL, Vina J. Decreasing xanthine oxidase-mediated oxidative stress prevents useful cellular adaptations to exercise in rats. The Journal of physiology. 2005 Aug 15;567(Pt 1):113-20. PubMed PMID: 15932896. Pubmed Central PMCID: 1474177. Epub 2005/06/04. eng.

[116] Malm C, Lenkei R, Sjodin B. Effects of eccentric exercise on the immune system in men. Journal of applied physiology (Bethesda, Md : 1985). 1999 Feb;86(2):461-8. PubMed PMID: 9931177. Epub 1999/02/04. eng.

[117] Gulati M, Pandey DK, Arnsdorf MF, Lauderdale DS, Thisted RA, Wicklund RH, et al. Exercise capacity and the risk of death in women: the St James Women Take Heart Project. Circulation. 2003 Sep 30;108(13):1554-9. PubMed PMID: 12975254. Epub 2003/09/17. eng.

[118] Couillard A, Koechlin C, Cristol JP, Varray A, Prefaut C. Evidence of local exercise-induced systemic oxidative stress in chronic obstructive pulmonary disease patients. The European respiratory journal : official journal of the European Society for Clinical Respiratory Physiology. 2002 Nov;20(5):1123-9. PubMed PMID: 12449164. Epub 2002/11/27. eng.

[119] Gunduz F, Senturk UK. The effect of reactive oxidant generation in acute exercise-induced proteinuria in trained and untrained rats. European journal of applied physiology. 2003 Nov;90(5-6):526-32. PubMed PMID: 12905046. Epub 2003/08/09. eng.

[120] Moller P, Loft S, Lundby C, Olsen NV. Acute hypoxia and hypoxic exercise induce DNA strand breaks and oxidative DNA damage in humans. The FASEB journal : official publication of the Federation of American Societies for Experimental Biology. 2001 May;15(7):1181-6. PubMed PMID: 11344086. Epub 2001/05/10. eng.

[121] Santos-Silva A, Rebelo MI, Castro EM, Belo L, Guerra A, Rego C, et al. Leukocyte activation, erythrocyte damage, lipid profile and oxidative stress imposed by high competition physical exercise in adolescents. Clinica chimica acta; international journal of clinical chemistry. 2001 Apr;306(1-2):119-26. PubMed PMID: 11282102. Epub 2001/04/03. eng.

[122] Watson TA, Callister R, Taylor R, Sibbritt D, MacDonald-Wicks LK, Garg ML. Antioxidant restricted diet increases oxidative stress during acute exhaustive exercise. Asia Pacific journal of clinical nutrition. 2003;12 Suppl:S9. PubMed PMID: 15023594. Epub 2004/03/17. eng.

[123] Husain K, Somani SM. Interaction of exercise training and chronic ethanol ingestion on hepatic and plasma antioxidant system in rat. Journal of applied toxicology : JAT. 1997 May-Jun;17(3):189-94. PubMed PMID: 9250541. Epub 1997/05/01. eng.

[124] Bobillier Chaumont S, Maupoil V, Jacques Lahet J, Berthelot A. Effect of exercise training on metallothionein levels of hypertensive rats. Medicine and science in sports and exercise. 2001 May;33(5):724-8. PubMed PMID: 11323539. Epub 2001/04/27. eng.

[125] Cazzola R, Russo-Volpe S, Cervato G, Cestaro B. Biochemical assessments of oxidative stress, erythrocyte membrane fluidity and antioxidant status in professional soccer players and sedentary controls. European journal of clinical investigation. 2003 Oct;33(10):924-30. PubMed PMID: 14511366. Epub 2003/09/27. eng.

[126] Ma J, Liu Z, Ling W. Physical activity, diet and cardiovascular disease risks in Chinese women. Public health nutrition. 2003 Apr;6(2):139-46. PubMed PMID: 12675956. Epub 2003/04/05. eng.

[127] Galan AI, Palacios E, Ruiz F, Diez A, Arji M, Almar M, et al. Exercise, oxidative stress and risk of cardiovascular disease in the elderly. Protective role of antioxidant functional foods. BioFactors (Oxford, England). 2006;27(1-4):167-83. PubMed PMID: 17012773. Epub 2006/10/03. eng.

[128] Meilhac O, Ramachandran S, Chiang K, Santanam N, Parthasarathy S. Role of arterial wall antioxidant defense in beneficial effects of exercise on atherosclerosis in mice. Arteriosclerosis, thrombosis, and vascular biology. 2001 Oct;21(10):1681-8. PubMed PMID: 11597945. Epub 2001/10/13. eng.

[129] Droge W. Free Radicals in the Physiological Control of Cell Function. PhysiolRev. 2002;82(1):47-95.

[130] Li G, He H. Hormesis, allostatic buffering capacity and physiological mechanism of physical activity: a new theoretic framework. Medical hypotheses. 2009 May;72(5): 527-32. PubMed PMID: 19211194. Epub 2009/02/13. eng.

[131] Reid MB, Khawli FA, Moody MR. Reactive oxygen in skeletal muscle. III. Contractility of unfatigued muscle. Journal of applied physiology (Bethesda, Md : 1985). 1993 Sep;75(3):1081-7. PubMed PMID: 8226515. Epub 1993/09/01. eng.

[132] Kang C, O'Moore KM, Dickman JR, Ji LL. Exercise activation of muscle peroxisome proliferator-activated receptor-gamma coactivator-1alpha signaling is redox sensitive. Free radical biology & medicine. 2009 Nov 15;47(10):1394-400. PubMed PMID: 19686839. Epub 2009/08/19. eng.

[133] Ji LL. Antioxidant signaling in skeletal muscle: a brief review. Experimental gerontology. 2007 Jul;42(7):582-93. PubMed PMID: 17467943. Epub 2007/05/01. eng.

[134] Teixeira VH, Valente HF, Casal SI, Marques AF, Moreira PA. Antioxidants do not prevent postexercise peroxidation and may delay muscle recovery. Medicine and science in sports and exercise. 2009 Sep;41(9):1752-60. PubMed PMID: 19657294. Epub 2009/08/07. eng.

[135] Ristow M, Zarse K, Oberbach A, Kloting N, Birringer M, Kiehntopf M, et al. Antioxidants prevent health-promoting effects of physical exercise in humans. Proceedings of the National Academy of Sciences of the United States of America. 2009 May 26;106(21):8665-70. PubMed PMID: 19433800. Pubmed Central PMCID: 2680430. Epub 2009/05/13. eng.

[136] Peternelj TT, Coombes JS. Antioxidant supplementation during exercise training: beneficial or detrimental? Sports Med. 2011 Dec 1;41(12):1043-69. PubMed PMID: 22060178. Epub 2011/11/09. eng.

[137] Alessio HM, Goldfarb AH, Cao G. Exercise-induced oxidative stress before and after vitamin C supplementation. International journal of sport nutrition. 1997 Mar;7(1): 1-9. PubMed PMID: 9063760. Epub 1997/03/01. eng.

[138] Davison GW, Ashton T, George L, Young IS, McEneny J, Davies B, et al. Molecular detection of exercise-induced free radicals following ascorbate prophylaxis in type 1 diabetes mellitus: a randomised controlled trial. Diabetologia. 2008 Nov;51(11): 2049-59. PubMed PMID: 18769906. Epub 2008/09/05. eng.

[139] Goldfarb AH, McIntosh MK, Boyer BT, Fatouros J. Vitamin E effects on indexes of lipid peroxidation in muscle from DHEA-treated and exercised rats. Journal of applied physiology (Bethesda, Md : 1985). 1994 Apr;76(4):1630-5. PubMed PMID: 8045842. Epub 1994/04/01. eng.

[140] Ryan MJ, Dudash HJ, Docherty M, Geronilla KB, Baker BA, Haff GG, et al. Vitamin E and C supplementation reduces oxidative stress, improves antioxidant enzymes and positive muscle work in chronically loaded muscles of aged rats. Experimental gerontology. 2010 Nov;45(11):882-95. PubMed PMID: 20705127. Pubmed Central PMCID: 3104015. Epub 2010/08/14. eng.

[141] Vincent HK, Bourguignon CM, Vincent KR, Weltman AL, Bryant M, Taylor AG. Antioxidant supplementation lowers exercise-induced oxidative stress in young overweight adults. Obesity (Silver Spring, Md). 2006 Dec;14(12):2224-35. PubMed PMID: 17189550. Epub 2006/12/26. eng.

[142] Vassilakopoulos T, Karatza MH, Katsaounou P, Kollintza A, Zakynthinos S, Roussos C. Antioxidants attenuate the plasma cytokine response to exercise in humans. Journal of applied physiology (Bethesda, Md : 1985). 2003 Mar;94(3):1025-32. PubMed PMID: 12571133. Epub 2003/02/07. eng.

[143] Lucotti P, Setola E, Monti LD, Galluccio E, Costa S, Sandoli EP, et al. Beneficial effects of a long-term oral L-arginine treatment added to a hypocaloric diet and exercise training program in obese, insulin-resistant type 2 diabetic patients. American journal of physiology Endocrinology and metabolism. 2006 Nov;291(5):E906-12. PubMed PMID: 16772327. Epub 2006/06/15. eng.

[144] Tauler P, Ferrer MD, Sureda A, Pujol P, Drobnic F, Tur JA, et al. Supplementation with an antioxidant cocktail containing coenzyme Q prevents plasma oxidative damage induced by soccer. European journal of applied physiology. 2008 Nov;104(5): 777-85. PubMed PMID: 18665388. Epub 2008/07/31. eng.

[145] Williams CA, Hoffman RM, Kronfeld DS, Hess TM, Saker KE, Harris PA. Lipoic acid as an antioxidant in mature thoroughbred geldings: a preliminary study. The Journal of nutrition. 2002 Jun;132(6 Suppl 2):1628S-31S. PubMed PMID: 12042475. Epub 2002/06/04. eng.

[146] Ryan MJ, Jackson JR, Hao Y, Williamson CL, Dabkowski ER, Hollander JM, et al. Suppression of oxidative stress by resveratrol after isometric contractions in gastro-

cnemius muscles of aged mice. The journals of gerontology Series A, Biological sciences and medical sciences. 2010 Aug;65(8):815-31. PubMed PMID: 20507922. Pubmed Central PMCID: 2903786. Epub 2010/05/29. eng.

[147] Marquez R, Santangelo G, Sastre J, Goldschmidt P, Luyckx J, Pallardo FV, et al. Cyanoside chloride and chromocarbe diethylamine are more effective than vitamin C against exercise-induced oxidative stress. Pharmacology & toxicology. 2001 Nov; 89(5):255-8. PubMed PMID: 11881979. Epub 2002/03/08. eng.

[148] Maranon G, Munoz-Escassi B, Manley W, Garcia C, Cayado P, de la Muela MS, et al. The effect of methyl sulphonyl methane supplementation on biomarkers of oxidative stress in sport horses following jumping exercise. Acta veterinaria Scandinavica. 2008;50:45. PubMed PMID: 18992134. Pubmed Central PMCID: 2586020. Epub 2008/11/11. eng.

[149] Olinescu R, Talaban D, Nita S, Mihaescu G. Comparative study of the presence of oxidative stress in sportsmen in competition and aged people, as well as the preventive effect of selenium administration. Romanian journal of internal medicine = Revue roumaine de medecine interne. 1995 Jan-Jun;33(1-2):47-54. PubMed PMID: 8535352. Epub 1995/01/01. eng.

[150] Panza VS, Wazlawik E, Ricardo Schutz G, Comin L, Hecht KC, da Silva EL. Consumption of green tea favorably affects oxidative stress markers in weight-trained men. Nutrition (Burbank, Los Angeles County, Calif). 2008 May;24(5):433-42. PubMed PMID: 18337059. Epub 2008/03/14. eng.

[151] Goldfarb AH, Garten RS, Cho C, Chee PD, Chambers LA. Effects of a fruit/berry/ vegetable supplement on muscle function and oxidative stress. Medicine and science in sports and exercise. 2011 Mar;43(3):501-8. PubMed PMID: 20689455. Epub 2010/08/07. eng.

[152] Bailey DM, Williams C, Betts JA, Thompson D, Hurst TL. Oxidative stress, inflammation and recovery of muscle function after damaging exercise: effect of 6-week mixed antioxidant supplementation. European journal of applied physiology. 2011 Jun; 111(6):925-36. PubMed PMID: 21069377. Epub 2010/11/12. eng.

[153] Bloomer RJ, Canale RE, Blankenship MM, Fisher-Wellman KH. Effect of Ambrotose AO(R) on resting and exercise-induced antioxidant capacity and oxidative stress in healthy adults. Nutrition journal. 2010;9:49. PubMed PMID: 21040582. Pubmed Central PMCID: 2987350. Epub 2010/11/03. eng.

[154] Bloomer RJ, Falvo MJ, Schilling BK, Smith WA. Prior exercise and antioxidant supplementation: effect on oxidative stress and muscle injury. Journal of the International Society of Sports Nutrition. 2007;4:9. PubMed PMID: 17915021. Pubmed Central PMCID: 2131751. Epub 2007/10/05. eng.

[155] Williams CA, Carlucci SA. Oral vitamin E supplementation on oxidative stress, vita-
       min and antioxidant status in intensely exercised horses. Equine veterinary journal
       Supplement. 2006 Aug(36):617-21. PubMed PMID: 17402493. Epub 2007/04/04. eng.

[156] Gaeini AA, Rahnama N, Hamedinia MR. Effects of vitamin E supplementation on
       oxidative stress at rest and after exercise to exhaustion in athletic students. The Jour-
       nal of sports medicine and physical fitness. 2006 Sep;46(3):458-61. PubMed PMID:
       16998452. Epub 2006/09/26. eng.

[157] Viitala PE, Newhouse IJ, LaVoie N, Gottardo C. The effects of antioxidant vitamin
       supplementation on resistance exercise induced lipid peroxidation in trained and un-
       trained participants. Lipids in health and disease. 2004 Jun 22;3:14. PubMed PMID:
       15212697. Pubmed Central PMCID: 479696. Epub 2004/06/24. eng.

[158] Lamprecht M, Hofmann P, Greilberger JF, Schwaberger G. Increased lipid peroxida-
       tion in trained men after 2 weeks of antioxidant supplementation. International jour-
       nal of sport nutrition and exercise metabolism. 2009 Aug;19(4):385-99. PubMed
       PMID: 19827463. Epub 2009/10/16. eng.

[159] McAnulty SR, McAnulty LS, Nieman DC, Morrow JD, Shooter LA, Holmes S, et al.
       Effect of alpha-tocopherol supplementation on plasma homocysteine and oxidative
       stress in highly trained athletes before and after exhaustive exercise. The Journal of
       nutritional biochemistry. 2005 Sep;16(9):530-7. PubMed PMID: 16115541. Epub
       2005/08/24. eng.

[160] Nieman DC, Henson DA, McAnulty SR, McAnulty LS, Morrow JD, Ahmed A, et al.
       Vitamin E and immunity after the Kona Triathlon World Championship. Medicine
       and science in sports and exercise. 2004 Aug;36(8):1328-35. PubMed PMID: 15292740.
       Epub 2004/08/05. eng.

[161] Bryant RJ, Ryder J, Martino P, Kim J, Craig BW. Effects of vitamin E and C supple-
       mentation either alone or in combination on exercise-induced lipid peroxidation in
       trained cyclists. Journal of strength and conditioning research / National Strength &
       Conditioning Association. 2003 Nov;17(4):792-800. PubMed PMID: 14666945. Epub
       2003/12/12. eng.

[162] Childs A, Jacobs C, Kaminski T, Halliwell B, Leeuwenburgh C. Supplementation
       with vitamin C and N-acetyl-cysteine increases oxidative stress in humans after an
       acute muscle injury induced by eccentric exercise. Free radical biology & medicine.
       2001 Sep 15;31(6):745-53. PubMed PMID: 11557312. Epub 2001/09/15. eng.

[163] Balakrishnan SD, Anuradha CV. Exercise, depletion of antioxidants and antioxidant
       manipulation. Cell biochemistry and function. 1998 Dec;16(4):269-75. PubMed PMID:
       9857489. Epub 1998/12/19. eng.

[164] Venditti P, Di Meo S. Effect of training on antioxidant capacity, tissue damage, and
       endurance of adult male rats. International journal of sports medicine. 1997 Oct;18(7):
       497-502. PubMed PMID: 9414071. Epub 1997/12/31. eng.

[165] Venditti P, Di Meo S. Antioxidants, tissue damage, and endurance in trained and un-trained young male rats. Archives of biochemistry and biophysics. 1996 Jul 1;331(1): 63-8. PubMed PMID: 8660684. Epub 1996/07/01. eng.

[166] Kingsley MI, Wadsworth D, Kilduff LP, McEneny J, Benton D. Effects of phosphati-dylserine on oxidative stress following intermittent running. Medicine and science in sports and exercise. 2005 Aug;37(8):1300-6. PubMed PMID: 16118575. Epub 2005/08/25. eng.

[167] Leelarungrayub D, Khansuwan R, Pothongsunun P, Klaphajone J. N-acetylcysteine supplementation controls total antioxidant capacity, creatine kinase, lactate, and tu-mor necrotic factor-alpha against oxidative stress induced by graded exercise in sed-entary men. Oxidative medicine and cellular longevity. 2011;2011:329643. PubMed PMID: 21904641. Pubmed Central PMCID: 3163015. Epub 2011/09/10. eng.

[168] Medved I, Brown MJ, Bjorksten AR, Leppik JA, Sostaric S, McKenna MJ. N-acetylcys-teine infusion alters blood redox status but not time to fatigue during intense exer-cise in humans. Journal of applied physiology (Bethesda, Md : 1985). 2003 Apr;94(4): 1572-82. PubMed PMID: 12496140. Epub 2002/12/24. eng.

[169] Medved I, Brown MJ, Bjorksten AR, McKenna MJ. Effects of intravenous N-acetyl-cysteine infusion on time to fatigue and potassium regulation during prolonged cy-cling exercise. Journal of applied physiology (Bethesda, Md : 1985). 2004 Jan;96(1): 211-7. PubMed PMID: 12959960. Epub 2003/09/10. eng.

[170] Close GL, Ashton T, McArdle A, Maclaren DP. The emerging role of free radicals in delayed onset muscle soreness and contraction-induced muscle injury. Comparative biochemistry and physiology Part A, Molecular & integrative physiology. 2005 Nov; 142(3):257-66. PubMed PMID: 16153865. Epub 2005/09/13. eng.

[171] Urso ML, Clarkson PM. Oxidative stress, exercise, and antioxidant supplementation. Toxicology. 2003 Jul 15;189(1-2):41-54. PubMed PMID: 12821281. Epub 2003/06/25. eng.

[172] McGinley C, Shafat A, Donnelly AE. Does antioxidant vitamin supplementation pro-tect against muscle damage? Sports Med. 2009;39(12):1011-32. PubMed PMID: 19902983. Epub 2009/11/12. eng.

[173] Kingsley MI, Kilduff LP, McEneny J, Dietzig RE, Benton D. Phosphatidylserine sup-plementation and recovery following downhill running. Medicine and science in sports and exercise. 2006 Sep;38(9):1617-25. PubMed PMID: 16960523. Epub 2006/09/09. eng.

[174] Kaikkonen J, Kosonen L, Nyyssonen K, Porkkala-Sarataho E, Salonen R, Korpela H, et al. Effect of combined coenzyme Q10 and d-alpha-tocopheryl acetate supplemen-tation on exercise-induced lipid peroxidation and muscular damage: a placebo-con-trolled double-blind study in marathon runners. Free radical research. 1998 Jul;29(1): 85-92. PubMed PMID: 9733025. Epub 1998/09/11. eng.

[175] Calabrese EJ, Bachmann KA, Bailer AJ, Bolger PM, Borak J, Cai L, et al. Biological stress response terminology: Integrating the concepts of adaptive response and pre-conditioning stress within a hormetic dose-response framework. ToxicolApplPharmacol. 2007;222(1):122-8.

[176] Le Bourg E, Rattan SIS. Mild Stress and Healthy Aging: Applying hormesis in aging research and interventions. Dordrecht: Springer; 2008.

[177] Mattson MP. Hormesis defined. Ageing Res Rev. 2008;7(1):1-7.

[178] Goldfarb AH, McIntosh MK, Boyer BT. Vitamin E attenuates myocardial oxidative stress induced by DHEA in rested and exercised rats. Journal of applied physiology (Bethesda, Md : 1985). 1996 Feb;80(2):486-90. PubMed PMID: 8929588. Epub 1996/02/01. eng.

[179] Sterling P, Eyer J, Fisher S, Reason J. Allostasis: a new paradigm to explain arousal pathology. Handbook of life stress, cognition and health. New York: John Wiley & Sons; 1988. p. 629-49.

[180] Irrcher I, Adhihetty PJ, Joseph AM, Ljubicic V, Hood DA. Regulation of mitochondri-al biogenesis in muscle by endurance exercise. Sports Med. 2003;33(11):783-93.

[181] Menshikova EV, Ritov VB, Ferrell RE, Azuma K, Goodpaster BH, Kelley DE. Charac-teristics of skeletal muscle mitochondrial biogenesis induced by moderate-intensity exercise and weight loss in obesity. Journal of Applied Physiology. 2007;103(1):21-7.

[182] Starnes JW, Barnes BD, Olsen ME. Exercise training decreases rat heart mitochondria free radical generation but does not prevent Ca2+-induced dysfunction. JApplPhy-siol. 2007;102(5):1793-8.

[183] Guarente L. Mitochondria-a nexus for aging, calorie restriction, and sirtuins? Cell. 2008;132(2):171-6.

[184] Wallace DC. A mitochondrial paradigm of metabolic and degenerative diseases, ag-ing, and cancer: a dawn for evolutionary medicine. AnnuRev Genet. 2005;39:359-407.

[185] Ji LL. Modulation of skeletal muscle antioxidant defense by exercise: Role of redox signaling. Free RadicBiolMed. 2008;44(2):142-52.

[186] Wakshlag JJ, Kallfelz FA, Barr SC, Ordway G, Haley NJ, Flaherty CE, et al. Effects of exercise on canine skeletal muscle proteolysis: an investigation of the ubiquitin-pro-teasome pathway and other metabolic markers. VetTher. 2002;3(3):215-25.

Chapter 7

Real and Simulated Altitude Training and Performance

Michael J. Hamlin, Nick Draper and John Hellemans

Additional information is available at the end of the chapter

.

1. Introduction

The use of altitude training to compliment normal training at sea level is widely used by coaches and athletes. There are a number of different altitude training models which range from living and training at moderate and high altitude to breathing hypoxic gas while living and training normally at sea level. In this chapter we will briefly overview the history of altitude training and touch on the science and practice of the various models of altitude training. We also discuss the beneficial effects reported in the scientific literature and give first-hand accounts of the effectiveness of the various methods from high performance coaches. Benefits and drawbacks from each altitude method will be discussed along with advice on preparing athletes prior to altitude training.

Approximately 80% of the world's population lives at low altitude (< 500 m) [1] which has an optimal atmospheric pressure and oxygen concentration for the human body's functioning. However as we ascend in altitude, the air volume expands due to the lowering of atmospheric pressure, which results in the reduction of oxygen availability to the muscles. This drop in oxygen concentration results in decreased oxygen pressure in the inspired air (P_IO_2) and a subsequent drop in the amount of oxygen in the arterial blood (P_aO_2). A reduction in the concentration of oxygen in the circulating arterial blood results in a decreased ability to extract oxygen for the working muscles and a reduced oxygen uptake. This reduced oxygen uptake is a major problem for mountaineers at high altitude and is responsible for the steady decline in maximal oxygen uptake ($\dot{V}O_2$ max) and subsequent performance at high altitude. Traditional altitude training uses these oxygen concentration changes that occur with changes in elevation to induce beneficial adaptations in the performance of athletes either at altitude or closer to sea level.

Aviation physiology research has contributed significantly to the understanding of how the human body responds and adapts to a hypoxic (low oxygen concentration) environment. In the 1880's an Italian physiologist, Angelo Mosso, (1846-1910) was one of the first to conduct experiments in the Italian Alps on the physiological effects of altitude on humans. Mosso's studies on respirational changes at altitude made him a leader in the field and Mosso's work was soon followed by other scientists in the late 1800's and early 1900's who were particularly interested in the medical effects of high altitude. Last century a number of famous high altitude expeditions were designed to collect data on the physiological effects of high altitude. These included the 1911 Anglo-American Pikes Peak Expedition, the 1921-1922 International High Altitude Expedition to Cerro de Pasco, Peru, the 1935 International High Altitude Expedition to Chile, and the 1960-1961 Himalayan Scientific and Mountaineering Expedition (Silver Hut) [2]. Research into the effects of high altitude on the human body became of great interest during the race to conquer Mt. Everest and research into the effects of altitude, particularly on exercise performance, became popular after the Olympic Games were awarded to Mexico City (elevation 2,300 m, 7,544 ft). It was found that during the Games, athletes that came from sea-level countries were affected by the low oxygen concentration in the air at Mexico City and struggled to gain medals. In particular, the sea-level middle and long distance runners' performance times were significantly slower at Mexico City compared with their performance times at sea-level the same year. On the other hand, the athletes from high altitude-based countries won many of the medals available in the middle and long distance track events. For example, from the 800m through to the marathon, out of a possible 18 medals up for grabs, 9 (50%) were won by athletes from Kenya and Ethiopia. Since the Mexico City Olympic Games a plethora of research has occurred in the area of altitude training. The main focus of this research has been to answer important questions around what the ideal altitude and length of stay is and what the effects of altitude are on the physiology of the human body.

It is now well established that exposure to real altitude produces a drop in P_IO_2, P_aO_2 and subsequently arterial oxyhaemoglobin saturation (S_aO_2) resulting in a decrement in kidney oxygenation. This reduction in oxygen concentration stimulates the synthesis and release of erythropoietin (EPO), a hormone produced in the kidney, which subsequently stimulates erythropoiesis in the red bone marrow, finally resulting in red blood cell (RBC) and haemoglobin production. Over a period of time these haematological changes may significantly improve aerobic performance in endurance athletes by enhancing the delivery of oxygen to working muscles and the ability of the muscles to use oxygen to produce energy. Indeed Levine and Stray-Gundersen (2005) argued that the primary mechanism responsible for improved sea-level endurance performance following prolonged exposures to altitude is an enhanced erythropoietic response, which results in an elevated red blood cell volume and a resultant enhanced rate of oxygen transport [3]. However, in response to Levine and Stray-Gundersen (2005), Gore and Hopkins maintained that the improvements in submaximal oxygen efficiency, or even cardiovascular adaptation, rather than the haematological changes alone should be considered when assessing the mechanisms responsible for the improved sea level performance after altitude training [4].

Debate continues over the mechanisms involved in performance improvement after altitude training. While some studies have reported increases in haemoglobin mass (or red cell mass) after classical altitude training at altitudes of 1900m or above [5-8], others have reported no such change after training at such altitudes [9-13], or at slightly lower altitudes (1740-1800m) [14, 15]. Indeed, recent research has indicated that performance can actually improve as a result of altitude training in the absence of any significant increase in haemoglobin mass [16]. So what other mechanisms might explain the improvement in performance at sea level after altitude training. Gore and colleagues argue that altitude training improves exercise economy [17] through an increased ability to metabolise carbohydrate during oxidative phosphorylation, a decreased cost of ventilation, or by an increased ability of the muscle contractile machinery to produce work more efficiently [18]. Early reports from other researchers suggest an increase in muscle buffering capacity may be a possibility [19, 20]. An increase in buffering capacity of the muscle or blood would allow a greater build-up of acidity during exercise. Because a limiting factor to exercise is an increase in acidity, such a change would allow the athlete to exercise for longer before fatiguing.

More recently, research at a genetic level has started to uncover some more clues as to what may be happening during altitude training [21]. It has been shown that a transcription factor called hypoxia inducible factor-1 (HIF-1), which is present in every cell of the body, is the universal regulator of oxygen homeostasis and plays a vital role in the body's responses to hypoxia. During periods of normoxia the level of HIF-1 are very low, with the HIF-1 sub-units being quickly degraded, however, under hypoxic conditions the sub-units are not degraded as quickly and HIF-1 levels increase in the cells allowing it to transcribe specific genes. A summary of the genes HIF-1 activates gives us some idea of the plethora of ways in which altitude training may enhance performance. HIF-1 activates EPO, and transferrin involved in iron metabolism and erythropoiesis. HIF-1 also stimulates angiogenesis and glycolytic enzyme activity, cell glucose transporters, muscle lactate metabolism, carbonic anhydrase for enzymes that regulate pH and others that produce vasodilators such as nitric oxide [22, 23]. Since hypoxia causes a multitude of responses in the human body including but not limited to changes in red cell mass [5], angiogenesis, glucose transport, glycolysis, pH regulation, and changes in the efficiency of energy production at the mitochondrial level which could all potentially have a positive impact on exercise performance, potentially all of these mechanisms either solely or combined could be the cause of enhanced sea-level performance after altitude training. Further research is required to further elucidate the mechanisms involved.

Training at real altitude is expensive and time consuming and in some cases may in fact work to decrease rather than increase performance due to a number of problems occasionally encountered at altitude. These problems include weight loss (particularly lean body mass), diarrhoea, headaches, insomnia, immune suppression, appetite suppression, drowsiness, dehydration, and nausea. Perhaps one of the biggest problems athletes face when going to altitude is the drop in training velocity (pace) at training intensities comparable to those at sea level which can potentially result in detraining of the athlete. Because of the altitude-associated decrements in oxygen concentration which result in a reduction of the $\dot{V}O_2$max and P_aO_2 which ultimately reduces oxygen to the muscles it is difficult for athletes (particularly endurance athletes) to maintain their normal sea level training intensity. This drop in performance is particularly noticeable in the first few days after arriving at altitude and many coaches insist on reduced training loads during this period to reduce the risk of illness, injury or overtraining. Dr.

John Hellemans (currently the National Triathlon Coach for the Netherlands Team) gives great attention to this early period of acclimatization and suggests that endurance athletes should limit their high intensity intervals to repetitions of no more than 3 minutes, alternated with longer recovery periods than would normally occur at sea level [24]. In general, over the first week or so after arriving at altitude, athletes should somewhat decrease their training frequency and duration and reduce their training intensity considerably to avoid these problems.

2. The different models of altitude training

2.1. Conventional altitude training

2.1.1. Live high-train high model

The traditional and probably the most commonly practiced form of altitude training is the Live High-Train High (LHTH) approach, in which athletes live at altitude for a period of time and perform all their training and "living" in one location. It is suggested that the optimal altitude dose for such training is 2000-2500 m for 3-4 weeks [25]. Going to very high altitude is unproductive as the stress on the body and the resultant side effects from such high altitude usually outweigh any performance benefits. For example at high altitudes, the large drop in arterial oxyhaemoglobin saturation results in large decreases in $\dot{V}O_2$max which necessitates a decrease in training intensity which can therefore lead to detraining. Moreover, at higher altitudes athletes are more susceptible to acute mountain sickness, nausea, lethargy which may all effect training quality and quantity. Table 1. shows the various altitude classifications commonly used in the literature. Altitude above 5000 m is tolerated for relatively short periods of time and altitudes above 7500 are dangerous to health [26]. Most LHTH altitude training for athletes occurs at moderate altitude.

Death Zone	> 7500m
Extreme Altitude	5000- 7500m
High Altitude	3000- 5000m
Moderate Altitude	2000- 3000m
Low Altitude	1000- 2000m
Sea Level	< 1000m

Data adapted from Pollard and Murdoch 1998.

Table 1. Altitude classification

However, some coaches (such as John Hellemans) suggest the optimum altitude for this type of training is lower (1500-2000 m) since athletes suffer fewer side-effects at lower altitudes and are able to maintain training quality [24]. Examples of some of the world's altitude training bases are presented in Table 2.

Altitude Training Site	Country	Elevation (m/ft)
Thredbo Alpine Training Centre	Australia	1365/4478
Crans Montana	Switzerland	1500/4920
Snow Farm, Wanaka	New Zealand	1500/4920
Albuquerque, New Mexico	USA	1525/5000
Fort Collins, Colorado	USA	1525/5000
Davos	Switzerland	1560/5117
Issyk-Kull	Kirgizstan	1600/5248
Denver, Colorado	USA	1610/5280
Medeo	Kazakhstan	1691/5546
Tamga	Kirgizstan	1700/5576
Boulder, Colorado	USA	1770/5800
Ifrane	Morocco	1820/5970
St. Moritz	Switzerland	1820/5970
Nairobi	Kenya	1840/6035
Font Romeu Odeillo	France	1850/6069
Colorado Springs, Colorado	USA	1860/6100
Kunming	China	1895/6216
Pontresina	Switzerland	1900/6232
Zetersfeld/Linz	Austria	1950/6396
Piatra Arsa	Romania	1950/6396
Tzahkadzor	Armenia	1970/6462
Belmeken	Bulgaria	2000/6560
Kesenoy-Am	Russia	2000/6560
Sestriere	Italy	2035/6675
Flagstaff, Arizona	USA	2134/7000
Los Alamos, New Mexico	USA	2208/7240
Quito	Ecuador	2218/7275
Alamosa, Colorado	USA	2300/7544
Mexico City	Mexico	2300/7544
Sierra Nevada/Granada	Spain	2320/7610
Addis Ababa	Ethiopia	2400/7872
Park City, Utah	USA	2440/8000
Mammoth Lake, California	USA	2440/8000
Bogota	Colombia	2500/8200
Toluca	Mexico	2700/8856
La Paz	Bolivia	3100/10168

Adapted with permission from Wilber (2004)

Table 2. Commonly used altitude training bases throughout the world.

2.1.2. Live high-train low model

To overcome the problems associated with living and training at altitude, Benjamin Levine and James Stray-Gunderson investigated the effects of living at altitude but training much closer to sea level. In a comprehensive study they compared 3 groups of runners; one group lived low and trained low (San Diego, California, 150 m), another lived high (Deer Valley, Utah, 2500 m) and trained low (Salt Lake City, Utah, 1250 m), while the last group lived high and trained high (Deer Valley, Utah). Upon initial return to sea level runners in the Live High-Train Low group improved their 5-km time trial performance by 1.3% as a result of the altitude training, the Live High-Train High runners showed a small detrimental change (-0.3%), whereas the Live Low-Train Low runners got much worse (-2.7%) After 4 weeks back at sea level all groups improved but the Live High-Train Low and Live High-Train High groups remained significantly faster than the Live Low-Train Low group. While this ground-breaking study was the first to point towards the Live High-Train Low model as the most appropriate to enhance subsequent sea-level performance a number of problems within this study do not make the results clear cut. Firstly, the fact that the researchers used Salt lake City as the training base for the Live High-Train Low model when 1250 m is not strictly low altitude. In fact, Gore and associates found that altitudes as low as 580m can have an effect on performance [27]. Another major problem is that the control group (Live Low-Train Low) actually decreased performance during normal training at sea level which may suggest inadequate or improper training for this group compared to the other two groups. Finally, the groups were not blinded to the intervention, therefore we cannot rule out a placebo effect (positive in the case of the altitude groups, and negative in the control group). However, in theory the Live High-Train Low model has an advantage over the Live High-Train High model because high intensity training can continue at lower altitudes enabling the athlete to gain sport-specific peripheral and neuromuscular adaptations that are normally lost at high altitude.

2.1.3. High high low model

This is a slight modification on the Live High-Train Low model whereby athletes live at high altitude and perform low to moderate-intensity training at high altitude but travel down to low altitude to perform high intensity training sessions. This model was developed to overcome the difficulties of performing high intensity training in a hypoxic environment

2.2. Altitude simulation

In attempts to provide more convenient and time efficient but less expensive ways to train in low oxygen environments, a number of new technologies have been developed to simulate real altitude training. The main types of simulated altitude provide their hypoxic stimulus through pressure reduction (hypobaric chamber), nitrogen dilution (hypoxic apartments and rooms) or oxygen filtration (hypoxicator machines). These simulation devices have given rise to a number of new procedures that aim to improve athletic performance.

2.2.1. Altitude apartments

As a means of supplying a hypoxic stimulus, individual rooms, apartments or houses are sealed off and the concentration of oxygen within these rooms or apartments is lowered either via nitrogen dilution or oxygen extraction. In most cases these apartments are designed for comfortable living by the athletes for periods between 12 to 18 hours per day. Finnish sport scientist were probably the first to develop an altitude room or apartment solely for the use of athletes in the early 1990's. The hypoxic rooms (via Nitrogen dilution) were situated at the Research Institute for Olympic Sport in Jyvaskyla, Finland. Other examples of altitude apartments can be found all over the world including the Australian Institute of Sport in Canberra Australia, the Karolinska Institute in Stockholm in Sweden and the recently constructed National Altitude Training Centre at the University of Limerick, Ireland. However these apartments are expensive to build and run and are not always convenient for athletes. In addition, such apartments require close monitoring of oxygen and carbon dioxide concentrations to ensure a safe environment for all athletes.

2.2.2. Altitude tents

These are portable small altitude systems that allow the athlete to travel with the equipment and set up the altitude in their own rooms. These systems have a generator and an oxygen extraction unit which feeds hypoxic air through a series of hoses into a portable sealed tent which is normally placed over the bed. This allows athletes to sleep in the hypoxic environment. Examples of this type of equipment include the GO2Altitude® Tent from Biomedtech, Melbourne, Australia, and the Altitude Tent systems from Hypoxico, New York, USA. However a number of issues exist with this technology including the generator noise. The generator is normally required to be placed in the room with the tent and some generators can be quite noisy. The hypoxic environment inside the tent can be variable due to leaks and subject movement, and in some cases the inside of the tent can become warm and humid which can affect sleep quality. Because of the small size of the tent the build-up of carbon dioxide is even more dangerous in altitude tents and needs to be monitored carefully.

2.2.3. Intermittent Hypoxic Exposure (IHE)

Intermittent hypoxic exposure (IHE) is exposure to short periods of hypoxic air at rest (9-15% oxygen, equivalent to approximately 6600-2700 m) alternated with normoxic air (21% oxygen). This technique was originally trialled by Russian aviators in attempts to preacclimatize pilots to the high altitudes encountered during sojourns in open cockpit planes [28]. The technique was subsequently refined and used by researchers and clinicians in attempts to provide a means of treatment from medical conditions ranging from asthma to hypertension [28]. After the cessation of the cold war between the east and west and the unification of Germany many of these previously unknown techniques started to surface in the west along with their eventual use by coaches and athletes. Athletes typically use a hypobaric chamber or a hypoxicator (machines that extract oxygen from the ambient air) to generate the hypoxic air. A typical protocol for this type of training is to breathe 5 minutes of hypoxic air followed by 5 minutes of normoxic air for a period of between 60 and 120 minutes per day for 2-3 weeks. The intermittent nature of this type of training allows for the oxygen concentration to drop to much lower levels than could be tolerated safely in other altitude training models. The drop in the inspired oxygen concentration of the air being breathed results in a drop of P_aO_2 and subsequently arterial oxyhaemoglobin saturation (S_aO_2) which stimulates the body to adapt. However, it is thought by some researchers that such a short altitude stimulus is not sufficient to cause significant haematological benefits for athletes and is therefore unlikely to produce performance change [29]. Others have argued that improved performance with such training is likely to be non-haemtological (i.e. enhanced skeletal muscle performance, improved muscle and blood buffering capacity, or beneficial changes in exercise economy) [30]. Recently a number of portable IHE devices have become available. These devices (AltiPower, GO2Altitude®, Australia and AltoLab, AltoLab Nominees, Auckland) usually require carbon dioxide scrubbers and are used in conjunction with pulse-oximeters that measure the oxygen concentration in the blood (SpO_2). Typical protocols for IHE (and IHT, see below) indicate a gradual lowering of the SpO2 values over a 3 week period (Table 3).

	Week 1	Week 2	Week 3
Athletes	84-80%	82-78%	80-76%
Mountaineers	84-80%	84-80%	80-76%

Targets are SpO2 levels (indicating arterial oxygen saturation as measured by pulse oximetery).

Adapted with permission from Hellemans and Hamlin (2009)

Table 3. Target blood oxygen saturation levels during intermittent hypoxia.

2.2.4. Intermittent Hypoxic Training (IHT)

IHT consists of breathing hypoxic air intermittently with normoxic air, however unlike IHE the athlete exercises while breathing the hypoxic air. This is similar to living at sea level and conducting training sessions at altitude (LLTH). The extra stress of training under hypoxic conditions is suggested to cause increased adaptations resulting in improved performance. The effectiveness of IHT for the enhancement of sea level performance, however remain controversial. Several studies have reported an enhanced athletic performance following IHT [31, 32] although a number have failed to demonstrate any substantial alteration in post-IHT performance measures [33, 34].

3. Aerobic performance change with altitude training

Research into the effects of altitude training on subsequent sea level endurance performance is equivocal with some researchers reporting significant improvements [5, 35-38] while others report decrements in performance [39] or in some cases no substantial change [40, 41]. A recent meta-analysis on the effect of various models of altitude training was published in

2009 and gives a good indication of what performance changes might be expected from the various methods (Table 4).

	Natural altitude models		Artificial altitude models			
	LHTH	LHTL	LHTL prolonged continuous	LHTL short continuous	LHTL intermittent (IHE)	LLTH (IHT)
Mean Power Output						
Elite	↔	↑	↔		↔	
Sub-elite	↔	↑	↑	↔	↑	↔
$\dot{V}O_2$max						
Elite	↓	↔	↔		↔	
Sub-elite	↑	↔			↔	↑

Data are very likely improvement in mean power output or $\dot{V}O_2$max (↑), very likely decrement (↓) and either trivial or unclear (↔) changes in variables. LHTH, Live High-Train High; LHTL, Live High-Train Low; LLTH, Live Low-Train High; LHTL prolonged continuous, spending between 8-18 hours per day in hypoxia uninterrupted; LHTL short continuous, spending between 1.5-5 hours per day in hypoxia uninterrupted; IHE, intermittent hypoxic exposure, which was typically less than 1.5 hours per day; IHT, intermittent hypoxic training, which was typically 0.5-2 hours per day. Missing data indicates insufficient research studies to calculate an effect.

Adapted with permission from Bonnetti and Hopkins (2009).

Table 4. Effects on sea level performance (mean power output) and maximal oxygen uptake following adaptation to hypoxia experienced by elite and sub-elite athletes in different models of natural and artificial altitude.

With the data published up until 2009, clearly Live High-Train Low is beneficial for elite athletes (Table 4). This model of altitude training typically produces a 4.0 ± 3.7% (mean ± 90% confidence level) improvement in performance at sea level. This indicates that the effect of this type of altitude training in more or less all elite athletes may be as small as 0.3% and as large as 7.7% improvement. Notice that such an improvement in performance is not always associated with an increase in $\dot{V}O_2$max indicating that other physiological measures may be causing the improved performance in elite athletes. Performance change in elite athletes as a result of other models of altitude training are either trivial or unclear or have not been tested to date (LHTL short continuous and IHT). For sub-elite athletes the Live High-Train Low method is again advantageous in terms of improving performance (4.2 ± 2.9%) along with the Live High-Train Low prolonged continuous (1.4 ± 2.0%) and the Live High-Train Low intermittent methods (2.6 ± 1.2%). There are obvious gaps in the research which require further investigation such as the effect of IHT on elite performance. Given this knowledge it is curious that many coaches and athletes continue to prefer the Live High-Train High model (see Table 5). Reasons for this choice are unclear but probably reflect practical issues such as adequate training venues, logistical and time issues required to travel up and down mountains, cost and proximity to high-class competition. This meta-analysis however, also highlights the applicability of new models of altitude training, particularly the use of Live High-Train Low prolonged continuous and Live High-Train Low intermittent models on sub-elite athletic performance. While there is undoubtedly a number of factors contributing to the conflicting results reported in the research literature (i.e. methodological differences including the duration and intensity of the hypoxic stimulus, type and intensity of training, subject training status and time-points following altitude exposure when re-retesting was completed), there remains a need for further investigation into the effects of all models of altitude exposure, particularly on elite athletic performance.

4. Anaerobic performance change with altitude training

The scientific rationale supporting the use of altitude training for anaerobic performance is less compelling than aerobic performance. Altitude-induced increments in RBC mass and haemoglobin are physiological adaptations which probably do not significantly affect the anaerobic performance in athletes. However, altitude training may also benefit anaerobic exercise performance, possibly via increases in muscle buffering capacity [42] and glycolytic enzyme activity [43]. IHE has been found to increase repeated kayak sprint power for mean and peak power [44] and repeated sprint run times [45] 3 days following hypoxia exposures. Similarly, 10 days of IHT at a simulated altitude of 2500 m improved anaerobic mean and peak cycling power at 9 days post-intervention compared to the placebo sea-level training group [46]. Our research group has also reported substantial increases in anaerobic power two (3.0%) and nine days (1.7%) post IHT training [47]. Conversely, some researchers have reported no beneficial effect of IHT [33] or IHE [48] on anaerobic performance over and above that of training closer to sea-level.

5. The current usage and effectiveness of altitude training by elite sportspeople

Debate into the effectiveness of altitude training continues with some coaches using altitude training 2-3 times per year [49], while others believe that the effects of altitude training are not conclusive and encourage coaches to invest their scare resources into other aspects of athlete development [50]. In a round table discussion on altitude training four international experts indicated that they used altitude training regularly with their athletes (average of 3 times per year), and during this training they went to an altitude of about 2200m for approximately 4 weeks [49].

In 2005-2006 a survey was given to 21 New Zealand coaches and high performance managers to assess the popularity and effectiveness of the various models of altitude training. Data was collected from 15 respondents representing approximately 40 separate altitude sojourns or interventions. The sports identified included triathlon, athletics, cycling, kayaking, snow-sports and rugby. Live High-Train High was the most popular altitude training method used, followed by the simulated altitude method Live High-Train Low intermittent (or IHE). Using altitude tents was the least popular method (Figure 1).

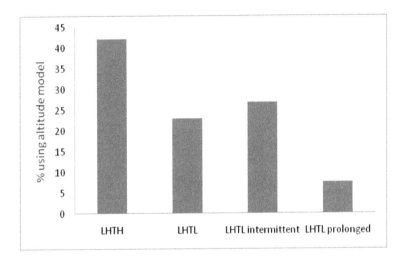

Figure 1. The proportion of respondents using the various methods of altitude training. LHTH, Live High-Train High; LHTL, Live High-Train Low; LHTL prolonged continuous, spending between 8-18 hours per day in hypoxia uninterrupted; LHTL intermittent, intermittent hypoxic exposure, which is typically less than 1.5 hours per day; *Adapted with permission from Sport New Zealand.*

Those coaches and high performance managers that indicated they used real altitude sojourns were then asked to rate the effectiveness of their altitude interventions on athletic performance (Table 5). In most cases altitude training at real sojourns was rated as moderately or very effective. Training sojourns ranged in elevation from 1100 m to 2500 m. Unfortunately the altitude model (LHTH or LHTL) was not examined in this question; therefore we cannot examine which of these methods is more effective from the coaches and managers perspective. The association between altitude elevation and the perceived effectiveness of the training camp is illustrated in Figure 2. The correlation between elevation and effectiveness score was -0.02 which indicates the effectiveness of the altitude camps is not solely due to the elevation. Indeed some very useful altitude camps were held at relatively low levels (e.g. Leutasch, Austria). 5

Altitude Venue	Altitude (m)	No. of Athletes	Sport Involved	No. of Weeks at Altitude	Effectiveness Score[a]
Aguascalientes, Mexico	1900	8	Cycling	2	5
Albuquerque, NM, USA	1525	10	Triathlon	4	2-4
Alp du Aez, France	1900	1	Triathlon	6	5
Bogota, Columbia	2500	10	Cycling	5	4
Boulder, CO, USA	1770	13	Triathlon	4-9	4-5
Davos , Switzerland	1560	6	Athletics	3	4
Flagstaff, Co, USA	2134	35	Triathlon	3-8	3-5
Font Romeau, France	1850	36	Triathlon Athletics	2-6	3-5
Gunnison, CO, USA	2300	2	Athletics	2	5
Leutasch, Austria	1100	1	Athletics	20	5
Los Alamos, NM, USA	2208	5	Athletics Triathlon	3-9	3-5
Quito, Equador	2218	8	Cycling	4	4
Sestriere, Italy	2035	12	Athletics	3	5
Sierra Nevada, Spain	2320	1	Athletics	3	4
Snow Farm, New Zealand	1500	38	Triathlon	2-3	4-5
St. Moritz, Switzerland	1820	18	Triathlon Athletics	2-9	5
Whakapapa, New Zealand	1730	1	Athletics	4	3

[a]Effectiveness was rated on a scale from 1 to 5; 1, don't know; 2, adverse effect; 3, no effect; 4, moderately effective; 5, very effective. Adapted with permission from Sport New Zealand.

Table 5. Effectiveness of real sojourns to altitude for elite athletes as described by their coaches and high performance managers.

Bonetti and Hopkins (2009) in a recent meta-analysis on altitude training found that both elite and non-elite athletes that live at altitude and train closer to sea level (LHTL) benefited from such training (by about 4.0%), whereas performance improvement in athletes (elite and non-elite) that trained and lived at altitude (LHTH) was unclear. However, due to the conflicting reports, uncontrolled studies, poor study design and variation in physiological adaptations found a consensus on the effects of altitude training is some way off.

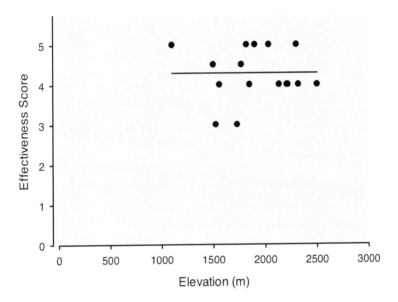

Figure 2. The association between altitude elevation and perceived effectiveness of the training sojourn. Effectiveness was rated on a scale from 1 to 5; 1, don't know; 2, adverse effect; 3, no effect; 4, moderately effective; 5, very effective. For effectiveness scores with a range we have calculated the mean score and inserted this into the above figure. Adapted with permission from Sport New Zealand.

In addition, coaches and high performance managers were also asked to rate the effectiveness of any simulated altitude training they had used previously. This produced some mixed responses with some reports of such devices even having a negative effect on performance (Table 6). However as with real altitude training the duration, hypoxic dosage and timing of the stimulus can have a substantial effect on results and therefore should be considered when deciding on altitude methods.

Type of Altitude Simulation	No. of Athletes	Sport Involved	Protocol Used	Effectiveness Score[a]
Hypoxicator	80+	Triathlon Athletics Cycling Kayaking Rugby	3 weeks duration for 60-90 minutes per day for 5-6 days per week. 5 minutes hypoxia interspersed with 5 minutes normoxia. Fraction of inspired oxygen 12-9% (▢4500-6600 m)	Mixed responses with a relatively equal proportion at 5, 3, 2 and 1.
Altitude Tents	12	Triathlon Cycling	2-3 weeks duration sleeping for 8-10 hours per night at fraction of inspired oxygen of 14.5-16.5 (▢3000-2000 m)	3-4
AltiPower or AltoLab	25	Triathlon Athletics Rugby	3 weeks duration for 60-90 minutes per day for 5-6 days per week. 5 minutes hypoxia interspersed with 5 minutes normoxia.	4 (Triathlon, Athletics), 2 (Rugby)

[a]Effectiveness was rated on a scale from 1 to 5; 1, don't know; 2, adverse effect; 3, no effect; 4, moderately effective; 5, very effective. Adapted with permission from Sport New Zealand.

Table 6. Effectiveness of simulated altitude training for elite athletes as described by their coaches and high performance managers.

Responders versus non-responders to altitude training

It is clear that there is considerable individual variation in the response to altitude (or hypoxia) [6, 51, 52]. This is clearly observed in mountaineering with some climbers having to use supplemental oxygen at moderate-to-high altitudes while others can climb just as high while breathing ambient air exclusively. Similarly, the response to altitude training in athletes can be just as variable. In a recent study the authors reported that some athletes significantly improved sea-level performance, while others showed a decrement after 28 days of Live High-Train Low training (LHTL) [51]. Similar levels of variation have also been reported after simulated Live-High-Train Low training via intermittent hypoxia [30]. While the mechanisms behind performance change with altitude training remain controversial it seems clear that not all athletes benefit from such training. It has been suggested that non-responders show a limited erythropoietin response in comparison with responders and therefore little improvement in $\dot{V}O_2$max and subsequent performance improvement [51]. However, other mechanisms must be at play since performance improvement after altitude training is not always related to positive changes in red blood cell indices or $\dot{V}O_2$max [10].

Our research group as well as others [53] have recently uncovered differences suggestive of neuro-vegetative imbalance in non-responders to altitude training. While still controversial, some researchers believe that ideal endurance training results in an increase in performance alongside a shift towards more parasympathetic activity as measured via heart rate variability (i.e. increased high frequency, HF) [54], whereas inadequate or ineffective training results in less parasympathetic and more sympathetic activity. Our research group has found that responders tend to have a decrease in sympathetic activity compared to non-responders, who have an increase in sympathetic activity (Figure 3).

We think that the effects of heavy training loads in association with the hypoxic stress of living at altitude may have a cumulative effect, whereby the normal adaptation processes are overwhelmed and athletes cannot cope, resulting in an increase in sympathetic stress. If recovery is not adequate and training and hypoxia continue, the athlete may move into a vicious cycle of inevitable stress resulting in an overtraining or overstress-type condition resulting in loss of performance. However more data needs to be collected over a longer period of time on a number of different athletes before we can be certain about this hypothesis.

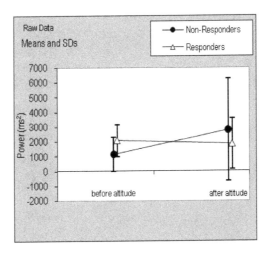

Figure 3. Low frequency component (sympathetic branch) of the heart rate variability: changes in standing position in non-responders and responders to 3 weeks of altitude training. Data are raw means ± SD of low frequency (0.04 – 0.15 Hz) reflecting sympathetic predominance. Pre, day 1 of altitude training; Post, day 20 of altitude training at 1550m.

We believe that in order to make the most of altitude training and to identify athletes who are perhaps not responding effectively to altitude training a number of subjective and physiological variables should be monitored over the training period. These variables range from subjective assessments of the athletes perception of how hard they are training along with their fatigue, stress and muscle soreness levels. We also record the athletes sleep quantity and quality which provides additional information on the adaptation to altitude. In many cases sleep disturbances may indicate overstress, and poor sleep quality can interfere with athletic training. Figure 4 shows a number of subjective variables collected on two elite athletes during a 20-day Live High-Train Low altitude camp. One of the athletes improved performance after the camp and was recorded as a responder, while the other failed to improve and in fact went backwards in terms of performance (non-responder).

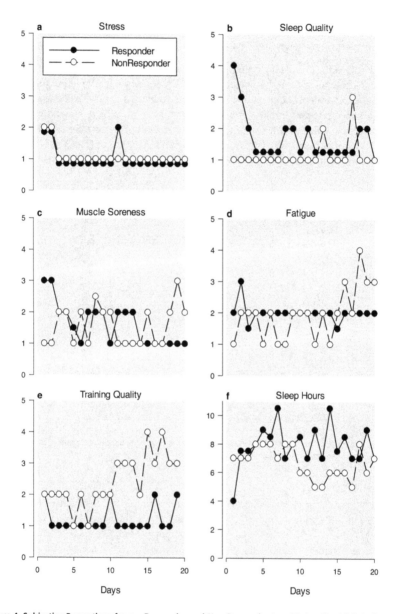

Figure 4. Subjective Perceptions from a Responder and Non-Responder to a 20-day Live High-Train Low Altitude camp. Subjective stress (a), sleep quality (b), muscle soreness (c), fatigue (d), training quality (e) and hours of sleep (f) in a responder (closed circles) and non-responder (open circles) throughout the 20-day altitude camp. Values are 1, excellent; 2, very good; 3, normal; 4, poor; 5, very poor.

It is apparent from Figure 4 that the non-responder to altitude training had increased feelings of fatigue, poorer training quality and fewer overall sleeping hours than the responder. Each of these parameters along with daily training schedules can give invaluable insight into whether athletes are coping with the altitude training or not.

6. Preparing the athlete for altitude training

As mentioned earlier in this chapter, altitude training provides an additional physiological stress in an attempt to enhance the athlete's response to training. However, there are a number of other stresses in the lives of athletes which need to be taken seriously when considering the use of altitude training, including, but not limited to; training, family, relationships, and psychological stress. Because of this added stress it is recommended that athletes decrease their training volume and intensity over the first few weeks of altitude [55], however there are also a number of other training and health-related factors that should be considered prior to any altitude training. It is suggested that athletes should only add the stress of altitude to their training when they have optimal nutritional status, and are free of illness, injury, and fatigue. Increasing the stress of altitude training on an already damaged or fragile athlete can result in inhibited performance.

One of the most important considerations is iron status, as adequate iron stores are necessary to develop new red blood cells. Iron supplementation with altitude training has been used for improved performance in athletes [56], whereas in some occasions exposure to altitude without a supplemental dose of iron, results in a marked decrease in serum ferritin [57]. Theoretically, iron is a requisite component of the haemoglobin molecule and serves as the exclusive site for oxygen binding and release. Iron is necessary for red blood cell multiplication which is part of erythropoetic process [55]. Ferritin, the storage form of iron, is significantly decreased after three weeks altitude exposure at 2,225 m in elite male swimmers [58]. Similar results were reported in elite female speed-skaters who lived at 2,700 m for 27 days and trained at an altitude between 1,400 m and 300 m [59]. These reports suggest that the hypoxic environment of altitude may exacerbate the requirement for iron among well-trained athletes [60]. In addition, recent studies have shown that endurance performance was decreased due to iron insufficiency in well trained non-anaemic athletes [61] signifying even if athletes meet guidelines for iron levels they may be disadvantaged if iron levels are not sufficient for their individual turnover rates.

In a recent randomised controlled study we examined the effect of iron supplementation (equivalent to 105 mg element iron, with vitamin C 500 mg as sodium ascorbate [FERRO-GRAD® C, Abbott Laboratories (NZ) Ltd, Naenae]), or a placebo tablet on 800-m swim performance in a group of elite triathletes completing a 20-day Live High-Train Low altitude camp (Live 1500m, train 300m). The performance measures before and after the altitude training camp can be seen in Figure 5. Compared to the placebo group, the triathletes who took the iron supplementation improved performance by 3.3% which suggests that coaches and athletes need to consider iron supplementation prior to altitude training. Low iron levels do not allow for the enhanced erythropoietic effect normally witnessed at real altitudes and therefore the athlete's body may take longer to adapt to the hypoxic environment and subsequently improve performance. We have also found that supplemental iron tablets helped to improve haematological parameters during IHE and IHT. After 2-3 weeks of either IHE [30], or IHT [47] athletes taking iron supplementation showed improved haematological indicators (Figure 6).

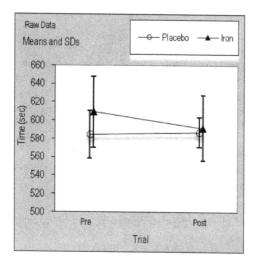

Figure 5. swim time trail performance (sec) in the triathletes who took iron supplementation or placebo tablets 1 week before (pre) and 1 week after (post) the LHTL altitude training camp.

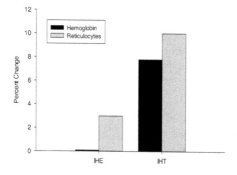

Figure 6. Change in blood variables in the simulated altitude versus control groups 2 days after a 2-3 week intermittent hypoxic intervention.

Altitude may also compromise the immune system and slow down the recovery from illness, so athletes with an illness are not recommended to go to altitude and close monitoring of athletes' wellbeing at altitude should be mandatory. We encourage a range of blood parameters including iron status, red and white cell count and EPO if available. In addition to monitoring changes in the haematological and immune responses other variables should be monitored including body weight, resting and exercise heart rate and haemoglobin saturation levels. Such monitoring is less subjective and gives a good indication of adaptation progress. For example, notice the overall lower haemoglobin saturation levels (S_pO_2) in the non-responder compared to the responder. Such a change probably reflects the inadequate ability of the non-responder to adjust to the hypoxic environment.

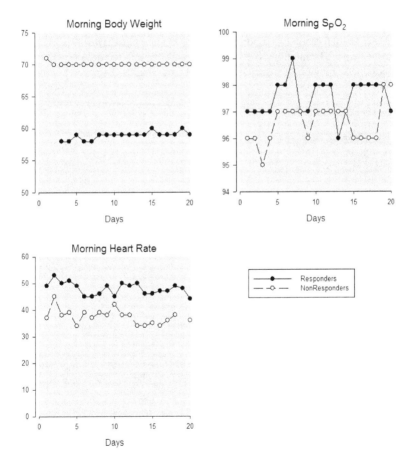

Figure 7. Physiological monitoring of a Responder (closed circles) and Non-Responder (open circles) to a 20-day Live High-Train Low Altitude camp.

7. Conclusion

We conclude that there is sufficient evidence to suggest that all methods of altitude training can benefit athletic performance in some way, however to gain improvement in sea-level performance for the top elite athletes, a Live High-Train Low method is recommended. Nevertheless, performance enhancement for athletes as a result of altitude training is not guaranteed. Indeed, some athletes may be unable to handle the extra stress that accompanies hypoxia, especially when they may be already working close to their physical limits. In such cases maladaptation and detraining may occur and the athlete's performance may decrease rather than increase. Through rigorous preparation, adequate training and recovery and thorough planning, the coach or performance manager can make altitude training sojourns successful. Maintaining detailed longitudinal data on individual athletes including subjective and objective measures of stress and performance will allow the early detection of problems and increase the chances of a positive altitude training block. However, questions still remain to be answered including; what is the most effective hypoxic dosage, what is the best way to monitor adaptation during hypoxia, and discovering the best way to delineate responders from non-responders.

Author details

Michael J. Hamlin[1*], Nick Draper[2] and John Hellemans[1]

*Address all correspondence to: mike.hamlin@lincoln.ac.nz

1 Department of Social Science, Parks, Recreation, Tourism & Sport, Lincoln University, Christchurch, New Zealand

2 School of Sciences and Physical Education, University of Canterbury, Christchurch, New Zealand

References

[1] Cohen JE, Small C. Hypsographic demography: The distribution of human population by altitude. Proceedings of the National Academy of Sciences of the United States of America 1998;95:14009-14014.

[2] West JB. Archival collections in physiology. News in Physiological Science 1999;14:268-270.

[3] Levine BD, Stray-Gundersen J. Point: Positive effects of intermittent hypoxia (live high:train low) on exercise performance are mediated primarily by augmented red cell volume. Journal of Applied Physiology 2005;99:2053-2055.

[4] Gore CJ, Hopkins WG. Counterpoint: Positive effects of intermittent hypoxia (live high:train low) on exercise performance are not mediated primarily by augmented red cell volume. Journal of Applied Physiology 2005;99:2055-2058.

[5] Levine BD, StrayGundersen J. "Living high training low": Effect of moderate-altitude acclimatization with low-altitude training on performance. Journal of Applied Physiology 1997 Jul;83:102-112.

[6] Friedmann B, Frese F, Menold E, et al. Individual variation in the erythropoietic response to altitude training in elite junior swimmers. British Journal of Sports Medicine 2005;39:148-153.

[7] Heinicke K, Heinicke I, Schmidt W, et al. A three-week traditional altitude training increases hemoglobin mass and red cell volume in elite biathlon athletes. International Journal of Sports Medicine 2005;26:350-355.

[8] Svedenhag J, Piehl-Aulin K, Skog C, et al. Increased left ventricular muscle mass after long-term altitude training in athletes. Acta Physiologica Scandinavica 1997;161:63-70.

[9] Dill DB, Braithwaite K, Adams WC, et al. Blood volume of middle-distance runners: effect of 2300-m altitude and comparsions with non-athletes. Medicine and Science in Sports 1974;6:1-7.

[10] Gore C, Craig N, Hahn A, et al. Altitude training at 2690m does not increase total haemoglobin mass or sea level VO2max in world champion track cyclists. Journal of Science and Medicine in Sport 1998;1:156-170.

[11] Ashenden MJ, Gore CJ, Dobson GP, et al. Simulated moderate altitude elevates serum erthyropoietin but does not increase reticulocyte production in well-trained runners. European Journal of Applied Physiology 2000;81:428-435.

[12] Ashenden MJ, Gore CJ, Dobson GP, et al. "Live high, train low" does not change the total haemoglobin mass of male endurance athletes sleeping at a simulated altitude of 3000 m for 23 nights. European Journal of Applied Physiology and Occupational Physiology 1999 Oct;80:479-484.

[13] Ashenden MJ, Gore CJ, Martin DT, et al. Effects of a 12-day "live high, train low" camp on reticulocyte production and haemoglobin mass in elite female road cyclists. European Journal of Applied Physiology 1999;80:472-478.

[14] Gore CJ, Hahn AG, Burge CM, et al. VO$_2$max and haemoglobin mass of trained athletes during high intensity training. International Journal of Sports Medicine 1997;18:477-482.

[15] Friedmann B, Jost J, Rating T, et al. Effects of iron supplementation on total body hemoglobin during endurance training at moderate altitude. International Journal of Sports Medicine 1999;20:78-85.

[16] Saunders P, Telford R, Pyne D, et al. Improved running economy in elite runners after 20 days of simulated moderate-altitude exposure. Journal of Applied Physiology 2004;96:931-937.

[17] Gore CJ, Clark SA, Saunders PU. Nonhematological mechanisms of improved sea-level performance after hypoxic exposure. Medicine and Science in Sports and Exercise 2007 Sep;39:1600-1609.

[18] Green H, Roy B, Grant S, et al. Increases in submaximal cycling efficiency mediated by altitude acclimatization. Journal of Applied Physiology 2000;89:1189-1197.

[19] Saltin B, Kim CK, Terrados N, et al. Morphology, enzyme activities and buffer capacity in leg muscles of Kenyan and Scandinavian runners. Scandinavian Journal of Medicine and Science in Sports 1995 Aug;5:222-230.

[20] Mizuno M, Juel C, Bro-Rasmussen T, et al. Limb skeletal muscle adaptation in athletes after training at altitude. Journal of Applied Physiology 1990;68:496-502.

[21] Zhu H, Bunn HF. Oxygen sensing and signaling; impact on the regulation of physiologically important genes. Respiration Physiology 1999;115:239-247.

[22] Clerici C, Matthay MA. Hypoxia regulates geneexpression of alveolar epithelial transport proteins. Journal of Applied Physiology 2000;88:1890-1896.

[23] Sasaki R, Masuda S, Nagao M. Erythropoietin: multiple physiological functions and regulation of biosynthesis. Bioscience, Biotechnology, and Biochemistry 2000;64:1775-1793.

[24] Hellemans J, Hamlin M. Intermittent Hypoxic Training. In: Kwong CP, Leahy T, So R, Mei TY, editors. Recent Advances in High Altitude. Hong Kong: Hong Kong Sports Institute; 2009. p. 4-11.

[25] Levine BD, Stray-Gundersen J. Dose-response of altitude training: how much altitude is enough? Adv Exp Med Biol 2007;588:233-247.

[26] Pollard AJ, Murdoch DR. The High Altitude Medicine Handbook. 3rd ed. Oxon, United Kingdom: Radcliffe Medical Press Ltd; 2003.

[27] Gore CJ, Little SC, Hahn AG, et al. Reduced performance of male and female athletes at 580 m altitude. European Journal of Applied Physiology 1997;75:136-143.

[28] Serebrovskaya TV. Intermittent hypoxia research in the former Soviet Union and Commonwealth of Independent States: history and review of the concept and selected applications. High Altitude Medicine and Biology 2002;3:205-221.

[29] Julian CG, Gore CJ, Wilber RL, et al. Intermittent normobaric hypoxia does not alter performance or erythropoietic markers in highly trained distance runners. Journal of Applied Physiology 2004;96:1800-1807.

[30] Hamlin MJ, Hellemans J. Effect of intermittent normobaric hypoxic exposure at rest on haematological, physiological and performance parameters in multi-sport athletes. Journal of Sports Sciences 2007;25:431-441.

[31] Dufour SP, Ponsot E, Zoll J, et al. Exercise training in normobaric hypoxia in endurance runners. I. Improvement in aerobic performance capacity. Journal of Applied Physiology 2006 Apr;100:1238-1248.

[32] Ponsot E, Dufour SP, Zoll J, et al. Exercise training in normobaric hypoxia in endurance runners. II. Improvement of mitochondrial properties in skeletal muscle. Journal of Applied Physiology 2006;100:1249-1257.

[33] Morton JP, Cable NT. The effects of intermittent hypoxic training on aerobic and anaerobic performance. Ergonomics 2005;48:1535-1546.

[34] Roels B, Bentley DJ, Coste O, et al. Effects of intermittent hypoxic training on cycling performance in well-trained athletes. European Journal of Applied Physiology 2007;101:359-368.

[35] Martino M, Myers K, Bishop P. Effects of 21 days training at altitude on sea-level anaerobic performance in competitive swimmers. Medicine and Science in Sports and Exercise 1995;27:S7.

[36] Adams WC, Bernauer EM, Dill DB, et al. Effects of equivalent sea-level and altitude training on VO_{2max} and running performance. Journal of Applied Physiology 1975;39:262-266.

[37] Dill DB, Adams WC. Maximal oxygen uptake at sea level and at 3,090-m altitude in high school champion runners. Journal of Applied Physiology 1971;30:854-859.

[38] Daniels J, Oldridge N. The effects of alternate exposure to altitude and sea level on world-class middle-distance runners. Medicine and Science in Sports 1970;2:107-112.

[39] Jensen K, Nielsen TS, Fiskerstrand A, et al. High-altitude training does not increase maximal oxygen uptake or work capacity at sea level in rowers. Scandinavian Journal of Medicine and Science in Sports 1993;3:256-262.

[40] Buskirk ER, Kollias J, Akers RF, et al. Maximal performance at altitude and on return from altitude in conditioned runners. Journal of Applied Physiology 1967;23:259-266.

[41] Faulkner JA, Daniels JT, Balke B. The effects of training at moderate altitude on physical performance capacity. Journal of Applied Physiology 1967;23:85-89.

[42] Gore CJ, Hahn AG, Aughey RJ, et al. Live high:train low increases muscle buffer capacity and submaximal cycling efficiency. Acta Physiologica Scandinavica 2001 Nov; 173:275-286.

[43] Katayama K, Sato K, Matsuo H, et al. Effect of intermittent hypoxia on oxygen uptake during submaximal exercise in endurance athletes. European Journal of Applied Physiology 2004;92:75-83.

[44] Bonnetti DL, Hopkins WG, Kilding AE. High-intensity kayak performance after adaptation to intermittent hypoxia. International Journal of Sports Physiology and Performance 2006;1:246-260.

[45] Wood MR, Dowson MN, Hopkins WG. Running performance after adaptation to acutely intermittent hypoxia. European Journal of Sport Science 2006;6:163-172.

[46] Hendriksen IJM, Meeuwsen T. The effect of intermittent training in hypobaric hypoxia on sea-level exercise: a cross-over study in humans. European Journal of Applied Physiology 2003;88:396-403.

[47] Hamlin MJ, Marshall HC, Hellemans J, et al. Effect of intermittent hypoxic training on a 20 km time trial and 30 s anaerobic performance. Scandinavian Journal of Medicine and Science in Sports 2010;20:651-661.

[48] Tadibi V, Dehnert C, Menold E, et al. Unchanged anaerobic and aerobic performance after short-term intermittent hypoxia. Medicine and Science in Sports and Exercise 2007;39:858-864.

[49] Baumann I, Bonov P, Daniels J, et al. NSA Round Table: high altitude training. New Studies in Athletics 1994;9:23-35.

[50] Rushall BS. The future of swimming: "myths and science'. Swimming Science Bulletin 2009;37:1-34.

[51] Chapman RF, Stray-Gundersen J, Levine BD. Individual variation in response to altitude training. Journal of Applied Physiology 1998;85:1448-1456.

[52] Jedlickova K, Stockton DW, Chen H, et al. Search for genetic determinants of individual variability of the erythropoietin response to high altitude. Blood Cells, Molecules & Diseases 2003;31:175-182.

[53] Schmitt L, Hellard P, Millet GP, et al. Heart rate variability and performance at two different altitudes in well-trained swimmers. International Journal of Sports Medicine 2006;27:226-231.

[54] Lee CM, Wood RH, Welsch MA. Influence of short-term endurance exercise training on heart rate variability. Medicine and Science in Sports and Exercise 2003;35:961-969.

[55] Wilber RL. Altitude Training and Athletic Performance. Champaign, IL: Human Kinetics; 2004.

[56] Nielsen P, Nachtigall D. Iron supplementation in athletes: current recommendations. Sports Medicine 1998;26:207-216.

[57] Cornolo J, Mollard P, Brugniaux JV, et al. Autonomic control of the cardiovascular system during acclimatization to high altitude: effects of sildenafil. Journal of Applied Physiology 2004;97:935-940.

[58] Roberts D, Smith DJ. Training at moderate altitude: iron status of elite male swimmers. The Journal of Laboratory and Clinical Medicine 1992;120:387-391.

[59] Pauls DW, Duijnhoven H, Stray-Gundersen J. Iron insufficient erythropoiesis at altitude-speed skating. Medicine and Science in Sports and Exercise 2002;34:S252 [Abstract].

[60] Stray-Gundersen J, Alexander C, Hochstein A, et al. Failure of red cell volume to increase to altitude exposure in iron deficient runners [Abstract]. Medicine and Science in Sports and Exercise 1992;24:S90.

[61] Friedmann B, Weller E, Mairbaurl H, et al. Effects of iron repletion on blood volume and performance capacity in young athletes. Medicine and Science in Sports and Exercise 2001;33:741-746.

Permissions

The contributors of this book come from diverse backgrounds, making this book a truly international effort. This book will bring forth new frontiers with its revolutionizing research information and detailed analysis of the nascent developments around the world.

We would like to thank Michael Hamlin, for lending his expertise to make the book truly unique. He has played a crucial role in the development of this book. Without his invaluable contribution this book wouldn't have been possible. He has made vital efforts to compile up to date information on the varied aspects of this subject to make this book a valuable addition to the collection of many professionals and students.

This book was conceptualized with the vision of imparting up-to-date information and advanced data in this field. To ensure the same, a matchless editorial board was set up. Every individual on the board went through rigorous rounds of assessment to prove their worth. After which they invested a large part of their time researching and compiling the most relevant data for our readers. Conferences and sessions were held from time to time between the editorial board and the contributing authors to present the data in the most comprehensible form. The editorial team has worked tirelessly to provide valuable and valid information to help people across the globe.

Every chapter published in this book has been scrutinized by our experts. Their significance has been extensively debated. The topics covered herein carry significant findings which will fuel the growth of the discipline. They may even be implemented as practical applications or may be referred to as a beginning point for another development. Chapters in this book were first published by InTech; hereby published with permission under the Creative Commons Attribution License or equivalent.

The editorial board has been involved in producing this book since its inception. They have spent rigorous hours researching and exploring the diverse topics which have resulted in the successful publishing of this book. They have passed on their knowledge of decades through this book. To expedite this challenging task, the publisher supported the team at every step. A small team of assistant editors was also appointed to further simplify the editing procedure and attain best results for the readers.

Our editorial team has been hand-picked from every corner of the world. Their multi-ethnicity adds dynamic inputs to the discussions which result in innovative outcomes. These outcomes are then further discussed with the researchers and contributors who give their valuable feedback and opinion regarding the same. The feedback is then collaborated with the researches and they are edited in a comprehensive manner to aid the understanding of the subject.

Apart from the editorial board, the designing team has also invested a significant amount of their time in understanding the subject and creating the most relevant covers. They scrutinized every image to scout for the most suitable representation of the subject and create an appropriate cover for the book.

The publishing team has been involved in this book since its early stages. They were actively engaged in every process, be it collecting the data, connecting with the contributors or procuring relevant information. The team has been an ardent support to the editorial, designing and production team. Their endless efforts to recruit the best for this project, has resulted in the accomplishment of this book. They are a veteran in the field of academics and their pool of knowledge is as vast as their experience in printing. Their expertise and guidance has proved useful at every step. Their uncompromising quality standards have made this book an exceptional effort. Their encouragement from time to time has been an inspiration for everyone.

The publisher and the editorial board hope that this book will prove to be a valuable piece of knowledge for researchers, students, practitioners and scholars across the globe.

List of Contributors

Kelc Robi, Naranda Jakob, Kuhta Matevz and Vogrin Matjaz
Department of Orthopedic Surgery, University Medical Center Maribor, Slovenia

Alexander Golant, Tony Quach and Jeffrey Rosen
New York Hospital Queens, Flushing, NY and Weill Medical College of Cornell University, New York, USA

Chariklia K. Deli and Athanasios Z. Jamurtas
Department of Physical Education and Sport Science, University of Thessaly, Trikala, Greece
Institute of Human Performance and Rehabilitation, Center for Research and Technology -Thessaly, Trikala, Greece

Ioannis G. Fatouros
Institute of Human Performance and Rehabilitation, Center for Research and Technology -Thessaly, Trikala, Greece
Department of Physical Education and Sport Science, University of Thrace, Komotini, Greece

Yiannis Koutedakis
Department of Physical Education and Sport Science, University of Thessaly, Trikala, Greece
Institute of Human Performance and Rehabilitation, Center for Research and Technology -Thessaly, Trikala, Greece
School of Sports, Performing Arts and Leisure, University of Wolverhampton, United Kingdom

Hilde Grindvik Nielsen
University College of Health Sciences – Campus Kristiania, Oslo, Norway

Guolin Li
College of Life Sciences, Hunan Normal University, Changsha, Hunan, China

Michael J. Hamlin and John Hellemans
Department of Social Science, Parks, Recreation, Tourism & Sport, Lincoln University, Christchurch, New Zealand

Nick Draper
School of Sciences and Physical Education, University of Canterbury, Christchurch, New Zealand

Printed in the USA
CPSIA information can be obtained
at www.ICGtesting.com
JSHW011423221024
72173JS00004B/660